RHEUMATOLOGY *for* CLINICIANS

W. Jeffrey Fessel, M.D., F.A.C.P., F.R.C.P.

*Rheumatologist, Kaiser-Permanente Medical Center,
San Francisco, California; Consultant to the
Rheumatic Disease Group, University of California
Medical Center, San Francisco, California*

STRATTON INTERCONTINENTAL MEDICAL BOOK CORPORATION
New York

Contents

Acknowledgments

Few readers may realize how comparatively small is the effort of an author in contrast to the cumulative work of his many helpers. The first drafts of this manuscript were typed by Miss Fran Freeman. Mrs. Ruth Straus not only gave invaluable editorial help and advice on the organization of the book but voluntarily, as an act of self-sacrificial kindness, typed the final version. Miss Anne-Marie Bandoni checked the accuracy of the bibliography. My sincerest thanks go to each of these ladies, without whom I would have failed.

Doctors Morris Collen, Derek Crawford, Robert Feldman, and Edmund Van Brunt have been mainly responsible for the administrative aspects of collecting, computerizing, and maintaining the data from Multiphasic Health Checkups and the computerized medical records of our clinics and hospitals; this treasure trove has been an inestimable source of knowledge in my studies. My thanks go to each of them, as well as to Dr. Bruce Sams, Jr., Physician-in-Chief, Kaiser Foundation Hospital, San Francisco, and to Dr. Joseph Sender, Physician-in-Chief, Kaiser Foundation Hospital, Oakland, for allowing me access to the computerized data. Doctors Morris Collen and Gary Friedman made available the material cited in Table 10-6; Dr. Gary Friedman arranged for several searches of the computerized records that enabled calculations to be made of many of the incidences and prevalences listed in this book. Dr. George Barr has given enormous assistance in other computer retrievals and analyses; the data in Table 12-1 are from ongoing collaborative studies with Dr. Barr. Dr. George Matula kindly gave me the figures concerning the results of NBT tests cited in Chapter 15. Dr. Alan Levin gave helpful advice in the construction of Figure 6-1. Dr. John Howard abstracted from the patients' records, the information cited in Tables 2-1 and 2-2.

Dr. John Talbott encouraged me in the preparation of this book: I am also obliged to him for permission to use material previously published in *Seminars in Arthritis and Rheumatism,* in Chapters 4 and 11. Parts of the texts of Chapter 10, and Tables 10-1 to 10-5 are reprinted, by permission, from *Archives of Internal Medicine.*

Last but not least, I am deeply grateful to all of my colleagues of the Kaiser-Permanente Medical Centers in Northern California, most especially those at the San Francisco facility, for sending me the patients who taught me much of what appears in this book.

—W. J. F.

To my wife, Nicole; and Jason, my son.

Introduction

The major texts on Rheumatology are derived from a background of university arthritis clinics, and reflect this by being concerned primarily with problems of rheumatoid and collagen disease in their most severe forms. As encountered in the general community, these diseases tend to be milder, sometimes more subtle in their expression, and almost always more benign; moreover, the collagen diseases are of far less numerical and economic importance than are soft-tissue rheumatism and osteoarthritis.

Table i-1 shows a computer-assisted tabulation of 45,602 visits made by 27, 636 patients during a six-month period to the Department of Medicine of The Permanente Medical Group's clinic in San Francisco, which takes care of the medical problems of approximately 100,000 adult residents of this city who subscribe to the Kaiser Foundation Health Plan. The tabulation probably represents one of the most accurate assessments presently available of an urban community's need for rheumatological services. The diagnoses listed are those made by the examining physicians of the Department of Medicine, most of whom are internists, about one-half of whom are "Board certified" and almost all the remainder of whom are "Board eligible." It is immaterial whether or not the diagnoses listed as present in the Table are totally accurate from a nosologic standpoint: the important observation is that disorders of the musculoskeletal system accounted for more than 10 per cent of all visits to a Department of General Internal Medicine during this period of six months. It is also noteworthy that the so-called "collagen diseases" caused only 1.2 per cent of all visits, a figure that includes only 0.9 per cent for rheumatoid arthritis; while osteoarthritis, disc disease, and "soft-tissue rheumatism" of various sorts accounted for 8.4 per cent of all visits. Conditions labeled by the examining physicians as "musculoskeletal pain, not further specified" accounted for 3.1 per cent of all visits; half of these were for pain in the neck or lower part of the back (Table i-2).

In the United States about 10 per cent of the population suffers from some form of arthritis or rheumatism. These diseases are responsible for about 14 million days lost from work each year, at a cost to the nation's economy that exceeds 3.5 billion dollars annually [524]. In the United States Health Examination Survey performed during the years 1960–1962 [176], osteoarthritis was found in the hands or feet of 37 per cent of the adult population. About 23 per cent of these adults with osteoarthritis had a moderate or severe form of the disease. Rheumatoid arthritis, defined as the presence of three or more of the American Rheumatism Association (ARA) criteria [585] and thus probable, definite, or classic rheumatoid arthritis, was found in 3.2 per cent of the adults of the United States, one-third of the identified patients having either definite or classic disease [176].

Table i-1. Frequency of Rheumatological Diagnoses Listed as Present in 45,602 Visits Made by 27,636 Patients to a Department of Medicine in San Francisco, July-December 1969

	Number of visits	Percentage of 45,602 visits
Musculoskeletal pain NFS*	1421	3.1
Osteoarthritis	1307	2.9
Rheumatoid arthritis	405	0.9
Gout	353	0.8
Periarthritis of shoulder	324	0.7
Postural back pain	185	0.4
Lumbar disc disease	160	0.4
Cervical disc disease	140	0.3
Neck sprain	109	0.2
Muscle cramps	95	0.2
Systemic lupus erythematosus	82	0.2
Elbow epicondylitis	34	0.07
Ankylosing spondylitis	29	0.06
Internal derangement of knee	23	0.05
Trochanteric bursitis	23	0.05
Ankle sprain	21	0.05
Myopathy NFS	20	0.04
Polymyositis	20	0.04
Total†	4751	10.4

* NFS = not further specified.

† Diagnoses omitted whose frequency was less than 20 in this period.

Yet all of the standard rheumatological texts and journals devote the majority of their space to rheumatoid arthritis and the collagen diseases, and pay disproportionately small attention to the problems that cause most of the disability in community practice.

The present text is an attempt to describe rheumatology as it is seen in an urban community, and is written for the general internist practicing in the com-

Table i-2. Sites of "Musculoskeletal Pain, Not Further Specified" in 50 Patients

	Per cent
Neck	24
Low back (muscular or postural)	24
Chest wall	20
Shoulder	6
Knee	6
Other joints	6
Limb, miscellaneous	14

munity. It may also be of some help to the rheumatologist in training, by providing a perspective that is not readily available elsewhere. The book takes for granted much background knowledge, and is not intended to be as comprehensive as the standard American text edited by Hollander and McCarty [313]. It contains, inevitably, many viewpoints that are biased by parochial experience; they are derived from having seen the rheumatological problems of 100,000 adults annually for ten years.

CHAPTER 1

Common Pain Syndromes

CERVICAL AND LUMBAR SYNDROMES

Pain in the neck, and pain in the lower part of the back present problems of diagnosis and treatment that are among the most common of those encountered in the office practice of rheumatology in the community. These are, too, among the most difficult conditions with which to deal, because the underlying mechanisms of causation are poorly understood. The usual presumption that these pain syndromes result from impingement on nerve roots, either by protruded intervertebral discs or by osteoarthritic spurs, is an oversimplification. That this is so, is shown by those patients who have severe radiological changes in the vertebrae without symptoms at any time; by those patients who have severe local pain but no radiologic changes in the vertebrae; by the frequent absence of neurological physical signs to support the presence of impaired function of nerve roots, and by the common presence of physical findings that show local muscle spasm. Spasm of paravertebral muscles is at least as common a cause of cervical and lumbar pain as is nerve root irritation. The pain from osteoarthritis in general, moreover, cannot result directly from degeneration of cartilage because this tissue has no nerve supply. Nerve endings that conduct pain are present in the joint capsule, in ligaments, and around vessels within the synovium. The pain derives from alteration in tension on the capsule and ligament, from distension of the blood vessels by inflammation, and from spasm of the surrounding muscles.

The observations of Lewis and Kellgren [420] are very important to the interpretation of clinical pain syndromes that originate in the neck and lower portion of the back. They found that, unlike pain arising from the skin, that which arises from deep structures is usually felt diffusely, is poorly localized, and is often felt at some distance from the stimulated point. They anesthetized the skin, then stimulated the underlying ligaments or muscles with injections of 6 per cent saline solution. Such injections induced a steady pain that lasted for several minutes. When the regions of the vertebral laminae and articular processes were injected, the segmentally referred areas of deep pain did not correspond exactly with the areas of segmental innervation of the skin. There were usually one or two areas of maximal pain within the full area of segmental distribution; if the pain was slight, only those points of maximal pain sensation were appreciated. In the limbs, these points of maximal pain were often in the joints; while in the trunk, they were in those areas of the deep fascia that have a rich nerve supply. When muscles were injected with the hypertonic saline solution, pain was strikingly referred to the joints moved by the injected muscle. Thus, pain derived from the anterior tibial muscle was felt at the ankle, and pain derived from the quadriceps was felt in the knee. Referred deep pain was accompanied by tenderness of the deep structures within the distribution of this pain. For example, stimulation of the infraspinatus by saline injections caused referred pain in the shoulder and tenderness of the deltoid muscle. Similarly, after stimulation of the fifth lumbar vertebra by the injections, the lateral side of the buttock, the posterior thigh, and the outer calf were painful and tender to deep palpation. The work of Lewis and Kellgren has been largely forgotten, which is a pity because it has direct relevance to the examination and treatment of patients with pain syndromes. The following experience is probably best understood on the basis of their observations:

Case 1-1. A 73-year-old woman with longstanding osteoarthritis affecting her neck, lumbar spine, and hands complained of pain in both sides of the neck. Physical examination showed that severe pain was elicited by pressure over the right acromioclavicular joint, and there was palpable and painful spasm in both midtrapezius muscles. Injection of lidocaine into the acromioclavicular joint induced immediate and total relaxation of both midtrapezius muscles.

The physical examination of patients who complain of pain in the neck that radiates into the head or arms should include not only a careful assessment of neck motion, but also examination of the state of the muscles of the shoulder girdle. If the pain syndrome results from impingement upon a nerve root, one may expect it to be reproduced or enhanced by maneuvers that aggravate the degree of impingement; e.g., ipsilateral flexion of the neck or telescoping the neck by downward pressure on the head. If the pain derives from muscle spasm, one may expect it to be reproduced or enhanced by maneuvers that irritate the muscle which is in spasm; e.g., contralateral flexion of the neck or squeezing the muscle. Spasm of the trapezius, especially its middle, or transverse, portion, or of the sternomastoid muscle is commonly responsible for pain in the neck. Spasm at the site of origin of levator scapulae is another frequent cause. Palpation of these muscles gives easy and convincing evidence of their tightness or spasm and of the fact that pain may be caused to radiate from them into the head and arm. Painful areas in the middle portion of the trapezius muscle cause pain that may be referred to the side of the head, the temple, or the arm; such areas in the upper portion of the trapezius cause pain that is referred to the back of the head; painful areas in the sternomastoid muscle cause pain referred to the region of the ear and sometimes to the throat.

The importance of differentiating between muscle and nerve root as the primary source of pain in the neck or arm lies in the diametrically opposite therapeutic approaches required for these mechanisms. Nerve root impingement by osteoarthritic spurs or by a prolapsed intervertebral disc requires immobilization of the neck by a collar and, sometimes, cervical traction. Muscle spasm requires local heat and stretching exercises; the exercises are especially inappropriate for nerve root impingement.

The decision that low back pain is caused by muscle spasm rather than by impingement on a nerve root is an extremely difficult one because the lumbar spine is not so freely mobile as is the cervical spine; and because severe protective muscle spasm is a frequent secondary phenomenon in lumbar disc disease. Thus,

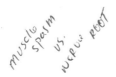

in the case of lumbar pain, the presence or absence of physical signs relating to impaired nerve root function is the most important physical finding. Again, the importance of determining which of the two mechanisms is the primary cause of the pain lies in the different therapeutic approaches required: strict immobilization for herniated discs; exercises and mobilization for muscle spasm. In either the lumbar or the cervical area, the use of local heat, local injections with lidocaine or corticosteroid preparations, and orally administered muscle relaxants may be useful.

BURSITIS AND TENOSYNOVITIS: A MULTIPLICITY OF PAIN SYNDROMES

According to Bywaters [80], there are some 156 bursae in the body. Some of these are at the frictional point where a muscle belly overlies a bony prominence; others, where muscle glides over muscle. In addition to bursae, there are many tenosynovial sites of potential inflammation and pain. For example, a woman complained of pain in the distal portion of the right thigh when she walked or sat for awhile. There was no pain in the knee or elsewhere in the lower limb. Physical examination showed that the pain occurred only with flexion of the knee against resistance. It was possible to demonstrate point tenderness in the tendon of the semitendinosus muscle in the distal portion of the thigh, about four inches above the popliteal fossa. Injection of this site with corticosteroid mixed with lidocaine induced complete and permanent relief. The following are common instances of tenosynovitis and bursitis of which the internist should be aware.

Trigger finger, a very common complaint, is due to tenosynovitis of the flexor tendons of the fingers, with nodular expansion of the tendon itself; when the tendon sheath undergoes circumferential fibrosis and contracture, the tendon nodule impedes free movement of the tendon during either its contraction or its relaxation. The jerky motion of the tendon nodule past the constricted portion of the tendon sheath causes the phenomenon known as trigger finger. In trigger thumb, the nodule is on the tendon of flexor pollicis longus; the patient frequently complains of pain in the interphalangeal joint of the thumb; but the palpable click felt in this joint when it is actively or passively moved is the clue that directs attention to the long flexor tendon.

Humeral epicondylitis is another common cause of discomfort. Although its precise pathological basis is not certain, this presumably results from tenosynovitis of the common flexor or extensor tendons of the forearm, from partial rupture of the tendon, or from inflammation of underlying bursae. Lateral humeral epicondylitis is more common than medial epicondylitis. The pain derived from lateral humeral epicondylitis is very typical, extending from the lateral aspect of the elbow down the dorsum of the forearm, over the back of the hand and into the fingers. The pain is mostly felt during motions that place considerable stress upon the extensor or flexor muscles that cross the wrist, e.g., lifting a heavy kettle or hammer, or twisting a doorknob. The pain may radiate upwards toward the shoulder or, rather rarely, into the scapular region. In lateral humeral epicondylitis, pain is induced in the epicondylar region by local pressure over the epicondyle or over the common extensor tendon, by performing a hand-grip while the wrist is flexed, and sometimes by resisted active extension of the fingers. In contradistinction to this diffuse radiation of pain from lateral humeral epicondylitis, the pain from medial epicondylitis is usually more localized to the medial aspect of the elbow. Both of these forms of epicondylitis are treated efficiently by local injections of corticosteroids. One should be careful, in medial epicondylitis, to inject only soluble steroid preparations, lest a crystalline preparation track posteriorly to the vicinity of the ulnar nerve and induce chemical neuritis.

Tenosynovitis of the extensor tendons on the dorsum of the wrist occurs frequently in rheumatoid arthritis, accounting for much of the obvious wrist swelling seen in that condition. It may be a troublesome problem to the patient. It is efficiently treated by local cortisone injections. Orthopedic surgeons often stress the important role of tenosynovectomy in preventing the complication of tendon erosion and rupture; but I have seen few such ruptures.

Achilles tenosynovitis is caused by Reiter's syndrome, ankylosing spondylitis, gout, or local pressure from ill-fitting shoes. Local injection of steroids is usually quite effective unless persistent friction by footwear is an important predisposing factor.

Tenosynovitis of the inferior tendon of the biceps brachii is an occasional manifestation of acute gout. It may lead to diagnostic confusion unless one is aware of this association.

Olecranon bursitis, a common problem, is most often caused by local trauma, gout, or rheumatoid arthritis. When the bursitis is of acute onset, and the bursa is tensely swollen and bright red, gout is its most likely cause; this diagnosis may be readily made by needle aspiration of the bursa and examination of the aspirate for uric acid crystals. The treatment for olecranon bursitis that is due to acute gout is the same as that for acute gouty arthritis. Rheumatoid arthritis may cause a chronic olecranon bursitis characterized by palpable nodules within the bursal sac. Rarely, the sac is infected; this may complicate needle aspiration and steroid injection.

Prepatellar bursitis, housemaid's knee, was most commonly of traumatic origin in the old days when floors were scrubbed on the hands and knees. Nowadays this is rare, and acute gout is its most frequent cause. Prepatellar bursitis may occur as an unusual manifestation of rheumatoid disease. The knees shown in Figure 1-1 are those of a patient with rheumatoid arthritis who had chronic prepatellar bursitis; the bursal sacs contained palpable nodules.

Although there are many causes of pain in and around the shoulder joint, including tenosynovitis of the superior tendon of the biceps, and small tears or inflammatory lesions of the rotator cuff, *the most common nontraumatic source of shoulder pain is subacromial bursitis.* The shoulder joint is extremely complex and it is difficult to be sure of the precise origin of pain coming from it; but I have found that the subacromial bursa is the most effective place for an injection in this area. This bursa is very easily injected by inserting a needle under the posterolateral aspect of the tip of the acromion process, while slightly separating the humeral head from the acromion tip by downward traction on the arm.

Trochanteric bursitis is a frequently assumed diagnosis for pain localized to the region of the greater trochanter. Although the diagnosis may be accurate in some instances, most often the pain may be elicited by deep palpation along the

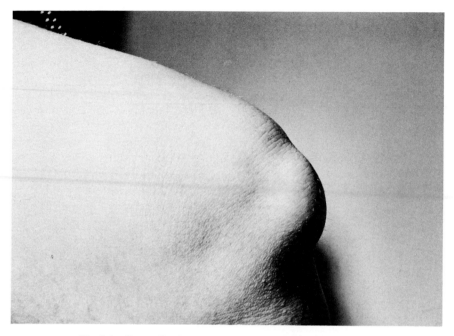

Fig. 1-1.   Prepatellar bursitis in patient with rheumatoid arthritis.

entire lateral aspect of the thigh, from the iliac crest downwards: it is then more likely to represent acute spasm in the muscle of the iliotibial band. As treatment for this pain syndrome it is usually inadequate to inject corticosteroids in the region of the greater trochanter alone. The entire region of the iliotibial band and its muscle requires infiltration with a dilute mixture of lidocaine and corticosteroid. Where unilateral spasm in the iliotibial band is recurrent, I have often found that the pelvis is tilted upward on the affected side; a heel lift on the contralateral shoe, sufficient to level the pelvis, usually suffices to prevent recurrence of the pain.

Anserine bursitis ("pes anserina" bursitis). The tendons of the sartorius, semimembranosus, and semitendinosus muscles cross the lower medial end of the femur in very close apposition, separated from one another and from the bone by a series of bursae. The three tendons are inserted into the upper and medial aspects of the shaft of the tibia via a common tendon, the so-called "anserine" tendon, beneath which is yet another bursa, which resembles a goose's foot in shape, hence is commonly called the *pes anserina* bursa. Any one of these various bursae may become inflamed and cause pain at the medial aspect of the knee. This is usually termed anserine bursitis, but it is often impossible to be sure precisely which of the various individual bursae is inflamed. The pain is usually felt diffusely in the medial side of the knee; the physical findings include tenderness over the sites of the aforementioned bursae, and absence of pain with motion of the knee. Sometimes the pain is reproduced by active contraction of the medial hamstrings or sartorius against resistance. It is important to differentiate between this pain syndrome and pain derived from the knee joint itself, so that a local injection of corticosteroids may be most effectively placed.

Several common pain syndromes may occur simultaneously. Sometimes more than one mechanism for pain in a limb may be simultaneously present.

Case 1-2. A 65-year-old woman complained of pain and numbness over the dorsal and ventral surfaces of the entire left hand, which radiated throughout the forearm to the elbow. Although the discomfort was worst in the second, third, and fourth fingers, the first and fifth were definitely affected. The symptom was present mostly by day, and had never awakened her. Although continuous, the complaint was aggravated, as in isolated epicondylitis, by grasping objects; moreover, the pain extended upwards from the elbow to the shoulder and into the side of the neck. Physical examination showed full cervical motion; but when the neck was flexed to the left, downward pressure on the head induced pain in the side of the neck and the left arm, together with numbness in the forearm and hand. These physical signs indicated radicular irritation in the neck as a source of pain. This conclusion was supported by the roentgenographic demonstration of osteophytes on the left side of cervical vertebrae, intruding into the nerve root foramina at the levels of $C_{3/4}$ and $C_{4/5}$. There was, too, a painful trigger point in the left midtrapezius muscle: this was possibly secondary to the root irritation. Pressure over the left lateral humeral epicondyle in the region of the common extensor tendon caused severe pain, confirming the presence of epicondylitis. There was definite hypalgesia in the median nerve distribution on the left side, where a positive Tinel's sign was elicited; Phalen's maneuver, i.e., hyperflexion of the wrist for one minute, reproduced the entire pain syndrome, causing a sensory disturbance in the hand, pain in the forearm, arm, midtrapezius region, and left neck region. During Phalen's maneuver, the patient reported numbness localized to the median nerve territory. These latter physical signs indicated carpal tunnel syndrome, and were confirmed by nerve conduction studies which demonstrated that latencies across the wrist of the distal motor and sensory fibers of the median nerve were greater on the left than on the right side (see Chapter 2 for discussion of carpal tunnel syndrome).

A second example is given to reemphasize the fact that elderly patients are likely to have several different underlying pathologic conditions.

Case 1-3. A 67-year-old woman was referred with the possible diagnosis of polymyalgia rheumatica, because she complained of pain in the neck and head, and had been observed to have a fast erythrocyte sedimentation rate. In fact, her pain was found to be in one side of the neck only, and radiated to both the head and arm on the same side. Laboratory findings included an erythrocyte sedimentation rate of 85 mm/hr (Westergren), fibrinogen level of 370 mg/100 ml; alkaline phosphatase level of 220 units/ml (normal, less than 90 units/ml), with normal levels of calcium, phosphorus, and α_2-globulin. Serum glutamic oxalacetic transaminase was borderline at 41 units (normal, less than 40 units) per 100 ml.

The high alkaline phosphatase was explained when review of x-rays that had been made at the referring clinic showed early Paget's disease of the skull. The pains in neck and arm were explained by the finding of osteophytic intrusion into the $C_{5/6}$ intervertebral foramen (Fig. 1-2A). Normal intervertebral foramina are shown for contrast (Fig. 1-2B).

The fast erythrocyte sedimentation rate was still a puzzle. The γ-globulin level was 36.8 g/100 ml, but the electrophoretic pattern did not show a monoclonal spike to suggest paraproteinemia. At first, the patient denied excessive alcohol intake; indeed, she claimed to have virtually abstained from ethanol for the past 30 years. However, she later admitted that approximately 40 years previously she had drunk liquor very excessively, and had frequently been inebriated. Sulfobromphthalein retention was 18.5 per cent at 45 minutes. Thus, the fast erythrocyte sedimentation rate was explained by cirrhosis; it was later discovered that this rate had been elevated for several years.

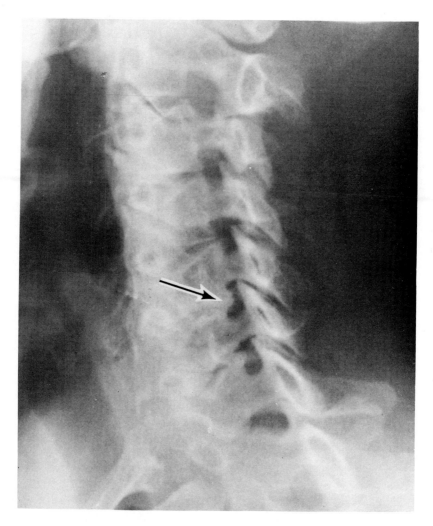

Fig. 1-2. A (above), oblique view of cervical spine showing osteophytes intruding into interverte-bral foramina at $C_{5/6}$ (arrow) and $C_{6/7}$. B, oblique view of normal cervical spine; normal shape and pa-tency of intervertebral foramina.

UNEQUAL LENGTHS OF LOWER LIMBS

Pain in either the knee or the hip may result from ipsilateral increase in limb length. Although well described [149], this cause of pain seems not to be widely appreciated. It is not rare; in a busy rheumatological practice, I see about one patient every month whose complaints clearly derive from this condition.

Case 1-4. A 36-year-old woman complained of pain in the left knee. Physical and roentgenologic examinations showed no abnormality in that knee. There was a very ob-vious discrepancy in the length of her legs, the right measuring, clinically, one inch shorter than the left. This was reflected by a considerable downward tilt of both the right shoulder and the right side of the pelvis. The discrepancy in leg lengths was confirmed by x-ray

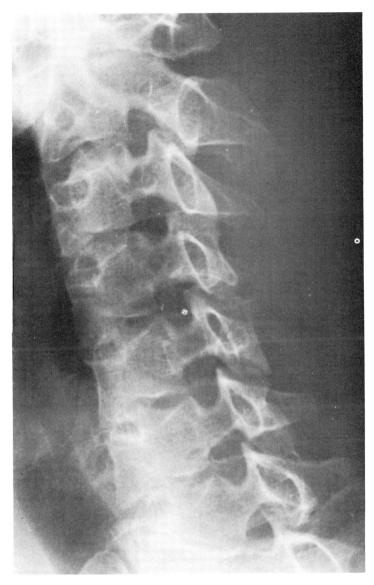

Fig. 1-2. B.

"scanograms" (Fig. 1-3), which showed a difference of 1 cm in length. After the right shoe sole had been built up by that amount, there was prompt relief of pain in the knee.

Unusual symptoms from asymmetric leg lengths were seen in the following patient.

Case 1-5. For the previous 15 years, a 52-year-old man had experienced a cold sensation in his right sole when stepping into water, even when he wore shoes; he had resorted to wearing fur-lined boots. More recently he had experienced pain in the entire right side of the body. In the upper limb, a sensation like an electric shock, starting in the

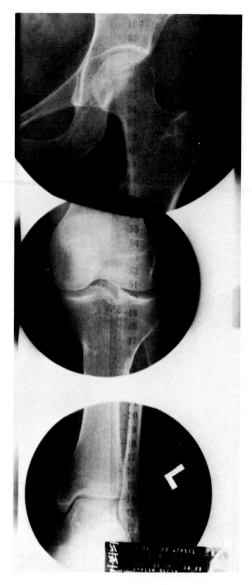

Fig. 1-3. Scanogram of legs enables one to measure the distance between the top of the femoral head and the bottom of the tibia so that the precise discrepancy between the two sides may be assessed.

lateral two digits of the hand, radiated up the arm to the neck and occiput. In the lower limb, a peculiar electrical sensation started in the toes and traveled up the leg to the right side of the belly. Physical examination showed a considerable downward tilt of the right shoulder and right side of the pelvis; there was evident compensatory kyphoscoliosis. Neurological examination revealed a heightened response to cold on the dorsal aspect of the anterior half of the right foot. Roentgenography revealed narrowing of the disc spaces between $C_{4/5}$, $C_{5/6}$, $L_{4/5}$, and L_5/S_1. Scanograms of the lower limbs showed shortening of one-half inch on the right, due entirely to a discrepancy between the lengths of the two femurs. During the course of the next three months, the right shoe sole was gradually built up a total of one-half inch. All of his symptoms ceased.

Knee pain may represent hip disease. Pain originating in the hip joint may occasionally be felt only in the knee.

Case 1-6. An intelligent man of 64 years had complained for at least two years of pain in the left knee, for which no cause had been found by internists or orthopedists. When I saw him, both knees were normal to physical examination; but motion of the hip in such a way as to stress the hip but not the knee reproduced pain in that knee and also caused pain in the hip. All of the hip motions were full. X-rays showed changes of severe osteoarthritis in the left hip.

Another patient, with severe Paget's disease in the hips (Fig. 1-4), had no pain in those hips during the eight years in which I treated her—only pain in the knees, which were clinically and radiologically normal!

POLYMYALGIA RHEUMATICA AND TEMPORAL ARTERITIS

Polymyalgia rheumatica and temporal arteritis are given consideration here in addition to the brief mention in the chapter on muscle diseases, because of the serious emergency that may develop when either of these is present. In all of the large reported series of patients with temporal arteritis, blindness developed in approximately 50 per cent of the patients. This tragic outcome may be prevented by use of corticosteroid drugs.

The incidence of classic temporal arteritis was estimated by Hauser and coworkers [297] in Rochester, Minnesota, as being approximately two cases per 100,000 per year. This is closely similar to our experience in the city of San Francisco, where we undertake the prepaid health maintenance of some 100,000 adults. Kurland and coworkers [394] demonstrated that the occurrence rises dramatically with increasing age: during the sixth decade of life the incidence of temporal arteritis was 1.7 per 100,000 per year; during the ninth decade it rose to 55 cases per 100,000 per year. In addition, we see approximately six new cases per year of polymyalgia rheumatica without clinically evident temporal arteritis.

In classic temporal arteritis there are swelling and tenderness over the superficial temporal artery, usually over the main branch just anterior to the ear. Later, the vessel may be palpable as a nonpulsatile cord. During the acute phase the entire scalp on that side may be extremely tender so that the patient dislikes sleeping with the affected side of the scalp against a pillow, and the hair follicles may be so tender that brushing or combing may be very disagreeable. About a third of the patients have accompanying polymyalgia. Loss of weight may be very prominent, often amounting to 20 or 30 pounds during four to six weeks. Two features of the illness are so frequent that nonconformity with them should raise doubts as to the accuracy of the diagnosis: virtually all patients are older than 50 years, and the erythrocyte sedimentation rate as measured by the Westergren method is over 50 mm/hr. Any major artery may be affected by the granulomatous arteritis; but there is an unexplained predilection for certain cranial vessels; namely, the superficial temporal, the ophthalmic, the posterior ciliaries, and the vertebral arteries. Rarely, the mandibular or lingual arteries are affected, inducing a dramatic symptom: claudication in the act of chewing and,

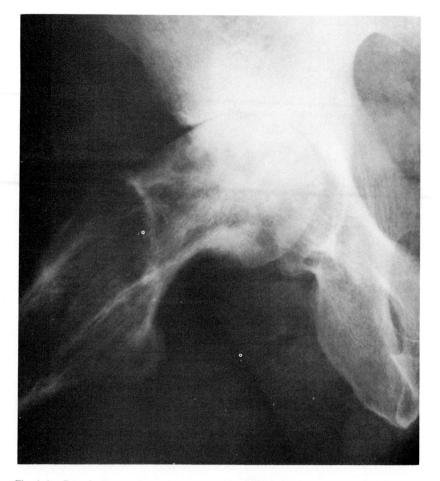

Fig. 1-4. Paget's disease of the hip. In this patient, all pain was referred to the knee; the hip itself was painless.

sometimes, blanching of the tongue. While the histopathological changes are classically those of granulomatous arteritis with giant cells (Fig. 1-5), a nonspecific arteritis without giant cells may occur (Fig. 1-6).

In the series of 154 patients reported from the Mayo Clinic [314], 50 per cent of the patients became blind in one eye within three months after onset of symptoms in the superficial temporal artery; among that group, a further 50 per cent became blind in the second eye within one month after occurrence of the original amaurosis. The administration of corticosteroid has dramatically reduced the incidence of blindness in both the first and second eye. If the second eye is to be saved, *it must be held as axiomatic that sudden blindness in a patient older than 50 years is caused by giant cell arteritis until proved otherwise.*

Two laboratory findings are worth emphasizing. First, the anemia may be marked and, on occasion, may occur in isolation. In an elderly patient with achrestic anemia accompanied by a rapid erythrocyte sedimentation rate, it is worth while making a superficial temporal artery biopsy even in the absence of other symptoms, because occasionally this may demonstrate arteritis as the underlying cause of the anemia [303]. Second, the level of α_2-globulin may be strikingly high. In almost all patients it is above normal (13 per cent of the serum proteins), and in some it accounts for 25 per cent of the total serum proteins. There are few other conditions in which the α_2-globulins are so remarkably high without an accompanying elevation in the γ-globulin fraction.

Polymyalgia rheumatica, another constitutional feature of giant cell arteritis, may appear separately from clinical temporal arteritis. Here again, the patients are almost invariably over the age of 50 years. The onset is often explosively sudden, with pain in the shoulder and pelvic girdle muscles, sometimes extending into the forearms and calves. There is often cervical and lumbar myalgia. Besides the pain, a prominent feature is stiffness of the muscles, which leads to a peculiar, stifflegged, penguin-like gait and difficulty in elevating the shoulders. As in clinical temporal arteritis, the accompanying loss of weight may be severe. Despite the marked muscle disorder and weight loss, all laboratory findings that ordinarily reflect a muscle disorder, i.e., serum enzyme levels, electrical testing and biopsy findings, show no abnormalities; indeed, when abnormalities are found by these examinations, the diagnosis of polymyalgia rheumatica must be discarded. Hematocrit readings, erythrocyte sedimentation rate, and α_2-globulin levels are the same as in clinical temporal arteritis. Biopsy of the superficial temporal artery reveals giant cell arteritis in 30 to 50 per cent of the patients. It can-

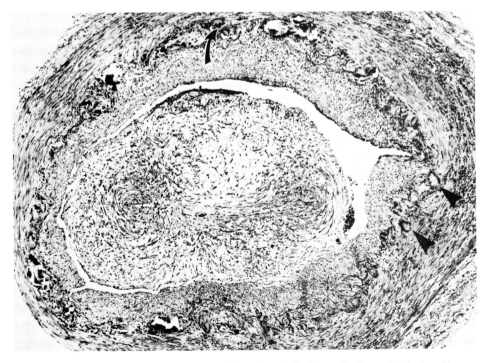

Fig. 1-5. Temporal artery from patient with polymyalgia rheumatica but no headaches. Biopsy taken after 2 weeks on prednisone 20 mg daily. Extreme fragmentation of internal elastic lamella which, in places, has disappeared; several multinucleated giant cells (arrows) adjacent to internal elastic lamella; moderate lymphocytic infiltrate persists in media to right of photograph. Hematoxylin and eosin, ×52.

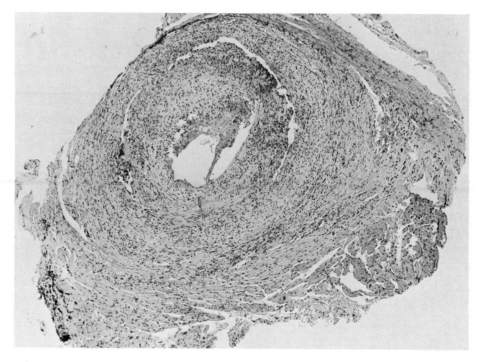

Fig. 1-6.   Acute temporal arteritis: intense infiltration of lymphocytes and plasma cells in media and adventitia, but no giant cells. Compare with Fig. 1-5.

not be too strongly emphasized that the biopsy may demonstrate giant cell arteritis even though there is no headache in the patient's history, and even though the temporal artery pulsates normally and no local tenderness is demonstrable. It has been shown by means of temporal arteriography that this type of arteritis does not affect the entire length or distribution of the vessel, but leaves unaffected many "skip" areas [246]. For this reason, bilateral biopsies of the temporal arteries should be done in every case because when positive this establishes the diagnosis as polymyalgia rheumatica. In one of our patients, two of three biopsies from different portions of the temporal artery gave negative findings. The temporal arteriogram is not a practical alternative, because it is tedious to perform and has not shown its superiority over biopsy as a means of detecting arteritis [323].

If both of the temporal artery biopsies give negative findings, then the case should be labeled as one of polymyalgia *syndrome,* and the label changed to polymyalgia rheumatica only after various other possible causes of the syndrome have been excluded. These include the following: hypothyroidism, which may cause marked myalgia and a very fast erythrocyte sedimentation rate; occult neoplasm (where this is suspected, early biopsy of the temporal artery may be important since, if positive, it clearly identifies the polymyalgia as part of giant cell arteritis and eliminates the need for tedious and costly work-up to exclude underlying neoplasm); systemic lupus erythematosus (SLE) (especially in elderly persons, a polymyalgia syndrome may be a prolonged prodrome of SLE) [210], and rheumatoid arthritis, where there may be an early anarthritic phase [26].

Only after an appropriate period of follow-up may one eliminate the latter possibilities with sufficient certainty to permit the diagnosis of polymyalgia rheumatica where the temporal artery biopsy is negative.

The response of the polymyalgia symptoms to corticosteroid drugs may be a helpful point in the differential diagnosis. Although many authors recommend using 20 or 30 mg. of prednisone daily as the therapeutic test, our experience shows that many cases of polymyalgia *syndrome* respond to these levels of prednisone. An approximately 50 per cent reduction in polymyalgic symptoms within the first 48 hours after only 5 mg of prednisone daily is a better clue to the likelihood of polymyalgia rheumatica. However, the danger of sudden blindness is too great to risk using tiny doses of prednisone before the results of the arterial biopsy are available, and higher preliminary doses are recommended (see below).

The frequency of blindness as a complication of polymyalgia rheumatica is difficult to assess because a case classified by one observer as polymyalgia rheumatica may be classified by another as being clinical temporal arteritis if, for example, there is a history of temporal headache or if there is tenderness over the superficial temporal artery. We have seen blindness develop in three patients among approximately 50 with polymyalgia rheumatica. Each of these three patients became bilaterally blind. In each, the superficial temporal artery biopsy showed giant cell arteritis.

Because the prevalence of blindness in polymyalgia rheumatica is not clearly defined, the question of treatment is not uniformly agreed upon. My approach is based upon the results of bilateral temporal artery biopsies of all patients. If the results of the biopsies show arteritis, then I treat the patient as I would any patient with temporal arteritis, i.e., with a moderate dose of prednisone—40 mg daily—for three months or until the erythrocyte sedimentation rate is normal, whichever period is longest. If the results of all biopsies are negative for arteritis, then I use symptomatically effective doses of prednisone and modify them according to the erythrocyte sedimentation rate. Because there is a danger, admittedly slight, that blindness may supervene before the biopsy has been performed or has been interpreted, I treat all patients with 40 or 60 mg daily of prednisone until the results of the biopsy are known.

The following case illustrates many interesting facets of classic giant cell arteritis.

Case 1-7. In a 61-year-old woman, rheumatoid arthritis developed in association with a background of psoriasis. About 10 years previously there had been a brief episode of acute polyarthritis, which had cleared after about six months. The rheumatoid arthritis was of such severity as to require small doses of prednisone for five years; the arthritis then became quiet and it was possible to withdraw the corticosteroid. About 15 months after the prednisone had been stopped, severe pain occurred in the right side of the neck, radiating into the right temple. Physical examination showed that both temporal arteries pulsated fully and were not tender; there was palpable spasm in the middle and upper portions of the right trapezius muscle. Because the erythrocyte sedimentation rate was 69 mm/hr (Westergren method), biopsy of the right superficial temporal artery was performed; the tissue had normal histopathological appearances. The pain in the neck and head ceased, but suddenly recurred about four months later, together with pain in both sides of the jaws accompanying chewing. Physical examination showed definite thrombosis in a peripheral branch of the left superficial temporal artery. Biopsy of that peripheral branch and the main portion of the left superficial temporal artery showed normal histologic patterns in the main portion of the vessel, but typical giant cell arteritis in the thrombosed peripheral portion. The symptoms cleared with prednisone therapy, but this was withdrawn after only five months because moderately severe hypertension developed, as well as a myopathy that was presumed to be secondary to the steroids. Two months later, she complained for the first time of intermittent claudication. Although the four pulses in her feet were all palpable, loud bruits were heard over both femoral arteries, and the brachial and radial pulses were absent in both arms. The blood pressure was not measurable in either arm. Loud bruits were heard over each subclavian, axillary, and brachial artery. Simultaneously with this episode, the erythrocyte sedimentation rate and fibrinogen level rose considerably. An arch aortogram revealed irregular narrowing of the right subclavian artery, extending into the proximal brachial vessel (Fig. 1-7). Restoration of the brachial and radial pulses, and of the blood pressure readings in the arms, was achieved by resumption of prednisone therapy.

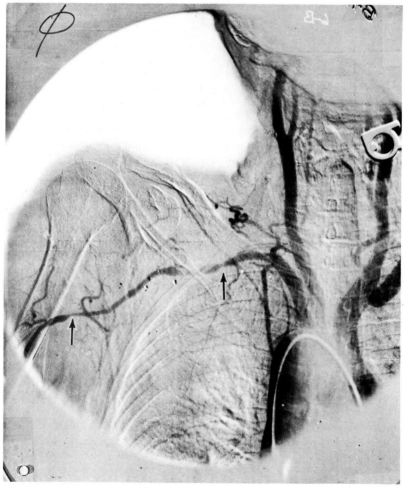

Fig. 1-7.   Case 1-7.   Arteriogram in giant cell arteritis; lesions (arrows) affecting subclavian artery.

A final interesting feature of this case has been the new appearance of antinuclear antibody in the serum, with negative LE cell preparations, a finding that I have observed in one other patient with giant cell arteritis proved by biopsy.

STRANGULATION OF MUSCLE

The anterior tibial syndrome is well known. It comprises pain in the anterior aspect of the leg, occurring after exercise and relieved by rest. It is considered to be the result of an excessively tight enclosure of the muscles in the anterior tibial compartment of the leg by a strong fascia. Rarely, there may be so much swelling of the muscles, induced by obstruction to the veins that drain the muscles and perforate the fascia, as to cause actual muscle necrosis.

The same mechanical problem may affect other muscles.

Case 1-8. A 25-year-old man complained that when he played his guitar he very rapidly experienced severe pain, stiffness, and swelling in the web of his left thumb, upon which he placed great strain in holding the guitar. It was possible to reproduce his syndrome by isometric contraction of the adductor pollicis brevis muscle. The adductor pollicis brevis is enclosed by a tight fascia in the lateral palmar space. His pain syndrome in the hand was analogous to the anterior tibial syndrome in the leg.

CHAPTER 2

Neurophysiology, Neurology, and Psychiatry in Rheumatologic Practice

Melzack and Wall [471] reviewed in 1965 the classic two opposing theories of pain, the *specificity theory* and the *pattern theory,* and proposed a new one of a *gate control system.*

According to the *specificity theory,* there is a mosaic of specific pain receptors in body tissue, which projects to a pain center in the brain. The pain impulses are carried by the A and C fibers in peripheral nerves, and by the lateral spinothalamic tract in the spinal cord, to a pain center in the thalamus. According to Melzack and Wall, the weakness of the specificity theory is its assumption that there is a direct, invariable, one-to-one relationship between stimulus and sensation. They pointed to the difficulties posed to this theory by causalgia, where surgical lesions of the peripheral and central system fail to abolish the pains; where light touch and other non-noxious stimuli may trigger excruciating pain; where new trigger zones for the pains may spread unpredictably to unrelated parts of the body where no abnormality exists, and in which pain from hyperalgesic skin often follows the stimulus after long intervals and continues beyond the removal of the stimulus. Among the psychological evidence that failed to support the assumption of a one-to-one relationship between pain perception and intensity of the stimulus, the most convincing example cited was that of wounded soldiers who entirely denied pain from their extensive wounds.

According to the *pattern theory* of pain, stimulus intensity and central summation are the two critical determinants. Within the framework of this theory, specific neural mechanisms have been suggested to account for the remarkable summation phenomena in clinical pain syndromes. Intense pathological stimulation of the body is conceived as setting up reverberating circuits in spinal internuncial pools, or as evoking spinal cord activities such as those reflected by the dorsal root reflex, which may then be triggered by normally non-noxious inputs and generate abnormal volleys that are interpreted centrally as pain. Related to theories of central summation is the theory of a specialized input controlling system which normally prevents summation. This proposes the existence of a rapidly conducting fiber system which inhibits synaptic transmission in a more slowly conducting system that carries the signal for pain. These two postulated systems which are required by the pattern theory have been given several names: epicritic and protopathic; fast and slow; phylogenetically new and old, or myelinated and unmyelinated fiber systems. None has received any substantial experimental verification.

The *gate control theory* of pain proposed by Melzack and Wall derives from the fact that stimulation of the skin evokes nerve impulses that are transmitted to three spinal cord systems: the cells of the substantia gelatinosa in the dorsal horn, the dorsal column fibers that project toward the brain, and the first central transmission cells in the dorsal horn. The gate control theory proposes that 1) the substantia gelatinosa functions as a gate control system which modulates the afferent patterns before they influence the central transmission cells; 2) the afferent patterns in the dorsal column system act as a central control trigger which activates selective brain processes, which in their turn influence the modulating properties of the gate control system; 3) the central transmission cells in the dorsal horn activate neural mechanisms which comprise the action system for response and perception; 4) pain is determined by interactions among these three systems. Experiments showed that the effect of nerve impulses in large fibers upon the central transmission cells in the dorsal horn was reduced by a negative feedback mechanism; whereas impulses in small fibers activated a positive feedback mechanism which exaggerated the effect of arriving impulses. These feedback effects are apparently mediated by cells in the substantia gelatinosa of the dorsal horn. The substantia gelatinosa consists of small, densely packed cells which form a functional unit extending the length of the spinal cord. Activity in these cells modulates the membrane potential of the afferent fiber terminals, thereby determining the excitatory effect of arriving impulses.

The spinal cord is continually bombarded by incoming nerve impulses even in the absence of obvious stimulation: this ongoing activity, carried predominantly by *small myelinated and unmyelinated fibers* which tend to be tonically active and to adapt slowly, *holds the gate in a relatively open position.* Since many of the larger fibers are inactive in the absence of stimulus change, when stimulation occurs it induces an increase in large fiber activity which is disproportionately intense relative to the increase in small fiber activity. When a *gentle stimulus* is applied to the skin, the afferent volley contains mainly *large fiber impulses* which not only fire the central transmission cells, but also *partially close the presynaptic gate,* thereby shortening the barrage generated by the central transmission cells. If the stimulus intensity is increased, more receptor fiber units are recruited and the firing frequency of active units is increased. The resultant positive and negative effects of the large-fiber and small-fiber inputs then tend to counteract each other; therefore, the output of the central transmission cells rises slowly. With *prolonged stimulation, the large fibers begin to adapt,* inducing a relative *increase in small fiber activity; as a result, the gate is opened further* and the output of the central transmission cells rises more steeply. Thus, the effects of the stimulus-evoked barrage are determined by 1) the total number of active fibers and the frequencies of the nerve impulses that they transmit, and 2) the balance of activity in large and small fibers. The theory allows for a central control of pain because it is established that stimulation of the brain activates descending efferent fibers which can influence afferent conduction at the earliest synaptic levels. Thus, it is possible for central nervous system activities subserving attention, emotion, and memories of prior experience to exert control over the sensory input. The gate theory suggests that these central influences are mediated through the gate control system described. It is proper to note that doubts have been expressed recently about 1) the accuracy of the wiring diagram proposed by Melzack and Wall, as well as 2) the inapplicability, as required by the Melzack and Wall hypothesis, of the theory of specificity of the primary afferents [646].

The gate control theory has relevance for the clinical rheumatologist, to the understanding of referred pain, spread of pain, and trigger points at some distance from the original site of body damage. The central transmission cell in the dorsal horn of the spinal cord has a restricted receptive field which dominates its normal activities; in addition, there is a widespread, diffuse input to the cell which may be revealed neurophysiologically by electrical stimulation of distant afferents. The gate theory would propose that this diffuse input from widespread sources is normally inhibited by presynaptic gate mechanisms, but may trigger firing in the cell if the input is sufficiently intense or if there is a change in gate activity. Because the central transmission cell remains dominated by its receptive field, anesthesia of the area to which the pain is referred, and from which only spontaneous impulses originate, is sufficient to reduce the bombardment of the cell below the threshold level for pain. The gate can also be opened by activities in distant body areas, since the substantia gelatinosa at any level receives inputs from both sides of the body and from the substantia gelatinosa in neighboring body segments. Mechanisms such as these presumably explain the findings of Lewis and Kellgren [420] as described in Chapter 1, and may account for such observations as that stimulation of trigger points on the chest induces pain in the limbs.

Further support for the gate theory came from Wall and Sweet [702], who studied eight patients with chronic cutaneous pain. When the sensory nerves and roots supplying the painful areas were stimulated so as to produce impulses only in the large-diameter fibers and close the gate, pressure on previously sensitive areas no longer evoked pain; some patients experienced sustained relief for more than 30 minutes after stimulation for only two minutes. Franz and Iggo [215] found that the evoked dorsal-root potential from small C fibers was either small or absent when preceded by the evoked dorsal-root potential from large A fibers (this presumably closed the gate), but became larger as the A fiber dorsal-root potential was reduced by cold-block of the impulses up the A fibers. The conclusion that myelinated A fibers exert an inhibitory effect on C fibers is supported by the histopathological observation that in postherpetic neuralgia the affected peripheral nerve shows a gross reduction in numbers of A fibers [518].

The gate hypothesis is important to the clinical rheumatologist also in understanding mechanisms whereby pain relief may be attained. In patients who have local muscle spasm, often derived from nerve root involvement by spinal osteoarthritis, it is common to inject the locally painful muscles with solutions of anesthetic, anesthetic mixed with corticosteroid suspensions, or even saline solution. Pain relief may last for days or months. Another common technique is to freeze or chill the skin overlying the painful muscles with ethyl chloride or fluorimethane sprays. Daily observation shows that chilling of the skin with such sprays results in immediate release of painful muscle spasm. The beneficial effects from these various therapeutic maneuvers can be explained on the basis of their interference with an afferent input of importance for pain perception. In a series of patients reported by Kibler and Nathan [377], pain and paresthesiae associated with lesions in peripheral nerves, nerve roots, root entry zones, posterior columns, and spinothalamic tracts were prevented by blocking the nerves distal to the lesion. By blocking the impulses from only a part of the region supplied by the affected nerves, it was possible to remove the spontaneous pain from the entire region. One of their patients was of particular interest. He had pain derived from arachnoiditis affecting the second through the fifth lumbar roots. Blocking of impulses from the cutaneous distribution of either the second and third posterior lumbar nerve roots or the fourth root caused cessation of pain throughout the distribution of all the roots. In some patients with pain of central nervous origin, Kibler and Nathan found that the relief from pain induced by local anesthesia lasted for months.

One corollary of the gate theory is that the pain from nerve root involvement may be caused by a *partial block* of nerve impulses passing through the root rather than by irritative phenomena. This may help explain pain in the distribution of cervical or lumbar nerve roots without collateral evidence of disc protrusion or radiological evidence of osteophytic intrusion into the intervertebral foramina.

Common clinical observation implies that spinal interneurones must be influenced by efferent controls as well as by afferent nerve impulses. The origin of these controls includes the cerebral cortex, brain stem, and other segments of the spinal cord itself. In the following case, sciatica as part of pain from acute gallbladder disease must have been under the control of descending pathways from the thoracic level to lumbar spinal interneurones.

Case 2-1. A 31-year-old woman complained of pain that started in the right upper quadrant of the abdomen, then radiated sequentially across to the left lower abdominal quadrant, around to the left lumbar region, and down the posterior aspect of the left lower limb as far as the ankle. Both the abdominal and sciatic components of this pain syndrome occurred after eating fatty food. Physical examination showed no significant abnormal findings in either the abdomen or the lower limbs. The deep tendon reflexes at the knees and ankles were present and symmetrical. X-rays of the lumbar spine, hips, and knees showed no evidence of disc disease or osteoarthritis. On barium x-ray examination, the entire gastrointestinal tract also appeared normal. Cholecystogram, however, showed many gallstones. Cholecystectomy was performed; over the ensuing eighteen months of observation, there was relief from the entire pain syndrome.

It seems possible to explain such a radiation of pain from gallbladder disease only by postulating a descending influence of an upper upon a lower segment of the spinal cord. Gunn and Keddie [272] described symptoms from gallstones, which were occasionally bizarre and confusing. In their 107 patients the sites of severest pain were unusually widespread, including the left lower portion of the chest, lower posterior portion of the chest, the left groin, and the left lumbar region.

THE NEUROLOGICAL OVERLAP

Clinical rheumatology interfaces with several medical disciplines, especially immunology, orthopedics, physical medicine, and neurology. Without a passing knowledge of each one of these, errors will occur.

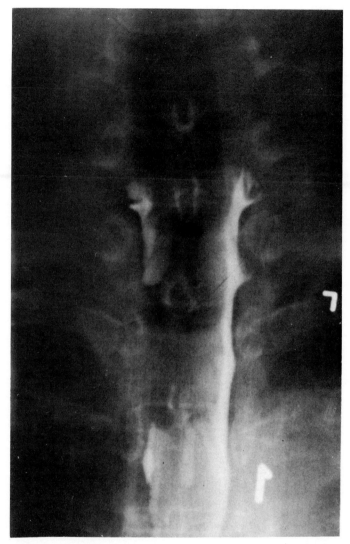

Fig. 2-1.   Case 2-2.   A (above), lumbar myelogram; block at level of C₇. B, cisternal myelogram; block commences at about level of C₂.

Cervical Cord Tumors

Case 2-2.   A 50-year-old woman had been seen by a rheumatologist elsewhere one year previously with the complaints of pain starting in the neck and radiating down both arms, and numbness in both hands. The pain was worse at night and disturbed her sleep. These symptoms had been present for 1½ years and had been accompanied by a loss of 20 pounds. The neck was found to have marked limitation of all motions; lumbar spine motion was also limited. Chest expansion was only 1½ inches. The tentative diagnosis of ankylosing spondylitis was not confirmed by x-rays of the sacro-iliac joints, which were normal; films of the cervical spine were not obtained at that time. During the next several months, her complaint of considerable weakness of the neck was considered to be probably hysterical.

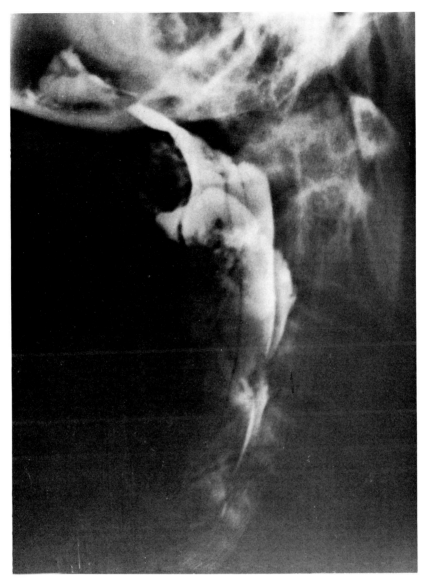

Fig. 2-1. B.

When seen at our clinic about 2½ years after onset of her symptoms, she stated that shortly after the pain had started in the neck and arms, numbness and tingling in her arms and hands had commenced, together with weakness and clumsiness of her hands. Later, both legs had become numb and she had experienced increasing difficulty in walking. During the previous months she had become so weak that she had had to hold to the bannister to ascend stairs. Neurological examination demonstrated exceedingly weak anterior neck muscles, so that she was barely able to raise her head off the couch. The biceps, triceps, deltoids, and muscles of the wrists and fingers were moderately weak. The hamstring and quadriceps muscles in the thighs were mildly affected. Temperature sensation in the hands and appreciation of vibration sensation in all four limbs were reduced. There were fasciculations in the right deltoid muscle. The biceps, triceps, and supinator reflexes were absent, and knee and ankle reflexes were hyperactive. Babinski responses were positive.

The above findings clearly indicated the presence of a cervical myelopathy. Combined lumbar and cisternal myelograms (Fig. 2-1A,B) demonstrated complete obstruction to the flow of dye between the levels of approximately C_3 to C_7. Neurosurgical exploration led to the complete removal of a benign ependymoma of the central cord. The patient made an uneventful recovery with rapid improvement in muscle strength.

Case 2-3. A 35-year-old man was referred by an orthopedist because of upper back pains that had started suddenly one year previously. Roentgenograms of the cervical spine had shown severe degenerative changes and the patient had received physiotherapy without improvement. Further historical detail included the intermittent occurrence of either electrical shock-like sensations or numb sensations that radiated from the fingers to the shoulders. For approximately a month he had noted progressive numbness of both feet and a tight sensation in the groin. More recently, both lower limbs had felt quite stiff. Pertinent physical signs included fasciculations of the triceps and forearm muscles, with wasting of the small muscles of the hand, spasticity of both lower limbs, hyperactive deep tendon reflexes, and positive Babinski reflexes.

Although the plain roentgenograms of the cervical spine (Fig. 2-2) showed marked degenerative changes, it was clear that this patient, also, had a cervical myelopathy. Cervical myelogram (Fig. 2-3) showed bar defects at the $C_{5/6}$ and $C_{4/5}$ levels. The sagittal diameter of the cervical canal at $C_{6/7}$ measured only 7.5 mm (normal would be approximately 14 to 17 mm).

Marked narrowing of the cervical canal and extensive osteophytosis impinging upon the canal were seen during the laminectomy.

Tumors of the foramen magnum, which account for only about 2 per cent of all spinal cord tumors, are important in rheumatological differential diagnosis because neck pain is one of their common manifestations. The early diagnosis of tumors in the region of the foramen magnum is difficult, because the cisterns at this level can accommodate a large quantity of neoplastic tissue before abnormal neurologic findings occur. Symptoms result from compression of the second cervical nerve root, inducing occipital pain; and from compression of the pyramidal or medial lemniscal decussations. Compression of the pyramidal decussation causes a mixture of upper motor neuron findings in the upper and lower extremities which may be difficult to trace to a single lesion; pressure on the medial lemniscal decussation gives rise to abnormalities in proprioception from one or all limbs, and sometimes to stereoanesthesia in one or more extremities. Stereoanesthesia from long tract lesions is distinguishable from the astereognosis of parietal lobe lesions by the absence, in stereoanesthesia, of such signs of parietal lobe dysfunction as extinction of double simultaneous stimuli or absent skin writing. Each of six patients with a benign tumor near the foramen magnum reported by Howe and Taren [317] underwent many months of inappropriate medical, surgical, and chiropractic therapy. These lesions were misdiagnosed as cervical spondylosis, multiple sclerosis, or ruptured discs. In four of the six patients, myelography was performed but did not demonstrate the tumors; in one other patient, the tumor was demonstrated only at the fourth myelogram. Another confusing aspect of this condition is that the spinal fluid protein is not always elevated.

CARPAL TUNNEL SYNDROME

The possibility of this condition is often overlooked by nonspecialists: patients with this syndrome are usually referred for rheumatological opinion with the diagnosis of "arthritis of the hands." Our studies of 50 patients with carpal tunnel syndrome show the diversity of symptoms. Patients describe the sensations in their hands in various ways, as numbness, tingling, ants crawling, tightness or bursting, a painful coldness, burning or scalding, throbbing or

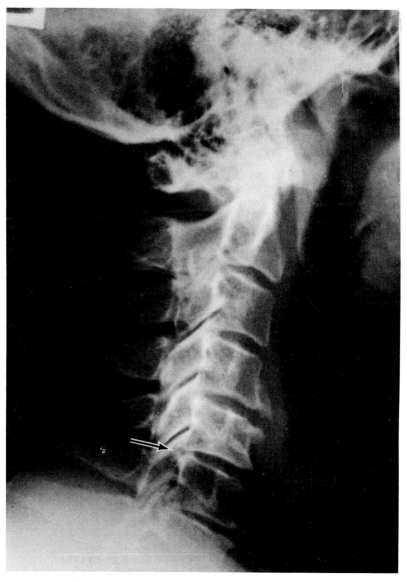

Fig. 2-2. Case 2-3. Lateral x-ray of cervical spine: minimal osteophytosis protruding posteriorly (arrow). Compare with Fig. 2-3.

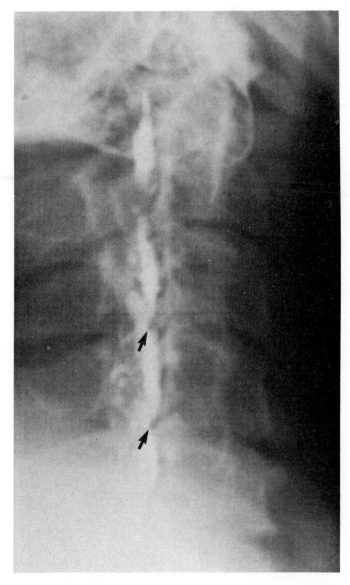

Fig. 2-3. Case 2-3. Lateral view of cervical myelogram with osteophytes indenting the column of dye (arrows). Compare with Fig. 2-2.

pulling. Among 50 patients analyzed (Table 2-1), 25 experienced radiation of the symptom above the wrist: six had radiation to the forearm, another six to the elbow, two to the upper arm, nine to the shoulder, one to the pectoral muscle, and one as far as the neck. Thirty-seven of the 50 patients experienced their symptoms at night as well as by day, and in 18 of these the symptoms were worse at night than during the day. A characteristic history includes relief from the symptoms when the hands are shaken, when the arms hang off the bed, or when the hands are massaged. Certain features—namely, occurrence of symptoms at night and relief by shaking the hands or hanging the arms down from the bed—suggest the diagnosis even before the patient is examined.

Sensory examination usually does not show marked defects of sensation in the distribution of the median nerve: most often there is no sensory abnormality, or merely a dysesthesia, i.e., an unusually unpleasant sensation resulting from a light scratch or stroke in the territory of the median nerve. Although the finding of muscle weakness is exceptional save in advanced cases, the motor examination is important because if weakness is present, surgical decompression of the carpal tunnel should not be long delayed. The muscles innervated by the median nerve

Table 2-1. Fifty Patients with Carpal Tunnel Syndrome

	No. of Patients
Symptoms	
Numbness, tingling, pain	29
Numbness, tingling	19
Pain	2
Clumsiness in fingers	5
Radiation of symptoms above wrist to	
Forearm	6
Elbow	6
Arm	2
Shoulder	9
Pectoral region	1
Neck	1
Time of symptoms	
Nocturnal or at first awakening	19
Night-time worse than daytime	18
Unspecified	13
Relief from shaking the hands, or hanging hands down from bed	14
Tinel's sign	
Positive	25
Negative	14
Unrecorded	11
Phalen's sign	
Positive	18
Negative	8
Unrecorded	24
Tourniquet test	
Positive (less than 2 minutes)	15
Equivocal (2 to 5 minutes)	5
Unrecorded	26
Median nerve motor latency across wrist	
Prolonged	18
Normal	6
Not measured	26

after it enters the carpal tunnel are 1) the abductor pollicis brevis, tested by the patient's ability to raise the thumb against resistance, toward the vertical position, with the hand supinated; 2) the flexor pollicis brevis, tested by the ability to flex the thumb at the metacarpophalangeal joint against resistance, and 3) the opponens pollicis, tested by the ability to oppose the thumb across the palm against resistance. Tinel's sign is elicited by tapping a reflex hammer over the median nerve at the wrist: the nerve enters the hand just medial to the tendon of palmaris longus. A positive Tinel's sign consists in sensations of electricity radiating into one or more of the lateral four digits: occasionally the sensory disturbance may radiate proximally toward the elbow as well as, or instead of, distally. Phalen's maneuver is hyperflexion at the wrist for 60 seconds; the response is positive if paresthesiae occur during this time in the distribution of the median nerve: if this test gives negative results, then hyperextension at the wrist for 60 seconds should be tried. If the above examinations fail to confirm carpal tunnel syndrome, the brachial artery should be occluded by a sphygmomanometer cuff for 5 minutes; aside from the discomfort of ischemia, this does not produce unpleasant symptoms except in carpal tunnel syndrome, where paresthesiae in the distribution of the median nerve occur—usually within 2 or 3 minutes. The final diagnostic test is measurement of the median nerve conduction velocity across the wrist, which is prolonged in carpal tunnel syndrome: unfortunately, the motor conduction time is not always prolonged in otherwise classic cases; and the more sensitive electrodiagnostic procedure, sensory nerve conduction, is not available in all laboratories.

Our own observations show that conservative therapy is effective in approximately 85 per cent of patients with carpal tunnel syndrome. In follow-up periods of up to 7 years (more than 1 year in 17 of the 50 patients), only 8 patients required surgical division of the retinaculum. Thiazide drugs were used as initial therapy in 35 of the 50 patients (Table 2-2); partial or complete relief was achieved with these alone in 22. In 8 patients, no other form of therapy was necessary. Before surgical decompression is recommended, a trial of corticosteroid injections into the carpal tunnel should be made.

ULNAR TUNNEL SYNDROME

Compression of the ulnar nerve as it passes through the ulnar tunnel in the palm of the hand is analogous to compression of the median nerve in the carpal tunnel syndrome. The ulnar nerve enters the hand by passing anterior to the flexor retinaculum and then lateral to the pisiform bone in the palm. At this point, it passes through a tunnel within the substance of the pisohamate ligament and is here subject to compression. Many patients who have median nerve compression within the carpal tunnel also complain of paresthesiae in the distribution of the ulnar nerve. Isolated ulnar tunnel symptoms, however, are extremely rare: I have recognized fewer than six instances during 10 years.

Case 2-4. A woman aged 35, with severe rheumatoid arthritis since her early teenage years, had marked rheumatoid deformities of the fingers and extensive radiological changes at the carpus. Her symptoms were painful paresthesiae in the fifth and

Table 2-2. Results of Hydrochlorothiazide Given as Initial
Therapy to 35 Patients with Carpal Tunnel Syndrome

		No. of Patients
Relief from hydrochlorothiazide		28
Complete relief lasting after cessation of therapy	8	
Complete relief only during continued thiazide therapy	6	
Marked improvement, followed by recurrence	3	
Partial relief, other measures necessary	11	
No relief from hydrochlorothiazide		7

fourth fingers of one hand, which awakened her at night. By shaking her hand vigorously she was able to rid herself of these symptoms as do persons with carpal tunnel syndrome. She had diminished sensation to pinprick in the fifth and fourth digits, but excellent strength in the abductor digiti minimi, and normal motor conduction velocity in the ulnar nerve.

TARSAL TUNNEL SYNDROME

The tarsal tunnel syndrome, in which the posterior tibial nerve is entrapped, either as it passes beneath the flexor retinaculum behind the medial malleolus of the ankle, or as it enters the foot through the substance of the abductor hallucis brevis, is quite uncommon. Yet if one is unaware of this entrapment syndrome, the symptoms it induces may suggest an incorrect diagnosis of arthritis. Pain, tingling, or numbness in the sole of the foot occurs in a distribution that depends upon whether the posterior tibial nerve, the medial plantar nerve, or the lateral plantar nerve is affected. Radiation of the symptoms into the calf sometimes occurs. A positive Tinel's sign may be elicited by tapping of the nerve behind the medial malleolus or in the posterior third of the abductor hallucis brevis. The sensation of pinprick may be impaired in the medial or lateral forefoot, depending upon whether the medial or lateral plantar nerves are affected. Soluble cortical steroids should be injected at the point where the positive Tinel's sign is obtained.

PSEUDOCLAUDICATION: CAUDA EQUINA SYNDROME: CYCLIC SCIATICA

Case 2-5. A 75-year-old man complained of pain that started in the lower part of the back and radiated down the posterior aspect of each thigh into the middle of the calf. The pain occurred only after he walked for two or three blocks and left almost immediately upon resting. The only pain that he experienced when not walking was in the back when he twisted in bed at night. Physical examination showed loss of the normal lumbar lordosis, with retention of approximately 75 per cent of the normal ranges of motion of the lumbar spine. The deep tendon reflexes at the knees and ankles were absent even with reinforcement. Sensation to pinprick was normal in both feet and there was only slight reduction in sensation to vibration at the ankles. All of the four pedal pulses were full and bounding; no bruit was heard over the femoral or carotid arteries. X-rays showed first-degree spondylolisthesis of L_4 on L_5, diminution of intervertebral disc spaces throughout the lumbar spine, and a considerable number of anterior and lateral osteophytes throughout the lumbar spine (Fig. 2-4).

The case just cited is an example of the so-called "pseudoclaudication syndrome" described in several publications by Kavanaugh and coworkers [370].

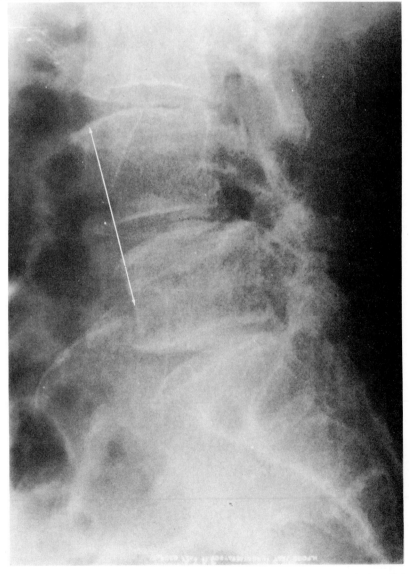

Fig. 2-4. Spondylolisthesis of L_4 on L_5, with narrowing of disc spaces, in Patient 2-5, with pseudoclaudication syndrome.

The clinical picture is quite characteristic, with pain in the lower limbs which is indistinguishable from that of intermittent claudication induced by peripheral vascular insufficiency; however, there is no evidence of vascular occlusion as in the typical patient with intermittent claudication. In the patients reported by Kavanaugh and coworkers, it was not until after arteriography had demonstrated complete patency of the peripheral arterial circulation that myelography was undertaken; it demonstrated disc protrusion. An occasional patient with this disorder has active ankle jerks at rest, which disappear after the patient has exercised to the point of pain.

A postulated mechanism for this syndrome is as follows: pressure by the herniated disc or the protruding osteophytes upon the lumbar venous plexus impairs its drainage. Under conditions of exercise, the plexus becomes engorged and either directly, or indirectly via the cerebrospinal fluid in the nerve root sleeve, causes pressure upon the nerve root, which leads to the pain syndrome. While the explanation is somewhat complex, the recognition of the clinical entity is of considerable importance to the selection of treatment.

Cauda equina syndrome. These patients with pseudoclaudication of the cord remind one of the cauda equina syndrome that has been described in patients with ankylosing spondylitis [258, 596]. In the patients with ankylosing spondylitis, however, the features suggestive of peripheral vascular disease are absent: the pains in the legs are persistent and are not particularly aggravated by exercise. Moreover, the usual features of cauda equina syndrome are present, with incontinence of urine or feces, or both, and sensory impairment in the distribution of the sacral nerve roots. A noteworthy feature has been the myelographic finding of diverticula of the lumbar sac. The importance of performing the myelogram with the patient in the supine position, so as to fill posterior lesions, has been emphasized. Arachnoiditis associated with ankylosing spondylitis has been proposed as responsible for these cases of cauda equina syndrome.

Cyclic sciatica. When ought one to consider the possibility of an obscure cause for a common symptom such as low back pain or sciatica? There are, obviously, many causes of these symptoms other than the common disc protrusions or arthritic degenerations of the spine. A careful history and physical examination will often suffice to suggest which patients might have some cause other than a common one. For example, when sciatica occurs intermittently, in close relation to the menstrual period, one may give strong consideration to the condition known as cyclic sciatica, where endometriosis occurs in or on the sciatic nerve or plexus [212].

On the other hand, even the common disc protrusion may require a careful history for its unmasking, as demonstrated by the following patient.

Case 2-6. A 23-year-old woman complained of cramps in one calf, present for two weeks, for which quinine had been unsuccessfully administered. Only after persistent questioning did she admit occasional paresthesiae in the fourth and fifth toes on that side as well as a recent, rare pain in the lower portion of the back on the same side. There had been no back injury or recent heavy lifting. Physical examination demonstrated loss of the ankle jerk, and mild weakness of dorsiflexion of the foot on the affected side. Although motions of the lumbar spine were full, hyperextension of the spine reproduced the pain in her calf. A myelogram showed a large defect in the L_5-S_1 interspace on the side of the pain; laminectomy with removal of the herniated disc cured her pain syndrome.

In the differential diagnosis of pain in the limbs, especially the lower limbs, one must remember that although tabetic lightning pains are uncommon, they are not rare.

Case 2-7. A 57-year-old woman had been seen by two general internists, a cardiologist, and another rheumatologist during the previous two years for her complaint of pain in the limbs. During the prior five years, three Venereal Disease Research Laboratory (VDRL) tests for syphilis had been negative. She stated that during the last two or three years there had been spasms of sharp pain that had started in the legs but now affected all four limbs as well as the trunk. These were intensely sharp and momentary. They did not radiate down the limb, but rather bore inwards. An uneducated woman, she gave a classic description: " . . . like my bones are trying to be broke (sic); like a knife has been put in there and twisted." For about five years she had experienced pain in the rectum, which lasted for a few minutes at a time and was very intense. More recently, there had been lower abdominal pains lasting from 10 minutes to 4 hours. Positive neurological physical signs included impairment of vibration and joint sense, and patchy impairment of temperature sensation in one lower limb. A VDRL blood test was again negative; but the fluorescent treponemal antibody blood test was positive. Unfortunately, she moved from the area shortly thereafter, and it was not possible to examine her cerebrospinal fluid.

In another patient with lightning pains in the lower limbs, responses to all serological tests for syphilis were negative, but there was a markedly abnormal glucose tolerance curve. I have also observed lightning pains in a further case of diabetic neuropathy, as well as in a patient with mononeuritis multiplex as part of the arteritis of severe rheumatoid arthritis. Almost any peripheral neuropathy may, rarely, be accompanied by lightning pains.

PARKINSONISM

The differential diagnosis of pain in the limbs must account for all possible affections of muscles, bones, joints, arteries, and nerves. Disease of the basal ganglia of the brain may be culpable, as in the following case.

Case 2-8. A 52-year-old Mexican American man had vague pains in his limbs for a few months before he was referred by his internist with a diagnosis of dermatomyositis. The situation had come to a head as a result of his recent dismissal from his work as a cook because he had become too slow. His face was remarkably plethoric and there was periorbital edema. All of his muscles were normal in strength. However, careful examination revealed a considerable increase in muscle tone, with so-called "lead-pipe" as well as "cog-wheel" rigidity in his right upper limb. He had lost the associated movements on the right side. Treatment with benztropine mesylate and levodopa induced dramatic improvement.

POSSIBLE CONTRIBUTIONS OF THE CENTRAL NERVOUS SYSTEM TO THE PATHOGENESIS OF CONNECTIVE TISSUE DISEASES

It is a matter of daily observation that a variety of circumstances contribute to any given instance of disease. Even an apparently simple infection is caused not only by the pathogenic organism that invades the body. Illustrating this point with the example of a man who had a cerebral thrombosis due to syphilitic endarteritis, Cohen [116] argued that the *Treponema pallidum* was a necessary but not sufficient cause of the man's disease, and that a host of causes—physical and psychological, acquired and hereditary—brought him to take the step that led to the hemiplegia. It seems probable that connective tissue diseases, multiple sclerosis, schizophrenia, arteriosclerosis, cancer, and most other major diseases of uncertain genesis have multiple causation. Christian [105, 106] hypothesized that in rheumatoid arthritis and systemic lupus erythematosus, genetic factors modify the host response, probably via altered immune mechanisms, allowing a ubiquitous environmental factor, e.g., a viral agent, to express itself in various ways.

The problem of multiple causation raises two important questions. The first concerns the component events and their relative importance; the second is the problem of how those events that are apparently unrelated in time or quality can be so integrated as to induce a disease picture. I have proposed a model for multiple causation that views pathogenesis as entailing three definite phases, each phase being contributed to by many factors, which are interrelated in a complicated way (Fig. 2-5) [198, 199]. In the early phase, a relationship between reacting factors is established; in the middle phase, the advent of a further constellation of factors sets in motion the tissue reaction of a general kind; in a final phase, clinical disease results as yet more factors precipitate chain reactions that arise from the background of the second phase. The proposed scheme can be justified in that it fits many of the known clinical and experimental facts about pathogenetic mechanisms, and many of its implications are open to experimental verification. This model seems particularly relevant to rheumatoid arthritis, and probably also to the other connective tissue diseases, where the possible pathogenetic categories of events include those of an infectious, endocrinologic, genetic, immunologic, and psychological nature [105].

Supporting this model is the evidence that experience of prior illnesses provides a background of pathogenetic determinants whose effects are cumulative. Jones [350], using mortality statistics derived from national population studies, concluded that each disease experience leaves permanent residua which tend to compound themselves and to make each subsequent disease experience more likely. He observed that individuals born and passing their childhood during years in which the infant and childhood death rates from infectious diseases were high had a greater-than-average tendency to incur internal disease during adult life; and that their death rates from these causes were higher than average. For example, in the populations of Sweden, Denmark, and Holland, Jones showed that increases and decreases in death risk in subpopulations defined by being at age 5 years in specific past years were strikingly paralleled by increases and decreases in death risk in the identical subpopulations when they reached age 50. Gibson and coworkers [243] studied the association between childhood leukemia and four other factors: 1) irradiation of the mother before conception of the child or 2) during pregnancy, 3) the mother's history of miscarriages and stillbirths before the child's conception, and 4) certain virus diseases contracted by the child more than 12 months before the diagnosis of leukemia. Their results showed that the current risk of leukemia rose with the increase in number of these factors occurring in the past. Statistical significance, however,

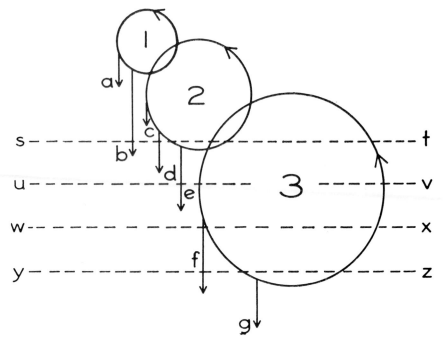

Fig. 2-5. The phases of pathogenesis. The circles represent the three phases of pathogenesis. Each phase is a constellation of many dynamically interrelated events and all phases are themselves interrelated. Linear chains eventuating from the separate phases are shown by arrows *a* to *g*.

   The symptoms, signs, and biochemical changes seen at a given time are a cross-section of all the events occurring at that time. The cross-sections are thus quite different, depending upon whether they are taken at times *s-t*, *u-v*, *w-x*, or *y-z*. (Reprinted by permission, from Arch Gen Psychiat 11:1–18, 1964 [198].)

was reached only if there had been a combination of irradiation with either virus disease in childhood or a maternal history of miscarriages and stillbirths. Another study showing that many antecedent events may participate in pathogenesis was made of multiple sclerosis by Currier and coworkers [130]. Sixty patients with multiple sclerosis had had significantly more of such antecedent events as infections, trauma, and surgical operations than had matched controls. A pertinent observation illustrating that a single pathogenetic event in the distant past may relate to serious disease in the present is the finding that stilbestrol given to the pregnant mother is associated with a high risk of genital cancer many years later in the female child born of that pregnancy [308].

   The remainder of this chapter considers the evidence that the central nervous system (CNS) participates in the pathogenesis of connective tissue diseases following the model of multiple causation just described. It is emphasized that a CNS dysfunction is not seen as a prime or sole pathogenetic factor, but as merely one *category* of pathogenetic event. Briefly discussed will be the influence of the CNS upon 1) immunogenesis, 2) the clinical course of certain connective tissue diseases, and 3) the development in animals of lesions resembling those seen in connective tissue diseases in humans. Some of the personality patterns that have been described in patients with connective tissue diseases will be mentioned.

INFLUENCE OF THE CENTRAL NERVOUS SYSTEM UPON IMMUNOGENESIS

There is considerable evidence that mental stress and disturbances of the hypothalamus and diencephalon affect blood protein levels [199]. Emotional stress was found to be associated with a significant rise of 19S proteins [199]. Lundin and coworkers [432] found that in rats, various forms of prolonged stress led to intense plasma-cell proliferation in several organs.

The role of the CNS in anaphylaxis has been studied for more than fifty years. For example, in 1910 Banzhaf and Famulener showed that anesthesia with chloral hydrate inhibited the anaphylactic response [29]. In a series of sensitized guinea pigs, the smallest dose of serum that regularly would kill any animal of the series was not lethal to those that had been properly anesthetized with chloral hydrate. Such studies have been continued and confirmed. Luk'yanenko [431] found that narcosis inhibited anaphylaxis, and Zakrividoroga [737] showed that reduction of parasympathetic tone delayed the primary immune response. The effect of the hypothalamus upon immunological reactivity was shown in an extensive series of reports by Szentiványi and his coworkers [666, 667]. Lesions in the region of the tuber cinereum, but not in other areas, gave protection against both active and passive anaphylactic shock. The tuberal lesion seemed to be associated with a reduction of both circulating and tissue-fixed antibodies and with increased resistance to histamine. Protection against both histamine shock and anaphylactic shock was induced by electrical stimulation of the tuberomammillary and anterior mammillary regions but not by stimulation of other areas of the hypothalamus. Freedman and Fenichel [218] were able to inhibit anaphylaxis by placing bilateral lesions in the reticular formation at the level of the superior colliculus; these authors found great variation in their ability to inhibit anaphylaxis, which seemed to depend upon the precise location of the lesions. They considered that the midbrain affected anaphylaxis by influencing smooth muscle tonus. A series of reports by Rasmussen and his coworkers [349, 570] described how the stresses of either high-intensity sound or avoidance-learning influenced passive anaphylactic shock and host resistance to viral infection.

Immune responses of the delayed type are also influenced by the CNS. Wistar and Hildemann [728] saw delayed skin homograft rejection after chronic avoidance-learning, and Levine and coworkers [415] observed a suppression of experimental allergic encephalomyelitis (EAE) by stress. EAE was inhibited also by reserpine treatment; this was postulated to result from interference with a central mechanism for control of immune response [339]. Mason and Black [446] were able to abolish positive skin test reactions to pollen allergens by hypnosis; the humoral basis for the hypersensitivity response remained, as shown by a positive Prausnitz-Küstner reaction in the skin of a volunteer who was ordinarily insensitive to the allergens.

Urbánek and Jansa [689] used the skin window technique to assess the inflammatory response at 24 hours after making a skin lesion: the results were considered normal if >60 per cent of the cells were macrophages, and severely abnormal if <20 per cent of the cells were macrophages. All of the 146 control subjects had normal responses. There were severely abnormal responses in 12 of the 19 patients who had lesions of cerebral cortical fields known to be related to the autonomic nervous system, i.e., the fronto-basal, fronto-polar, or insular regions. Other patients with severely abnormal results included seven of ten with Charcot-Marie-Tooth disease, and five of ten with amyotrophic lateral sclerosis. These findings give further evidence for a role of the nervous system in the inflammatory response.

The influence of stress upon the blood proteins and immunogenesis is presumably mediated by the CNS. A likely pathway is the limbic system, hypothalamus, pituitary and peripheral endocrine glands; however, the experimental evidence for such a link between CNS and immunogenesis is not substantial. Some of this evidence has been summarized elsewhere; [199] the work of Szentiványi and coworkers [667], and of Freedman and Fenichel [218] was mentioned above. Korneva and Khai [388] showed that lesions in the dorsal hypothalamus completely suppressed antibody formation and delayed elimination of antigen from the blood. Beardwood and coworkers [34] found that in baboons, hypophysectomy caused a considerable rise in γ-globulin; the level fell to normal after administration of hydrocortisone. One effect of altered hypothalamic function is upon the pituitary-adrenal axis, and this is presumably a way whereby the immune system is influenced. That adrenocortical hormones can modify the immune response is well known. It has been observed that steroid sex hormones also can modify the immune response: Kappas and coworkers [363] found that the injection of estrone together with thyroglobulin and complete Freund's adjuvant caused greatly diminished intensity of induration in the delayed skin reaction to both tuberculin and thyroglobulin. Estrone diminished the incidence of adjuvant-induced arthritis by 50 per cent, and testosterone clearly inhibited the development of autoimmune thyroiditis in rats. These findings are reminiscent of Szenberg and Warner's [665] observation that in some chick embryos the injection of testosterone caused complete atrophy of the thymus; in later life, these chickens showed a selective loss of immunologic responses.

The influence of stress upon the immune system might be mediated not only by hormones but also through proteolytic enzymes, which are increased by emotional and physical stress, adrenal steroids, adrenaline, acetylcholine, and histamine [196]. Many sorts of peripherally and centrally induced afferent stimuli were found by Schneck and Von Kaulla [604] to cause increased fibrinolysis; pitressin and pneumoencephalography were particularly effective in this regard. Some evidence suggests that plasmin may be under reflex control [392]. That emotional stress increases the turbidity that is induced by incubating dextran with plasma has been reported [196]. This effect was believed to result from increased fibrinolysis, altering the fibrinogen molecule. It seems possible that in conditions of stress, increased proteolysins could alter the structure of various body proteins so as to make them "foreign" and autoantigenic.

INFLUENCE OF THE CNS UPON THE COURSE OF SOME CONNECTIVE TISSUE DISEASES

Rheumatoid arthritis. Many authors have written about the personality characteristics of patients with rheumatoid arthritis. A prominent finding has been that the containment of a large volume of unexpressed hostile feelings seems to be associated with active rheumatoid arthritis [112]. An early example of this was given by McGregor [460]: A woman struggled to send her son both to a private school and to law school. He then married a girl of whom the mother disapproved. "She sought refuge in an extremity of grief and rage; while outwardly calm, internally she was literally beside herself." During this period, typical rheumatoid arthritis developed. Jelliffe [342], as long ago as 1936, expressed his viewpoint as follows: "Psychoanalysis has thus far only a slight look in on the unconscious pulling, hauling, muscular tensions of greed and grasping, the aggressive, hostile striking, kicking, beating tensions which are of significance in the arthritides. These deep psychological conflicts . . . help to bring about the changes that lock up the joints in fruitless arthritic bondage. Those unsuppressed hostile aggressive impulses which in the anti-social individual force society to lock him up in jail or hospital, in the repressed but unsublimated individual turn upon himself and through self punishment bring about a different kind of jail—the wheel chair." This eloquent and provocative metaphor of Jeliffe's seems rather extreme, especially since persons with various psychosomatic disorders have many psychosocial factors in common. Hippocrates' aphorism, that "judgment is difficult and experience fallacious," is particularly appropriate in the context of interpreting psychosomatic relationships. Clinical experience with patients who have rheumatoid arthritis certainly suggests that psychic trauma may sometimes play a role in the pathogenesis of exacerbations of the joint inflammation. Were the following events merely coincidental to the patient's rheumatoid tragedy or did they, like the gods in a Greek drama, give a stamp of inevitability to the subsequent events?

Case 2-9.   When I saw this 62-year-old white woman, she had been bedridden for almost seven years with the most vicious variety of rheumatoid arthritis, which had resulted in severe limitation of motion at the shoulders, elbows, wrists, all finger joints including terminal interphalangeal joints, hips, knees, ankles, and feet. X-rays showed advanced erosions in all of these locations. Her complete helplessness had been alleviated neither by total hip replacement on each side, nor by prosthetic replacements of the metacarpophalangeal joints.

The record showed that her arthritis had started quite suddenly in December 1966 and had given her only moderate discomfort for most of the following year. In October 1967 she had attended the funeral of a close friend, and recalls that, although the arthritis was quiet, "I could hardly walk out of the church because of worry."

A diagnosis of stomach cancer had been made in one of her brothers in 1965. He was still alive when, in November 1967, the patient received telephone calls informing her that a second brother in Los Angeles and a third brother in Alaska each had stomach cancer. She recalls that she flew to Los Angeles on November 4, 1967, and found herself unable to open her brother's door because of a sudden attack of pain and swelling in the finger joints; two days after visiting this brother she flew to Alaska, where she was stricken with such pain in the hips that she could hardly walk. She returned home, where all efforts by her doctors to relieve the acute inflammation in her joints were unsuccessful and she was in bed for most of the time. During the next few months all three brothers died. In November 1968 her daughter was murdered, apparently in error by the jealous husband of a friend. The record shows that the patient remained bedridden for the next six years, because the arthritis was generalized and relentlessly active.

The reader is referred to several articles by Moos and Solomon [487, 488, 644], who reviewed the extensive literature about the personality in rheumatoid arthritis and reported their own studies. They concluded that arthritics tend to over-react to their illness and to be self-sacrificing, masochistic, rigid, moralistic, conforming, self-conscious, shy, inhibited, perfectionistic, and interested in activity [487]. Moos and Solomon [488] found that those patients whose rheumatoid arthritis had progressed *slowly* scored highest in psychological test scales that reflect compliance-subservience, perfectionism, denial of hostility, capacity for social responsibility and social status. Those whose disease had progressed *rapidly* scored higher on scales that reflect physical malfunctioning, general maladjustment, anxiety, manifest hostility, and imperturbability. Moos and Solomon interpreted these observations as indicating that those patients whose disease had progressed more rapidly were experiencing ego disorganization and breakdown.

Meyerowitz and coworkers [474] made psychosocial studies in seven sets of identical twins discordant for rheumatoid arthritis. Their most striking finding was that the ultimately affected twin, but not the unaffected one, was involved for months or years before onset of rheumatoid arthritis in a series of life events which were inferred to be demanding and restricting. They chose the term *entrapment* to denote the particular nature of this psychologically stressful experience: it consists of circumstances in which the person feels totally responsible to meet the demands of a close object or of a situation. Such demanding situations eventually limit their own activity and at this point psychological stress is inferred to occur. Such psychological stress, with the quality of entrapment, was seen to precede the onset of rheumatoid arthritis in the affected sibling of each of the four sets of adult twins whom they studied, and was suggested in two of the three younger pairs of twins.

The outstanding question in all so-called "psychosomatic diseases" is to what extent the relevant personality characteristics were present before the physical illness, to what if any extent they may have contributed to the pathogenesis of the disease, and to what extent they are determined by the presence of a chronic illness. This is also a problem in interpreting the accompanying physiological abnormalities. For example, Lewis, Sinton, and Knott [417] found that among 13 patients with rheumatoid arthritis, seven had abnormal electroencephalograms. Four had cerebrospinal fluid abnormalities. Astapenko [21] observed abnormal responses of blood pressure and skin temperature to ephedrine in patients with rheumatoid arthritis; he considered this evidence of hypothalamic dysfunction. The reactions became normal after clinical improvement. Do such observations reflect an alteration of the CNS induced by the disease or are they due to a more fundamental CNS abnormality which plays a part in pathogenesis? It is impossible to answer this question with assurance. The paper by Thompson and Bywaters [679] is of great interest. They studied the influence of previous hemiplegia upon the course of subsequent rheumatoid arthritis. The hemiplegic limb was remarkably spared in their patients, one of whom even developed subcutaneous nodules on the contralateral arm but not on the hemiplegic arm.

Confirming that the nervous system has an influence upon the course of arthritis, but not entirely supporting the clinical observations of Thompson and

Bywaters [679], is the work of Courtright and Kuzell [125] on adjuvant arthritis of rats. They showed that spinal cord damage tended to lead to more severe and extensive arthritis in the paralyzed limb, but that sciatic nerve section before administration of adjuvant delayed the onset and diminished the extent of arthritis in the operated limb. Whatever the explanation of these experimental findings may be, they lend no support to the suggestion that the sparing of a hemiplegic limb by rheumatoid arthritis is the result of immobilization of the joints.

Systemic lupus erythematosus. These patients seem to have personality characteristics similar to those described for rheumatoid arthritis. McClary and coworkers [454], studying 14 patients with systemic lupus erythematosus (SLE), observed that the threat of the loss of a significant personal relationship regularly provoked an exacerbation of pain and disability. They found that the patients had made great use of activity to relieve anxious and depressed feelings, and considered that this need for hyperactivity was an outgrowth of early-life reaction to loss in the mother-child relationship, in which passive longings had been denied and hyperindependence had then developed.

Jessar, Lamont-Havers, and Ragan [344] observed that 20 per cent of their patients had had emotional upsets as possible precipitating factors in the causation of SLE. In my review with Solomon [205], we reported that the histories of patients with SLE regularly showed an inordinate amount of psychological difficulties long before SLE was clinically manifest, and described two patients who had had psychotic reactions some years before SLE developed; since that report I have seen many other similar instances. Psychotic reactions occur at some time in the course of SLE in about a quarter of all patients with this disease. It is noteworthy that in those cases where careful post-mortem study was performed, the amount of cerebral arteriolar or neuronal pathologic change was often very scant. In seven (35 per cent) of 20 cases the pathological findings were insufficient to explain the mental abnormalities. Atkins and coworkers [23] observed immune complex deposition in the choroid plexus in such cases, but this mechanism for mental illness has not been confirmed.

In a disease like SLE it is difficult to determine the extent to which the behavior disorder results from organic brain damage, from corticosteroid therapy, or from a pre-existing psychological disturbance. There is no question but that organic brain disease and corticosteroids account for many of the behavior disorders seen. It seems likely, on the basis of the evidence quoted above and the findings in the related diseases, rheumatoid arthritis, scleroderma, and Raynaud's disease, that psychological mechanisms play a role in the pathogenesis of SLE and that psychotic reactions may appear with less organic damage or a smaller steroid dose than would induce a mental disorder in unpredisposed individuals.

Our own studies (see chapter on SLE), as well as those made by Siegel and Seelenfreund [629], showed that the susceptibility to SLE was highest in Negroes, and least in white people. These differences seemed independent of poor housing, overcrowding, and migration [629]. It is possible that these racial differences in prevalences of SLE reflect different genetic predispositions; an equally tenable hypothesis is that they result from greater *stress* affecting the black minorities than the white population. As mentioned later in this chapter,

animal experiments have shown that overcrowding and social strife affect the incidence of several sorts of disease.

Raynaud's disease and scleroderma. Some physicians find it difficult to
reconcile a psychological mechanism with the pathogenesis of a major, life-
threatening disease such as SLE. It is re-emphasized that psychological and CNS
events are seen as only two among a host of pathogenetic determinants that
interact in the complex ways referred to earlier in this chapter. A one-to-one relationship between psychological or CNS activities and lesions of SLE—or of any
other psychosomatic disease—is not postulated to occur; it is for this reason that
the participation of the CNS is not always clear. In Raynaud's disease, however,
the effect of psychological and CNS activities is much more readily
demonstrated. Since Raynaud's phenomenon is so common in connective tissue
diseases and so-called "Raynaud's disease" sometimes evolves into scleroderma,
the example of the psychosomatic relationship in these two conditions is an important one.

Mittelmann and Wolff [482] described a patient with Raynaud's disease
who could maintain a normal finger temperature when emotionally secure and
relaxed. When stressful life situations were discussed there was a rapid fall in
finger temperature and finally a painful attack of Raynaud's phenomenon.
Graham [261] demonstrated increased tone in the cutaneous capillaries of
patients with Raynaud's disease at times of emotional disturbance and noted an
association between the Raynaud's phenomenon and an attitude of hostility,
namely, a wish to take directly aggressive action. Many other authors have made
similar psychological observations. Psychoanalysis of a patient with Raynaud's
phenomenon and scleroderma showed a general parallelism between increasing
emotional stress and the development of the disease; some attacks of vasospasm
were related to aggression and anger [576]. Three years after this patient stopped
intensive psychotherapy, catatonic schizophrenia developed. Another patient,
treated psychoanalytically by Millet [478], first manifested Raynaud's disease
two days after her father died. Millet thought that Raynaud's phenomenon was
induced by emotional stress and appeared primarily as a conditioned reflex
response to fear of contact with death. This fear, Millet believed, might be
generated by exposure to the actual or anticipated death of a loved person, or
might be transformed through guilty fears and be experienced as fear of dying.
Mufson [499] summarized seven case histories relevant to these considerations.
Each patient had a commensalistic personality which made him susceptible to
threats of death, indigence, or the loss of a significant love-object upon whom the
patient had for a long time been emotionally overdependent. The fulfillment of
such a threat to security was in each case promptly followed by the onset and
persistence of the manifestations of vasospasm and its sequelae. I have observed
a patient with Raynaud's phenomenon and keratoconjunctivitis sicca. On two occasions when close relatives died, the patient, who was unable to weep, instead
manifested vasospasm.

The following patients provide excellent examples of the role played by
emotional factors in the course of scleroderma.

Case 2-10. A 50-year-old woman had been referred with the question, whether
chloroquine should be used at this time; on a previous occasion, its use had been

associated with an apparent remission of her scleroderma. The letter of referral mentioned that the patient's mother had been an invalid for the past 12 years, with rheumatoid arthritis, Mediterranean anemia, and hemochromatosis; the father was also chronically ill, with lumbar disc disease. After my interview and physical examination of the patient were terminated, she recalled me into the room to express her own view that the previous remission was not attributable to the use of chloroquine. She described her parents as "two cords around my neck," and stated that the improvement in her scleroderma had commenced when she was persuaded to send her mother to a convalescent home. She had then felt, she said, as though one of the cords had been cut. Later, when her father died, she felt as though the second cord had been cut. At his funeral she had been unable to weep, barely able to restrain laughter.

Case 2-11. Severe Raynaud's phenomenon first developed in this woman at about age 20; at that time it was related more to feelings of anger than to cold. She made a happy marriage and her symptoms disappeared completely until about six months before I saw her, at age 29, when the Raynaud's phenomenon recurred after she was forced by financial circumstances to live in the home of her mother-in-law. Frank scleroderma then appeared and rapidly became severe. About three months after her first visit a cold, dead sensation developed in the anterior part of her tongue. A couple of months later, the whole tongue turned completely white and remained so for 15 minutes; this vasospastic condition persisted, and on a later occasion she stated that the anterior 2 inches of the tongue had turned as white as paper for approximately 10 minutes, then bright red for about one minute, with simultaneous tingling, after which the color had become normal. The attacks had not been precipitated by cold food; rather, they appeared during emotional stress—fear that her children might be in a traffic accident. It was not possible to induce an attack by holding an ice cube on her tongue tip for three minutes; but discussion of the possibility that her children might be killed by a car while playing in the street rapidly induced pallor of the anterior inch of the tongue, lasting about two minutes.

Case 2-12. A male school teacher, aged 44, had first manifested scleroderma one year before being seen by me, during his wife's terminal illness from lymphosarcoma. For five years his wife had had a severe schizo-affective reaction with a strong paranoid component, and had made many accusations about her husband's fidelity. He rarely lost his temper, commenting, "What's the use?" He was upset when she died but "relieved for her and the children." Within six months he made a happy remarriage and one year later there was marked improvement of the scleroderma.

Sydenham's chorea. The psychological disturbance that may occur in Sydenham's chorea is so prominent that until comparatively recently many observers held that in some patients this illness was entirely psychologically determined. Careful examination of 20 patients by Mathews and coworkers [450] showed a common personality pattern. The patients were selfconscious and insecure, overdependent on adults, and afraid of their own aggressive feelings, which they did not know how to handle. Their parents had serious emotional difficulties: the fathers were portrayed as punitive and the mothers as neglectful and rarely loving. Freeman, Aron, and coworkers [219], in a retrospective study of 40 patients with chorea, found a high incidence of psychological problems before onset of the illness. Unfortunately, it is difficult to find adequate controls for such studies, so that conclusions must be tentative. Restudying their 40 patients after an average of 29 years, those authors found a high incidence of serious psychoneurosis, and almost two-thirds of the subjects had personality disorders.

Electroencephalographic (EEG) studies made during chorea have shown ab-

normalities in many patients. However, the EEG in rheumatic fever uncompli-
cated by chorea is also abnormal in a high percentage of patients [417], serving
to emphasize a special difficulty in interpretation of the psychosomatic interrelationship. Can we say that chorea has an important psychogenic determinant; or
is it a special form of rheumatic encephalitis?

ANIMAL STUDIES RELATING CNS FACTORS TO PATHOGENESIS OF CONNECTIVE TISSUE DISEASES

There is little clinical evidence bearing upon the contribution of the CNS to
the pathogenesis of scleroderma, dermatomyositis, or polyarteritis; but the experimental evidence from Selye's studies in animals is considerable. His extensive
work has been collated in several books [613, 614], and is only briefly summarized here.

Many distinct forms of cardiopathy may be induced or prevented by various
combinations of electrolytes, steroids, and stress. According to Selye, these cardiopathies are due not to the effects of inherently cardiotoxic agents, but to the
creation or abolition of pathogenic situations. However, the effects of agents that
are inherently cardioactive—whether toxic or protective—may be markedly influenced by electrolytes, steroids, or stress. Moreover, depending upon the circumstances, stress may induce or prevent the same cardiopathy. A polyarteritis
affecting the coronary arteries and the medium-sized arteries and arterioles of
most other organs is a prominent feature of the so-called "hyalinizing cardiopathy"; this is most readily induced in animals by the combination of certain
steroids with electrolytes but may also be evoked by cold in rats that have been
sensitized by unilateral nephrectomy and 1 per cent salt solution as drinking
fluid.

Calciphylaxis has been defined [613] as a condition of hypersensitivity in
which—especially during a critical period after sensitization by a systemic calci-
fying factor—topical treatment with certain challengers causes an acute local
calcinosis followed by inflammation and sclerosis. There are many histological
resemblances between cutaneous calciphylaxis and scleroderma, both being
characterized by swelling of collagen tissue, with calcification and sclerosis. Polyarteritis, also, may be induced by means similar to those that cause cutaneous
calciphylaxis. Of considerable interest is the fact that exposure to severe stress,
such as restraint, may inhibit these calciphylactic responses. This inhibition is
presumably mediated by a neuroendocrine response which, however, is not
simply an adrenal one—despite being reproducible by administration of glucocorticoids—because it is not abolished by adrenalectomy.

Along different lines have been studies in animal populations showing the
influence of overcrowding upon the incidence of various diseases. For an extensive review of this topic, the reader is referred to the article published by
Christian in 1964 [107]. Deer that were overcrowded in their natural habitat
developed a severe, exudative glomerulonephritis; woodchuck, a non-exudative
intercapillary glomerulonephritis. The severity and rate of development of these
lesions were reduced when the social strife in the animal populations was
diminished. The mechanisms underlying these phenomena are probably complex

and connected with the CNS influence upon immune mechanisms and pathogenesis in general. A related observation by Vessey [695] was that in a grouped population of mice, antibody production was inhibited in all but the dominant animals.

CONCLUSION

The evidence cited above shows that the CNS has an important influence upon the development and course of connective tissue diseases. The CNS affects the immune response and thus, presumably, the course of events in diseases whose pathogenesis is considered to have an autoimmune component. There is ample evidence that the CNS influences the development in animals of experimentally induced lesions that resemble those seen in connective tissue diseases of man. Lesions of the CNS alter the rate of development of arthritis in man and animals. Finally, there are important psychological correlates of the connective tissue diseases.

The question may be posed, which is primary—the CNS dysfunction, or the systemic connective tissue disease? This is the same problem that requires an answer in the context of the general psychosomatic interrelationship. My bias is that primacy cannot be accorded to any of the component events of pathogenesis; the complexity of interplay between cause and effect is such that the various mechanisms are truly interdependent, the final clinical expression being the delicately balanced resultant of them all. Confusion arises because one rarely has accurate knowledge of the psychological status before onset of the connective tissue disease and because CNS and psychological activities may not only influence pathogenesis, but in turn be shaped by the disease itself.

CHAPTER 3

The Diagnosis of Acute Arthritis

The differential diagnosis of acute arthritis is the most difficult diagnostic challenge faced by the rheumatologist. Accurate diagnosis requires consideration of all the general medical conditions that may have occasional rheumatic manifestations. Misdiagnosis may have dire consequences: failure to recognize the acute arthritis that occurs during the treatment of a patient with leukemia or myeloma, as being from infection rather than from gout, may eventuate in destruction of the joint; failure to recognize severe arthralgia, myalgia, and a maculopurpuric rash on the hands and feet as possibly caused by Rocky Mountain spotted fever may result in a fatal outcome in this disease, where the mortality rate for untreated patients is 20 to 30 per cent.

A bedside approach is to consider the following aspects of the problem: the age and sex of the patient; the severity of the acute arthritis; the distribution of the involved joints; the duration of the arthritis, and the associated, nonarthritic manifestations.

AGE AND SEX OF PATIENT

In the young female, primary gout is exceedingly rare, and this low prevalence persists until the fifth decade of life; if analysis of synovial fluid demonstrates uric acid crystals, one should consider secondary gout, e.g., from underlying leukemia. Likewise, ankylosing spondylitis is rare in the female but should be considered as an underlying diagnosis in any male with polyarthritis— especially when the joints affected are central rather than peripheral. The older the patient, naturally, the more likely is degenerative arthritis, which occasionally may have an acute onset. If the patient who has acute arthritis gives a history of having had rheumatic fever in infancy, and especially if the present examination reveals no heart murmur, it is important to remember that rheumatic fever is extremely rare in children younger than four years. Since juvenile rheumatoid arthritis does affect infants, this history may be relevant in assessing the possible causation of the current acute arthritis in adulthood.

SEVERITY OF ARTHRITIS

As a rule of thumb, it is well to recall that the most severely inflamed joints are seen in gout and in acute infectious arthritis. Here, the factors of age and sex are important in differentiation. Primary gout is rare in females, especially in those younger than 45 years; in males, primary gout is rare before the age of 30

serum uric acid. It is possible that the appearance of gouty arthritis implies an adjuvant to tissue deposition of urate that is present in gout but not in asymptomatic hyperuricemia; but this has never been proved, or even strongly supported by inferential evidence. Thus, agents that reduce serum uric acid should be started only when acute attacks of gout become inconveniently frequent, when tophi or renal stones are present, or when renal function is impaired.

PSEUDOGOUT

Pseudogouty arthritis is caused by an inflammatory response to crystals of calcium pyrophosphate. Most cases of pseudogout are idiopathic but certain diseases have been associated with it, e.g., hemochromatosis, hyperparathyroidism, and diabetes mellitus. Pseudogout and classic gout may even coexist. The crystals in the synovial fluid of patients with pseudogout are considered to derive from preformed deposits in the articular cartilage or menisci. The prevalence of such crystal deposits in the general population is quite high: they were found in 3.2 per cent of cadavers by crystallographic analysis, and in 7 per cent of elderly patients in an x-ray survey [57, 453].

The clinical picture may vary from mild chronic arthralgias to recurrent episodes of acute arthritis, frequently resembling an acute attack of gout. Examination of joint fluid under the polarizing microscope is of considerable importance in establishing the diagnosis, most especially since 30 per cent of these patients may have hyperuricemia. The knee is the most commonly involved joint [495].

Case 4-1. The patient with articular chondrocalcinosis whose x-rays are shown in Figure 4-1 came to us from elsewhere, requesting more relief than had been afforded by oral penicillin. This had been given because the erroneous diagnosis of infectious arthritis had been made when the knee had suddenly become hot, swollen, and exquisitely tender. The synovial fluid contained 56,000 leukocytes per milliliter, 90 per cent polymorphonuclears, and 114 mg of glucose per 100 milliliters; it was sterile on culture. The polarizing microscope revealed numerous typical calcium pyrophosphate crystals that were lying both free and within the cytoplasm of leukocytes. Treatment with indomethacin was followed by rapid improvement.

HYPOPHOSPHATEMIA

Rheumatological accompaniments of hypophosphatemia are important to recognize because of their ready reversibility. Hypophosphatemia results most commonly from intravenously administered glucose, vomiting or gastric suction, antacid use, and liver disease; less common causes include hyperparathyroidism and hyperalimentation.

Case 4-2. A 54-year-old white man had been well until, eight months previously, he began to experience pain in the feet, ankles, sacroiliac joints, and thorax. On one occasion, his right ankle was seen to be pink, warm, and swollen. X-rays of the sacroiliac joints showed changes that were thought at the time to be consistent with the diagnosis of

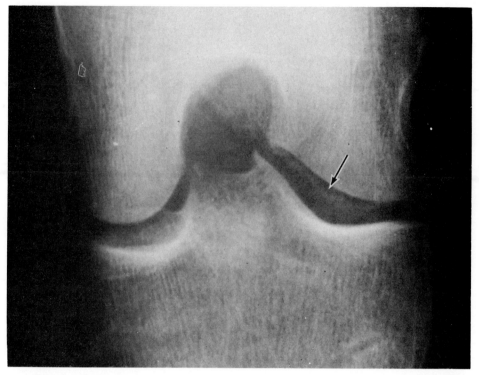

Fig. 4-1.   Case 4-1.   A (above), pseudogout with chondrocalcinosis of knee (arrow). B, pseudogout, chondrocalcinosis of patella.

ankylosing spondylitis. His symptoms did not respond to treatment with salicylates, indomethacin, phenylbutazone, or corticosteroids. After about a year of this treatment, the observation that his serum phosphorus level was 1.7 mg/100 ml caused his admission to the hospital.

The main finding on physical examination in the hospital was a firm subcutaneous lump measuring 1 × 1 cm, over the dorsal surface of the right great toe.

The urine pH was 5.0. The serum creatinine level was 0.9 mg/100 ml; serum calcium, 8.6 mg/100 ml, phosphorus 1.7 mg/100 ml; alkaline phosphatase, 22.5 King-Armstrong units/100 ml (normal, <13). No calcifications were seen on plain x-rays of the kidneys. Roentgenographic survey of the skeleton showed only mild, generalized demineralization. Films of the sacroiliac joints showed hazy articular margins and subchondral sclerosis.

On a diet that contained approximately 1500 mg of phosphorus daily, the 24-hour urine collection contained 624 mg. of phosphorus; simultaneously, the serum phosphorus level was only 1.6 mg/100 ml. Intravenous infusion of calcium demonstrated that he had good ability to conserve phosphorus: at the end of the infusion, the serum phosphorus level rose to 3.0 mg/100 ml. Urinary aminoacid levels were normal. Intestinal malabsorption was excluded by normal levels of stool fat and of serum carotene, by normal response to the D-xylose test, and by normal radiological appearances of the upper gastrointestinal tract.

The patient was given vitamin D, 50,000 units daily, and supplements of phosphate orally. His symptoms resolved and the serum phosphorus and alkaline phosphatase levels returned to normal; after 3 months he was virtually asymptomatic.

The lesion over the right great toe was excised and had the microscopic appearances of a benign mesenchymoma, identical to those described by Olefsky and coworkers [529]

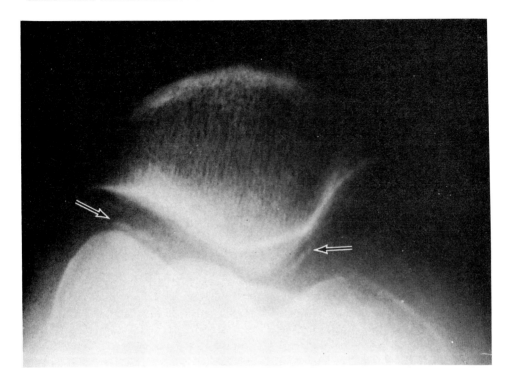

Fig. 4-1. B.

in a similar case. One year after removal of this tumor, the vitamin D and phosphate supplement were stopped. Skeletal symptoms did not recur, and after a brief initial fall in serum calcium and phosphorus levels, these became normal and have remained so after three years of follow-up.

Such disappearance of vitamin D resistance after removal of the tumor is consistent with previously reported experience [529].

Case 4-3. A 57-year-old woman was admitted to the hospital because of bleeding from a large duodenal ulcer, which had perforated and then spontaneously sealed. She was treated with 30 ml of magnesium-aluminum gel every half-hour. While in the hospital she complained of acroparesthesiae, which spread proximally to affect the trunk and, eventually, her lips and tongue. She complained of inability to walk, but was discharged because she was considered to be hysterical. Her complaints of weakness led to her readmission into the hospital 5 days later. Her speech was now slurred, and there was mild to moderate weakness of several of the proximal girdle muscles. Her serum phosphorus level was 0.7 mg, calcium 9.7 mg, and alkaline phosphatase 22 King-Armstrong units, per 100 ml. A 24-hour urine specimen contained 88 mg of phosphorus and 108 mg of calcium, at a time when the serum phosphorus level was 1.1 mg/100 ml and her diet contained approximately 1,500 mg of phosphate daily. Electromyogram was consistent with a myopathic disorder. Antacid treatment was stopped; within 5 days, her subjective complaints and objective evidence of muscle weakness disappeared, and the serum and urinary phosphorus levels became normal. Six weeks later, follow-up electromyogram gave normal results.

The first of these two patients had vitamin D-resistant rickets, presumably the result of the mesenchymoma. His complaints of pain in the lower back and hips, knees, and ankles, together with radiological changes in the sacroiliac joints, led to an initial diagnosis of ankylosing spondylitis; the occurrence of swelling in one of his joints contributed to this misdiagnosis. It is interesting in this regard that a rheumatoid-like arthritis and, even, joint erosions that heal after parathyroidectomy have been reported in primary hyperparathyroidism [745]. A patient with vitamin D-resistant rickets reported by Blackard and coworkers [51] had obliterated sacroiliac joint spaces and calcification of the anterior spinal ligaments. Patton [539], who studied seven patients with vitamin D-resistant rickets, saw radiological appearances almost indistinguishable from those of ankylosing spondylitis: there were roentgenographic squaring of the vertebral bodies, and calcification of the paravertebral ligaments, disc annulus, and ligaments within the sacroiliac joints. Of related interest was a patient with hypoparathyroidism reported by Chaykin and coworkers [101], who appeared clinically to have ankylosing spondylitis, with anterior flexion of the head and neck, complete clinical ankylosis in the thoracic and lumbar portions of the spine, chest expansion limited to only three-quarters of an inch, and restricted motions in the hips and shoulders. X-rays showed normal sacroiliac joints, but extensive calcification was seen in the posterior paraspinal ligaments, the apophyseal articulations, and the coracoid-acromial ligaments. A patient with vitamin D-resistant rickets who has been reported elsewhere [493, 529] was originally diagnosed as having ankylosing spondylitis and has obliterated sacroiliac joints (Fig. 4-2).

In Case 4-3, where the serum phosphate was depressed by excessive use of antacids, the major symptom was profound muscle weakness, as has been stressed in previous reports [24, 54, 429, 560, 696].

HYPOTHYROIDISM

This is a frequent cause of reversible rheumatic symptoms. Bland and Frymoyer [52] mentioned 11 patients with myxedema, all referred by internists with the diagnosis of "arthritis", who recovered completely on thyroid replacement therapy. As indicated in Table 11-1 (Chapter 11), hypothyroidism accounts for approximately 10 per cent of all acquired myopathic disorders.

Case 4-4. During the previous two years, a 65-year-old man had experienced severe cramping of the muscles of all four limbs and the trunk, of such duration as to cause contraction of the neighboring joints. Some careful observers had considered that he had myotonia, but the electromyogram failed to confirm this.

Physical examination revealed slight weakness of the shoulder girdle muscles and of both iliopsoas muscles. The thyroid gland was slightly enlarged and contained several small nodules. Serum creatine phosphokinase was elevated at 240 units/100 ml (normal, <12); protein-bound iodine levels were consistently low at 1.6, 1.9, and 2.0 μg/100 ml (normal, >4.5). Red blood cell uptake of triiodothyronine was depressed, at 23 per cent (normal, >25). Muscle biopsy showed mildly myopathic appearances, i.e., variation of muscle fiber size, increase in the numbers of sarcolemmal nuclei, an occasional basophilic

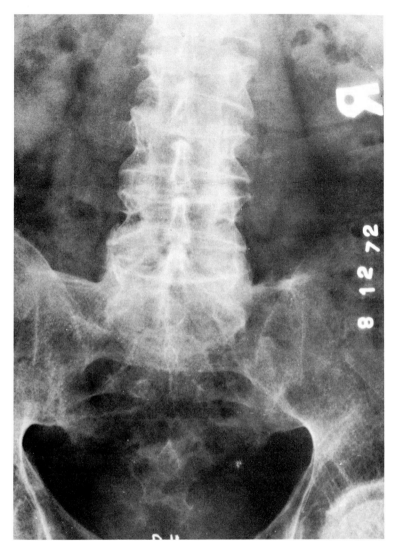

Fig. 4-2. Longstanding vitamin D-resistant rickets; almost total obliteration of the sacroiliac joints.

fiber, and a solitary focus of chronic interstitial inflammatory infiltrate. After 2 months of thyroid replacement therapy, the patient was without symptoms.

Pseudomyotonia is a well-known feature of hypothyroid myopathy. Both hypertrophy and atrophy of muscles may occur. Some patients have severe pain in the muscles [200]. In their 75 patients with hypothyroidism, Collins and coworkers [119] recorded muscle cramps or stiffness in 15 (20 per cent) and weakness in 33 (44 per cent). Thus, a muscle disorder is extremely common in hypothyroidism. Contrariwise, Ramsay [569] has shown that muscle weakness, while also very common in hyperthyroidism, is seldom its presenting manifestation (except in Oriental persons, who have an unexplained high rate of periodic paralysis caused by hyperthyroidism); whereas it may for many months be the sole feature of hypothyroidism.

HYPERLIPIDEMIA

Glueck and coworkers [247] emphasized the occurrence of acute bouts of tendinitis and synovitis in familial type II hyperlipoproteinemia. One of their patients whose serum uric acid level was normal had had numerous episodes of pain and swelling of a great toe, simulating podagra, recurring two or three times every year. Another had concurrent attacks in knees and ankles, the symptoms increasing over 12 to 24 hours to a point where the patient could not walk, and gradually resolving during the subsequent 72 to 96 hours. The joint fluid contained no uric acid or cholesterol crystals, 70 mg of cholesterol per 100 ml, and 5,400 white blood cells per cubic millimeter, mostly polymorphonuclear leukocytes. Several of their patients had recurrent inflammation in the Achilles tendons. Similar attacks in familial hypercholesterolemia, described by Khachadurian [376], varied in severity and duration from mild joint pains lasting a few days with no physical signs, to severe, incapacitating pain with redness and swelling, lasting as long as a month.

Musculoskeletal disorders associated with type IV hyperlipoproteinemia were described by Goldman and coworkers [250]. Their 12 patients were mainly of middle age; nine had morning stiffness; six complained of recurrent joint swelling, but only two had observed joint effusions. The arthralgias were usually asymmetrically distributed and affected variable numbers of both large and small joints. There was a suggestion that lowering the plasma lipids led to marked improvement in joint pain.

Polyarthritis was reported by Shagrin and coworkers [619] in seven of 31 patients who had been treated for obesity by jejunocolostomy. In the majority the articular manifestations lasted for less than 12 months, but in two patients the joint symptoms were severe and lasted for more than 24 months. The affected joints included the wrists in all seven patients, the fingers in five, the knees in three, and the ankles in three. There was actual swelling of joints, but no synovial fluid analyses were reported. All of the patients had tenosynovitis involving the fingers and hands. In two patients, x-rays showed small erosions of joints. None had antinuclear antibodies or rheumatoid factor in the serum; and all had normal blood levels of uric acid, calcium, phosphorus, and alkaline phosphatase. In one patient, the normal anatomical sequence of the bowel was restored because of the severe articular symptoms; she immediately had complete relief of her symptoms. The cause of the arthropathy in these patients, as in the more classic enteroarthropathies, is completely unknown.

HEMOCHROMATOSIS

A specific arthritis associated with hemochromatosis was first described by Schumacher [607] in seven patients, and a further excellent description in 16 patients was given by Hamilton and coworkers [284]. The arthritis affects especially the proximal interphalangeal and the metacarpo-phalangeal joints of the hands, causing firm enlargement without much soft tissue swelling. Eight of the patients studied by Hamilton and coworkers [284] had a history of acute episodes of arthritis; in one, crystals of calcium pyrophosphate were identified in the joint fluid taken during an acute attack. Radiological evidence of chondrocalcinosis was extremely common in their patients. The most frequent site was the menisci; sometimes the articular cartilage of the knees was also calcified. The iron content of articular cartilage and synovium was approximately the same as in controls, but calcium concentration was five to six times that in controls. Aside from these attacks of apparent pseudogout, the joint symptoms in hemochromatosis are fixed in nature and do not have the waxing and waning quality of rheumatoid arthritis. The onset of the arthritis usually coincides with the other first symptoms of hemochromatosis. X-ray changes are quite similar to those of osteoarthritis; chondrocalcinosis, as noted, is frequent. Examination of synovial tissue shows hemosiderin in the synovial lining cells without much, if any, inflammatory reaction.

ACROMEGALY

Arthritic symptoms are common in acromegaly, where they result from overgrowth of cartilage. There are hyperplasia and hypertrophy of the chondrocytes and an increase in matrix. This overgrown cartilage is highly susceptible to mechanical stress and its consequent degenerative changes. In addition, there is a noninflammatory fibrous hyperplasia of the periarticular and intra-articular soft tissue. Before the diagnosis of acromegaly is established, the articular symptoms may be deceptive; a patient reported by Good [254] was considered for 13 years to have rheumatoid arthritis before the correct diagnosis was made. The x-ray picture shows degenerative changes in and around the joints; also, there is often widening of the joint spaces, particularly the metacarpophalangeal ones, and an exostotic bony proliferation of the ends of the distal phalanges produces a so-called "arrowhead tufting" appearance (Fig. 4-3). Distally-directed exostoses at the bases of the distal phalanges are frequent. These changes are not pathognomonic; they are seen occasionally in the hands of heavy manual laborers; the x-rays shown in Fig. 4-4 are of a man in whom careful study yielded no evidence of acromegaly.

AMYLOIDOSIS

Amyloid joint disease is a rare cause of arthritis; here, amyloid deposits infiltrate the synovium, periarticular tissues, or marrow adjacent to the joint. There is usually a bilaterally symmetrical arthritis affecting large joints, as well as the small joints of the fingers and the wrists. Common complaints are pain, stiffness, and swelling; palpable nodules resembling rheumatoid nodules are present in more than 60 per cent of the patients [720]. This simulation of rheumatoid arthritis was emphasized by Davis and coworkers [134], two of

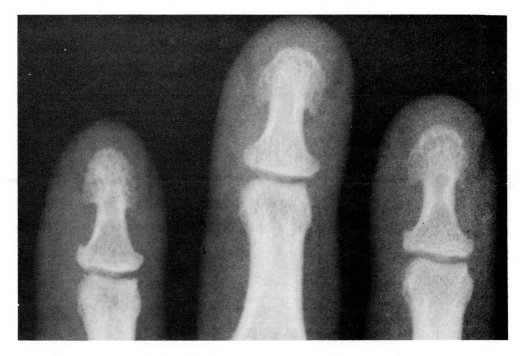

Fig. 4-3. Terminal phalanges and interphalangeal joints in case of acromegaly. Note mild "arrowhead" appearance and widened joint spaces. Compare with Figure 4-4.

whose patients were diagnosed and treated for a long period for rheumatoid arthritis. Where synovial fluid has been analyzed, the results have been characteristic of noninflammatory arthritis. Rarely, fragments of amyloid have been found floating free within the synovial fluid.

A PUZZLING CASE

The illness in the following patient is undiagnosed but offers a good opportunity to discuss some unusual disorders associated with lysis of bones.

Case 4-5. A woman first seen at age 31 complained of pain in the feet for the previous five years. The pain was mainly in the proximal interphalangeal joints of several toes and, more recently, in the fifth right metatarsophalangeal joint. The joints sometimes felt hot, but were never really swollen. During the previous year she had noted morning stiffness that lasted for many hours, affecting her elbows, hands, and knees. For several years she had been losing hair excessively. She had been diagnosed at another institution as having hypothyroidism but her hair continued to fall despite adequate thyroid hormone replacement.

Physical findings were entirely within normal limits, aside from mild tenderness in the fifth right metatarsophalangeal joint, and the presence of a white forelock.

Her mother was of Italian and Spanish parentage, her father of Irish and German descent. There was no family history of similar joint or bone disorder; no other members had a white forelock, and she knew of no family history of neurological or mental disorder.

Past history was interesting in that she had had recurrent, unexplained, abdominal pains and fevers in her youth, and at age 23 she had had an episode of dizziness and headache for which pneumoencephalography was performed after skull x-rays had revealed intracranial calcifications. Perusal of extensive past medical records showed that no abnormal findings had been made that would account for these illnesses.

X-rays taken at the time of initial evaluation and during the next two years showed multiple areas of bone lysis, giving the appearance of cysts, at the heads of the fifth and fourth right metatarsals (Fig. 4-5), at the outer end of the left clavicle, and at the head of the fifth left metacarpal. Radioisotopic scintiphotos of bone showed uptake of the injected isotope in the region of bone lysis in the foot (Fig. 4-6).

Blood alkaline phosphatase levels were abnormally low whenever tested during the following two years. By a method that gives normal levels in excess of 19 King-Armstrong units per 100 ml, the mean of seven separate determinations was 12 units/100 ml with a range of 4 to 18; by another method whose normal value exceeds 30 units/100 ml, the patient's blood level was 27. Alkaline phosphatase isoenzyme study showed that the predominating isoenzyme in her blood was of hepatic origin. The alkaline phosphatase in her peripheral leukocytes was not reduced. Phosphoethanolamine was undetectable in her serum and was not elevated in amount in her urine. Twenty-four hour urinary levels of calcium, phosphate, hydroxyproline, and total aminoacids were all normal. Blood alkaline phosphatase levels in her mother, father, and brother were normal.

The fourth metatarsophalangeal joint was removed from her right foot for diagnostic purposes. The cyst-like lesions detected roentgenographically were seen microscopically to result from replacement of the metatarsal head by fat. The area of fatty replacement abutted very closely upon the articular cartilage, where there was a microfracture. There was minimal inflammatory reaction of the synovium but no pannus formation. Several consultant pathologists examined the bone sections and were unable to offer a definitive diagnosis.

Rectal biopsy showed no evidence of amyloidosis.

The consistently low levels of alkaline phosphatase in this woman's serum,

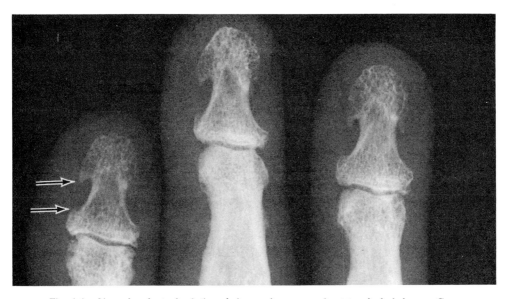

Fig. 4-4. Normal variant: simulation of changes in acromegaly at terminal phalanges. Compare with Fig. 4-3.

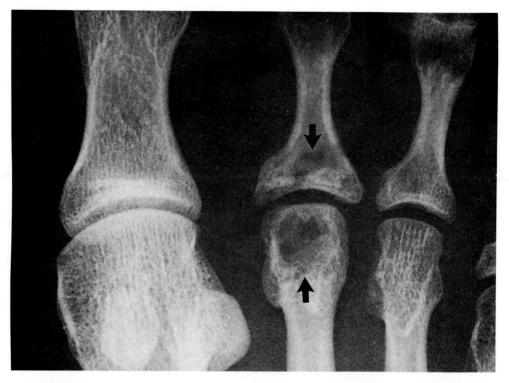

Fig. 4-5. Case 4-5. Arrows point to area of bone lysis in head of right second metatarsal and base of distal phalanx (see, also, Fig. 4-6).

and the failure of electrophoretic analysis to detect a bone-derived fraction in the enzyme suggest the possibility that her condition may be *familial hypophosphatasia*. This disease is usually seen in infants and children; Jardon [340] was able to find only 13 cases in adults. The pattern of bone involvement in this patient is not consistent with that seen in others with hypophosphatasia, where rickets predominates. Features that argue further against this diagnosis are the normal levels of serum and urinary phosphoethanolamine, each of which is raised in patients with hypophosphatasia. Moreover, her white blood cells contained normal levels of alkaline phosphatase; bone uptake of the radioisotope indicated metabolic activity, and her brother had normal serum levels of alkaline phosphatase.

Another interesting disease, sometimes termed "disappearing bone disease," must be considered in this patient. In this condition, entire bones or segments of a bone undergo atrophy and finally disappear. Gorham and coworkers [260] have reviewed this entity, reporting two of their own patients and summarizing 16 other cases from the previous literature. In their two patients the serum alkaline phosphatase was either elevated or normal. The most striking histopathological finding was an overgrowth of small, thin-walled vessels, apparently a form of angiomatosis.

In the *arthritis of familial Mediterranean fever,* which appears at some time during the course of the illness in approximately 70 per cent of patients with this disease, x-ray changes are usually minimal, consisting of osteoporosis in the protracted attacks; some patients show a remarkable lysis of the ends of the bones [305]. The arthritis is episodic, and usually affects one large joint at a time. Its onset is most often in early childhood or adolescence. The arthritic attack is abrupt, and marked by rapidly intensifying pain and tenderness as exquisitely severe as that of gout. Redness and local heat are frequently disproportionately less than the degree of swelling. There may be a transient synovial effusion. The attack often resolves in only two or three days, most commonly in a week. Some attacks are protracted, as long as nine months; but there is almost always complete functional and anatomical recovery. Synovial fluid changes are those of inflammation. Synovial biopsy findings are also those of low-grade, subacute inflammation. In three of 10 cases studied appropriately [305], small quantities of amyloid material were detected in vascular structures of the cap-

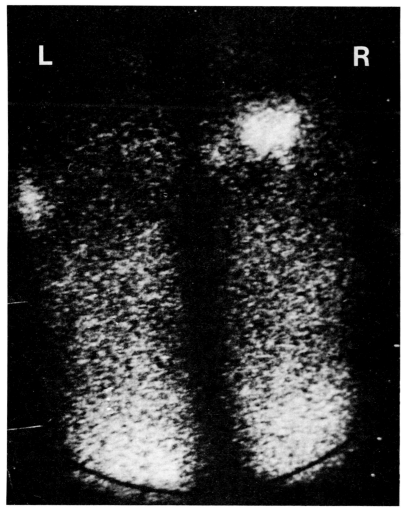

Fig. 4-6.   Bone scan in Case 4-5; accumulation of isotope in areas of bone lysis (compare with Fig. 4-5).

sular or subchondral tissues, although there was no evidence that the inflammatory joint disease had developed in relation to these deposits.

The Mediterranean ancestry of the patient described in Case 4-5, and the episodic fever and unexplained abdominal pains in her youth are all consistent with the diagnosis of familial Mediterranean fever; but the absence of amyloidosis, and of a strong family history of a similar illness make it difficult to convince oneself of this diagnosis.

Occupational acroosteolysis, described in detail in Chapter 12, is characterized by lysis of terminal phalanges and occasionally of other bones, Raynaud's phenomenon, and a sclerodermatous reaction; it occurs in workmen who clean the reaction chambers where vinyl chloride has been polymerized. A familial variety has also been described. There is no reason to suspect a similar illness in Case 4-5.

Sudeck's atrophy or reflex sympathetic dystrophy is accompanied by considerable pain of the affected part, which is often warm, red, and slightly swollen. Trauma may initiate this disorder but often it is spontaneous. The patient whose foot is illustrated in Figure 4-7 had suffered a fracture of the ipsilateral upper tibia some three months previously. Sympathectomy often alleviates pain in these patients, although mostly there is spontaneous recovery.

Transitory osteoporosis of the hip was described by Curtiss and Kincaid [131] as a painful condition occurring in pregnancy, but it is restricted neither to pregnancy nor to women [325]. It sometimes involves both hips and occasionally other joints. This peculiar, unexplained condition runs its course to complete

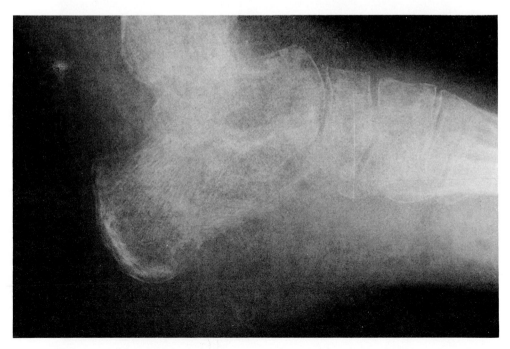

Fig. 4-7. Sudeck's atrophy. Generalized acute deossification simulates arthritis radiologically, but preservation of the articular cortex in Sudeck's atrophy distinguishes it from arthritis.

recovery within about six months. Hunder and Kelly [325] saw mild chronic inflammation in seven of nine synovial biopsies made in these patients. Where serum calcium, phosphorus, and alkaline phosphatase have been reported, values have been normal.

In many respects Case 4-5 resembles transitory osteoporosis, except that the patient's hips have been spared and the condition has lasted longer than two years. A migratory osteolysis of the lower extremities, described in three patients by Duncan and coworkers [164], differed from transitory osteoporosis in that there was a considerable inflammation of the overlying skin and the bone biopsy showed inflammatory cells.

Essential osteolysis with nephropathy is characterized by lysis of, especially, carpal and tarsal bones, and chronic glomerulonephritis [682]. Some, but not all, cases are hereditary [626].

Hypervitaminosis A: an occasional patient who takes excessive quantities of supplemental vitamin A may experience musculoskeletal discomfort. Frame and coworkers [214] reported three such patients, all of whom complained of pain in the muscles or bones. Serum vitamin A levels were high in all, and periosteal calcification was a prominent feature in two. The symptoms and radiological abnormalities subsided after vitamin A was stopped.

Muenter and coworkers [498] saw a patient who had such severe muscular stiffness and fatigue after exercise as to suggest the possibility of McArdle's syndrome (see Chapter 11). This patient also had pain in the bones and joints. Her physical findings included dry skin, angular stomatitis, enlargement of liver and spleen, and bilateral papilledema. All symptoms and signs regressed after withdrawal of vitamin A. Among the 17 case reports in the literature reviewed by Muenter and coworkers [498], 13 cited pain in the bones and joints, and seven cited muscle stiffness. The daily vitamin A intake in these 17 patients had ranged from 41,000 to 600,000 IU; they had taken the vitamin for periods of two months to two years.

The ready availability of vitamin A without prescription, and the widespread public belief in the value of vitamin supplements suggest that such cases as the above might not be uncommon; however, I have not yet identified similar instances in my own practice.

Kashin-Beck disease is a chronic, disabling, degenerative, generalized osteoarthrosis involving peripheral joints and the spine without associated systemic manifestations. It occurs principally in childhood and is endemic in eastern Siberia, northern China, and northern Korea. Although the occurrence of this disease has not yet been recognized in the United States or Western Europe, brief mention in the present context is justified by the fact that it is considered to result from a mycotoxin [513]. The fungus, *Fusarium sporotrichiella,* infects the grain used as human food in the regions in which the disease is endemic. Apparently, when experimental animals were fed grain contaminated by this fungus, changes developed in their articular cartilages resembling those of Kashin-Beck disease. It remains to be determined, whether this illness has any relevance to the common variety of osteoarthritis.

CHAPTER 5

Associations and Consequences of Hyperuricemia

For many years there have been discussions in the literature about associations of hyperuricema other than gout. Additional importance has been conferred on these associations by the widespread estimation of serum uric acid levels as part of automated biochemical analyses of blood of asymptomatic persons undergoing a routine health check. Asymptomatic hyperuricemia has greater numerical importance than clinical gout. By definition, 2.5 per cent of the population is hyperuricemic, i.e., has a uric acid value beyond 2 standard deviations from the mean; yet clinical gout affects 1.7 per cent or fewer of the population (see Chapter 4). The literature that will be reviewed in this chapter suggests that patients with gout not only develop renal disease and urolithiasis but have a strong tendency to hypertension, cardiovascular disease, and diabetes. For some years we have been concerned with whether persons with asymptomatic hyperuricemia have similar tendencies. We shall contrast findings in the literature with some of our own in 124 patients with asymptomatic hyperuricemia [204].

Our 124 patients with asymptomatic hyperuricemia [204] were identified as having two or more measurements of uric acid above 2 standard deviations from the mean of the white population of the appropriate sex and age group. All were white persons 20-49 years of age. When originally selected, none of them had gout, renal disease (abnormal creatinine or urine analysis), hypertension (blood pressure higher than 150/95), atheroma (as judged by retinal arteries, foot pulses, electrocardiogram; there were no arterial bruits), diabetes, rheumatoid arthritis, psoriasis, cancer, recent weight loss, or other conditions associated with hyperuricemia; and none used thiazides or aspirin. Normouricemic controls (224) were matched in all other respects with hyperuricemic patients. The hyperuricemic and control groups were all of the persons having appropriate characteristics among a population of about 150,000 persons who had taken an automated multiphasic health check at the San Francisco or Oakland clinic of The Permanente Medical Group. All subjects had been followed for a mean of $4\frac{1}{4}$ years. We compared the two groups for their baseline biochemical and other characteristics and for the incidence, during the follow-up period, of hypertension, cardiovascular disease, diabetes, renal disease, and urolithiasis.

THE PROBLEM OF NORMAL LIMITS, ILLUSTRATED BY SERUM URIC ACID

Before reviewing the associations and correlations of abnormal levels of uric acid, it is worthwhile to consider the concept of normal and abnormal, illustrating this by our experience with serum uric acid values. For a normally distributed variable, the range of normal values in a reference population may be defined in terms of the mean and standard deviations. A common practice is to place the upper limit of normal at the mean plus 2 standard deviations, which is at approximately the 97.5 percentile level. For factors the distribution of which is not of a gaussian sort, the normal range may be expressed in terms of percentile levels for the reference population, in which case it is common to use the 95th percentile level as the upper limit of normal. The reference population would ideally be described in terms of those factors known to affect the measurement. As an example of the important influence of race, age, and sex on serum uric acid, we have found that black women ages 60–69 have a mean serum uric acid level almost 0.5 mg/100 ml higher than white women of similar age. The high levels of serum uric acid normal in certain ethnic groups are described in a later section.

It is almost superfluous to mention the influence of thiazide drugs on serum uric acid, but it is obvious that, ideally, the use of these and other drugs by the reference population should be known. Other environmental influences of indeterminate sort may also be important and should be considered. For example, a study of Dreyfuss et al showed significantly lower mean serum uric acid values in Negev Bedouin than in Arab villagers or in Haifa Jews. The Arab villagers and Haifa Jews, however, had similar values [158].

When comparing a certain value with those obtained from a standard reference population, one must be certain that he has controlled for both individual and laboratory variations across time and for the use of different techniques. Individual variation was studied by Rubin et al in healthy, normally active, young adult males [593]. They found a small but statistically significant diurnal serum pattern, with highest levels occurring in the midafternoon. The variation over long periods in our laboratories is shown in Table 5-1. Between September 1964 and August 1966, the mean serum uric acid level was somewhat higher among San Francisco men aged 14–49 than in comparable Oakland men.

Table 5-1. Fluctuation of Serum Uric Acid Levels (mg/100 ml)

Test Period	San Francisco Men (14–49 Yr)			Oakland Men (14–49 Yr)		
	Number	Mean Serum Uric Acid	SD	Number	Mean Serum Uric Acid	SD
9/64–8/65	5256	6.12	1.16	5621	5.76	1.28
8/65–8/66	4944	5.90	1.23	5587	5.66	1.27
9/66–8/67	4913	5.28	1.35	5985	5.78	1.26
1/67–12/67	3359	5.16	1.35	4685	5.78	1.20
1/68–8/68	3571	5.83	1.30	4204	6.02	1.29
4/69–6/69*	941	5.43	1.16	1221	5.32	1.11

* Studies in this test period were made in the AutoChemist by the uricase method. In all other test periods, studies were made in the AutoAnalyzer by the phototungstic acid method. (Reproduced by permission from Fessel, Siegelaub, Johnson: Arch Intern Med 132:44, 1973)

Starting in September 1966, the mean serum uric acid level of Oakland men rose above that of San Francisco men, and this disparity persisted through September 1968. The importance of knowing the technique used is illustrated by the fact that all except the lowest row of the values reported in Table 5-1 were determined on a Technicon AutoAnalyzer by the phototungstic acid technique. Since January 1969, we have determined uric acid on an AutoChemist by the uricase method, which provides values approximately 1 mg/100 ml lower than those obtained on the AutoAnalyzer. A study of Bywaters and Holloway further emphasizes the importance of knowing the laboratory technique used in estimating serum uric acid [82]. Sera from each of three donors were sent to 36 centers in Great Britain for serum uric acid estimation. The 36 laboratories used three categories of methods: colorimetric (manual), colorimetric (AutoAnalyzer), and ultraviolet spectrophotometric (uricase). The least variation between laboratories was with the AutoAnalyzer colorimetric method, which gave ranges of 3.6–4.0, 3.6–4.6, and 5.2–6.1 mg/100 ml for each of the three sera. The manual colorimetric method gave the widest variation: 3.8–7.7 mg/100 ml in one serum.

Even allowing for the above influences on the normal range as obtained in a reference population, questions arise about the relevance of a single abnormal laboratory finding in a subject who has no appropriate clinical symptoms. The circumscription of a normal range necessarily results in a certain percentage of the population having values outside this range. The burden of proof rests upon us, as physicians, that the portion of the population that stands beyond the normal limits for a given measurement carries a higher risk of future illness than the larger portion of the population with values within the arbitrary normal range. The remainder of this chapter will consider the evidence as to whether some of those persons with hyperuricemia carry such a high risk.

GOUTY ARTHRITIS IS NOT THE MAJOR CONCERN

From the clinician's viewpoint, the problem engendered by the finding of apparently asymptomatic hyperuricemia is not whether the patient will develop gout but whether other associated conditions are likely to ensue, because gouty arthritis is itself easily treated with modern drugs. In Caucasian populations, gout seldom develops in persons with hyperuricemia. In an English population survey [403], none of the hyperuricemic people had gout; in a Finnish study [335], only 2 per cent of hyperuricemic persons had gout, and in a similar study from Canada [400], only three persons among the 106 found to be hyperuricemic had primary gout, although another six had secondary gout. An 18-year follow-up of 17 persons with asymptomatic hyperuricemia showed that gout had developed in only three (18 per cent), and that three (18 per cent) had become normouricemic [568]. In the Framingham study [282], the incidence of new attacks of gout has been dropping, in spite of the fact that most subjects with high blood urate levels have not yet had an attack. In our own studies, only three (2.4 per cent) of 124 hyperuricemic patients developed gout during 4¼ years of follow-up [204]. There are reports, too, that certain ethnic groups with hyperuricemia have a low prevalence of gout (e.g., the Australian aborigine, and the

Rarotongans), even though many ethnic groups (e.g., the Maori) have a high prevalence of both gout and hyperuricemia [175, 561, 562].

HYPERURICEMIA AND THE KIDNEY

This is an important topic for two reasons. First, since Garrod indicated the two possible explanations of hyperuricemia (increased formation or increased retention of uric acid) [234], the role of the kidneys has been subject to some controversy. Second, if it were shown that hyperuricemia per se is very likely to cause serious future renal disease, prophylactic drug therapy might be warranted for asymptomatic individuals. It is not my purpose to discuss in detail the evidence for and against a defect in the renal handling of uric acid in primary gout. The reader is referred to the excellent discussions of this problem by Gutman and Yü [273], Gutman et al [274], Nugent and Tyler [523], Rieselbach et al [579], and Steele and Rieselbach [655]. Steele and Rieselbach [655] found that in normal man, only 2 per cent of the filtered urate escapes tubular reabsorption, irrespective of the plasma level, and the tubular secretion of urate, which accounts for virtually all the urinary urate, is a direct function of the serum uric acid level. Gutman et al [274] made similar findings in gouty patients and held it unnecessary to postulate a specific renal defect in the elimination of uric acid in gout. However, when Rieselbach et al [579] separated gouty patients into normoproducers and overproducers of uric acid on the basis of ^{14}C uric acid turnover data, they were able to show that the acceleration of tubular secretion of uric acid was less pronounced in the normoproducers than in the overproducers, implying a renal defect in at least normoproducers with gout.

The development of modern concepts of the renal handling of uric acid has been aided by studies with pyrazinoic acid, which has been thought to suppress the renal secretion of uric acid. Some modification of these ideas may be necessary if the work of Fanelli et al [186, 187] is extended to man. Their evidence in Cebus monkeys and chimpanzees suggested that pyrazinoic acid has a dual effect on urate transport: blocking, although incompletely, tubular secretion of uric acid; and stimulating active tubular reabsorption. They also proposed that, in addition to tubular secretion, tubular cellular biosynthesis of uric acid might contribute to urinary uric acid. Although the renal handling of uric acid in different animals varies remarkably, Fanelli et al [187] considered that the chimpanzee is closest to man in this respect, so that their findings may be applicable to the human kidney.

The second question, regarding the potential for, and the degree of, future renal damage in the presence of hyperuricemia, is of very great practical importance. The fact that serious renal disease may develop in patients with gout does not necessarily apply to hyperuricemic persons without gout [671]. In this regard it is also important to note the observation of Talbott and Lilienfeld [670] that, despite the frequency of renal involvement in gouty patients, *critical* renal insufficiency is uncommon and does not bias the mortality data of gouty patients. We may divide this issue of the potential for future renal damage into two parts: the evidence for disordered renal function and anatomy in asymptomatic hyperuricemia and early gout, and the liability that hyperuricemia carries for urolithiasis.

DISORDERED RENAL FUNCTION AND ANATOMY IN ASYMPTOMATIC HYPERURICEMIA AND EARLY GOUT

Dornfeld et al [156] found abnormal maximal renal concentrating ability in five (26 per cent) of 19 subjects with asymptomatic hyperuricemia. Five of six patients with asymptomatic hyperuricemia showed defective renal response to an acute acid load. Gutman and Yü found normal renal clearances of inulin or creatinine (C_{inulin}, C_{cr}) and of para-aminohippurate (C_{PAH}) in 13 hyperuricemic members of 11 gouty families; none had had gout [273]. Likewise, we saw no differences in serum creatinine levels before and after onset of asymptomatic hyperuricemia (Table 5-2).

Other studies of patients with overt gout are open to criticism on the grounds that renal arterial and arteriolar lesions may already have been present and that these, rather than hyperuricemia per se, may have contributed to renal functional disorders. The same question applies to asymptomatic hyperuricemia, because no one has performed kidney biopsies to demonstrate normal vessels in such cases. Duncan et al [165] attempted to circumvent this difficulty by injecting uric acid intravenously into dogs and measuring the effect on renal clearances. Single injections of large amounts (40 and 100 mg/kg) of uric acid had no effect on the clearance of creatinine or PAH, but daily injections for 10 days induced a temporary decrease in them. The main histologic changes induced were dilation of glomeruli and tubules. However, the very high serum urate levels induced by these large injections of uric acid are not comparable to those in gout or asymptomatic hyperuricemia. The only analogous clinical situations occur in the drug therapy of myeloma, leukemia, or lymphoma, where renal tubular blockage by uric acid crystals is a well-known and serious complication. A similar criticism applies to the experiments of Stavric et al [653], who induced a urinary uric acid output 22 times the control level in rats and demonstrated uric acid deposition in the tubules. Gutman and Yü [273] saw generally normal

Table 5-2. **Mean Serum Creatinine Levels before and after Onset of Asymptomatic Hyperuricemia**

	Before Hyperuricemia Established	Last Value after Onset of Hyperuricemia
Males	N = 16	N = 16
Serum creatinine, mg/100 ml	1.13	1.14
Months before or after onset of hyperuricemia	17.6 (9–32)	31.0 (0*–67)
Females	N = 16	N = 16
Serum creatinine, mg/100 ml	0.86	0.91
Months before or after onset of hyperuricemia	20.9 (10–38)	39.1 (16–72)

* In 3 men, the final recorded creatinine level was the one obtained at entry to the study.
(Reproduced by permission from Fessel, et al: Arch Intern Med 132:44, 1973)

C_{inulin} in 150 gouty patients and only a moderate reduction in C_{PAH} in 110. They observed that C_{inulin} and C_{PAH} gradually fell with increasing age in both gouty and normal persons. While declining to speculate on the significance of the apparent fall in renal plasma flow indicated by the C_{PAH} findings, they considered that any fall in C_{inulin} that may occur in gouty subjects is usually ascribable not to the effects of gout per se but to degenerative changes in the renal vasculature associated with aging. It was their opinion that the predisposition to renal disease in gout is related to the degenerative vascular changes of advancing age, arteriosclerosis associated with hypertension, pyelonephritis resulting from calculus formation and infection, and direct injury by cumulative urate deposits in and around the renal tubules and collecting system.

Gonick et al [253] found that only seven (25 per cent) of 28 renal biopsy specimens from gouty patients were normal. They were struck, as have been others [75], by the observation that the arteries and arterioles were hyalinized out of proportion to the parenchymatous changes. Regrettably, however, 62 per cent of their patients were hypertensive. Although they confirmed the known finding of tubular atrophy and interstitial inflammation, they agreed with the earlier conclusion of Greenbaum et al [264] that the tubular atrophy and inflammation need not be attributable to infection, because polymorphonuclear cells were rare; the predominant reaction was in the neighborhood of the atrophic Henle's tubules rather than in the medulla and juxtamedullary cortex as is usual in pyelonephritis; and quantitative urine cultures in their gouty patients showed a low (4 per cent) prevalence of significant bacteriuria. Likewise, Greenbaum et al [264] obtained sterile cultures from the needles used in biopsy of the kidneys in five of their patients and only a saprophyte grew from a sixth. Gonick et al [253] emphasized the low prevalence of tophi in kidneys studied by biopsy and autopsy and concluded that gouty nephropathy is unlikely to be initiated by deposition of urates in collecting ducts. Rather, they suggested that the pathogenesis of gouty nephropathy is a reaction of the kidney to an increased filtered load of uric acid or some as yet unidentified urate precursor. This conformed with the observation of Greenbaum et al [264] that perhaps the earliest anatomic abnormality is a fine interstitial fibrosis and with Gutman and Yü's finding [273] that the main functional abnormality is an increased filtered urate load. Among the 12 kidneys examined at biopsy by Greenbaum et al [264] were four having entirely normal histopathologic appearances, four showing quite extensive changes, and four with intermediate abnormalities. Their tables show that the mean duration of gout (15.7 years) in those with the worst histopathologic changes was no different from that in those with normal appearances (17 years), but the mean age of the patients with the worst changes was greater (65 versus 46.5 years).

This rather confusing situation may be summarized by saying that in the approximate 30 per cent of gouty patients who are normoproducers of uric acid, tubular secretion rates of uric acid may be impaired; in asymptomatic hyperuricemia there are minor but definite renal function disturbances; the renal function disturbances in established gout are also relatively minor and are ascribable in part to arteriolonephrosclerosis; experimental studies show that similar depression of renal function is obtained only by intravenous injection of amounts of uric acid that almost never obtain in gout; vascular lesions tend to be striking in both biopsy and autopsy material; the earliest biopsy change is probably fine interstitial fibrosis; and there is some question whether uric acid deposition in the collecting tubules is an early pathogenic event.

HYPERURICEMIA AND UROLITHIASIS

The tendency to uric acid stone formation is an important consideration in assessing the risks of hyperuricemia, but these risks must be considered separately for gout and for asymptomatic hyperuricemia. It is noteworthy that primary gout is not the major cause of uric acid stones. In Melick and Henneman's [465] examination of 207 consecutive patients seen in a kidney stone clinic, 22 were found to have uric acid stones and only four (18 per cent) of these had primary gout. The liability to uric acid stones in gout has been variably assessed as between 10 and 30 per cent. Undoubtedly many factors contribute to this variable risk: genetic factors (Jews and Italians were found in one important study to have an increased risk) [465]; geographic location (in the tropics, dehydration leads to increased urinary concentration, and chronic diarrhea may cause metabolic acidosis and increased renal acidity); medical advice and treatment (undoubtedly the prevalence of stone will be less in those communities where gouty subjects are advised to maintain high urine volume and are given therapy to lower uric acid and alkalinize the urine).

Peters and Van Slyke [554] found that the solubility of uric acid in urine increased from 8 mg/100 ml at pH 5.0 to 1,520 mg/100 ml at pH 8.0. Fried and Vermeulen [221] confirmed this dramatic effect of pH on solubility and made the surprising observation that urine specimens from 20 of 50 normal persons were supersaturated with respect to uric acid and that this supersaturation could be maintained for a protracted time. Pak Poy [535] observed that gouty patients had lost the normal diurnal rhythm for urinary pH, excreting persistently acid urines with pH values below 6 throughout the day. Although 10 of Pak Poy's 13 patients had evidence of renal damage, this abnormality of urinary pH regulation would certainly enhance the tendency to uric acid lithiasis.

A somewhat separate problem is posed by the presence of asymptomatic hyperuricemia, because in this condition the prevalence and incidence of urolithiasis is unclear. In our 124 asymptomatic hyperuricemic patients followed for a mean of 4¼ years, only one renal stone occurred, and this was analyzed as calcium oxalate. By contrast, in the control group of 224 normouricemic patients followed for a similar period, renal stones developed in two patients; one of those stones was analyzed and found to contain 20 per cent uric acid [204]. In Framingham [283], 4.8 per cent of men had a serum uric acid level in excess of 7 mg/100 ml, and just over one in ten of these developed stones (unanalyzed for chemical composition) during 12 years. Of the men with a serum uric acid level of over 8 mg/100 ml, one of five developed stones during the 12 years. For 9 years, one of our patients has been known to have serum uric acid levels as high as 16 mg/100 ml, but neither gout nor renal disease has developed. Several factors may account for the differences between the findings in our study and in Framingham. The Framingham observers did not screen out patients who had hypertension or diabetes to start with and found that clinical evidence of renal disease developed in 3 per cent of patients with hyperuricemia. By contrast, none of our patients entered the study with renal disease, hypertension, or diabetes, and renal disease (other than stone) has developed in none.

The complexity of the problem of uric acid nephropathy is illustrated by two further studies. Duncan and Dixon [163] reported the family of a gouty propositus aged 19 years. All of the seven surviving first-degree relatives had hyperuricemia, and all but two had renal disease. One sister died at age 14 from hypertension and renal failure. His mother and two sisters had hypertension and preeclamptic toxemia. In contrast, Henneman et al [306] reported six patients who formed uric acid stones but did not have gout, hyperuricemia, or hyperuricuria. These patients were found to have increased acidity of their urine and depressed ability to increase ammonium excretion after acid loading.

HYPERLIPIDEMIA, ATHEROSCLEROSIS, VASCULAR THROMBOSIS, HYPERTENSION, OBESITY, AND DIABETES

Writing in 1897 on the "Cardio-Vascular and Renal Relations and Manifestations of Gout," Davis [135] considered that the complications he saw in gout were attributable to "accumulation in the blood of . . . uric acid . . . which produce[s] the vascular, cardiac, and renal changes. By removing the cause of these complications of gout their progress may be brought to a halt . . . " Since Davis wrote that, a large literature has confirmed that hyperuricemia may often accompany atherosclerosis, vascular thrombosis, and hypertension. Are these conditions merely additional causes of hyperuricemia? Is hyperuricemia a member of a constellation of abnormalities to which these belong? Does hyperuricemia play an indirect or a direct role in their causation, or is the hyperuricemia only a loosely related epiphenomenon? The therapeutic implications of these questions have led to many studies. Unfortunately, our relative ignorance of the general pathogenetic mechanisms of hypertension and atherosclerosis and of the tangled interrelation between these and obesity, hyperlipidemia, and diabetes makes it difficult to clarify the contribution made by uric acid. The confusion in the literature may be reduced by examining only those papers reporting work in which, as far as possible, the observations were well controlled and acute physiologic derangements and drug therapy were eliminated as causes of the hyperuricemia.

HYPERURICEMIA AND HYPERCHOLESTEROLEMIA

Authors of a number of uncontrolled studies, extensively reviewed by Marinoff et al [444], have asserted an association between hypercholesterolemia and hyperuricemia, and many well-controlled investigations confirm this. The careful observations of Schoenfeld and Goldberger [605] involved 14 patients who were seen weekly, six to ten times. At each visit, serum cholesterol and uric acid determinations were made. Each observation in this matched series of 98 pairs of cholesterol and 98 pairs of uric acid values was compared to the one preceding it for the magnitude and direction of change. There was a significant tendency for the changes in serum cholesterol and uric acid to parallel each other in magnitude as well as in direction. The mean values for cholesterol and uric acid in the individual patients during the study period were also positively correlated. In the Tecumseh Community Health Study [507], 8.8 per cent of the 588 men whose serum cholesterol distribution was at or above the 80th percentile, but only 6 per cent of the 603 men whose serum cholesterol distribution was at or below the 20th percentile were hyperuricemic. Similar differences were reported for the women in the study. The differences disappeared when the figures were corrected for age and body weight or build, but for reasons discussed in a later section of this chapter we consider that it is improper to make this correction. An early study by Gertler and Oppenheimer [241] had shown significant correlations between serum uric acid, serum cholesterol, lipid phosphorus, and Sf 10-20 lipoproteins in men but not in women. The correlation coefficient between serum uric acid and ponderal index was insignificant for the men but was the only significant one for the women. Our studies in highly selected, carefully matched groups of hyperuricemic and normouricemic individuals showed significantly higher levels of cholesterol in the hyperuricemic group [204].

There are some reports that deny this relation between uric acid and cholesterol. In the Framingham population of 2,172 male subjects, the mean serum uric acid was 5.1 mg/100 ml and mean cholesterol was 233 mg/100 ml; among the 65 patients with gout, the mean serum uric acid was 6.4 mg/100 ml and cholesterol 240 mg/100 ml, differences that were not significant although in the expected direction [283]. A tendency for the cholesterol to increase with increasing uric acid levels in the total population was not statistically significant. Fairly large groups of subjects were studied by Berkowitz [43], Dunn and Moses [167], and Benedek [39], and none of these investigators saw any relation between serum uric acid and cholesterol. Some subjects in small groups of patients with familial hypercholesterolemia have been found to have hyperuricemia, but examination of 185 members of 12 families with familial hypercholesterolemia demonstrated no statistically significant difference in uric acid levels and cholesterol between those individuals who had and those who did not have the trait [343]. The authors believed that previously reported, elevated uric acid levels in familial hypercholesterolemia should be regarded as unusual findings.

On the other hand, the relation between triglycerides and uric acid in gouty patients is clearcut. Berkowitz [43] observed hyperuricemia in 41 of 50 patients with hypertriglyceridemia. A notable study by Feldman and Wallace [192] was of 34 patients with gout who had never had angina, coronary insufficiency, myocardial infarction, congestive heart failure, electrocardiographic changes compatible with coronary artery disease, hypertension, diabetes mellitus, cerebrovascular, renovascular or peripheral vascular disease, or hypothyroidism. No patient had taken uricuric drugs for at least one month prior to study, and none was taking salicylates. The controls were 28 healthy men of similar age distribution. The mean serum triglyceride level in the patients with gout was 142 mg/100 ml; in the controls, 100 mg/100 ml. Hypertriglyceridemia (186 mg/100 ml or more) was present in 11 of the 34 patients with gout but in only one of the healthy men. Benedek [39] confirmed hypertriglyceridemia in gout and observed no relation between serum triglyceride level and ponderal index. Dunn and Moses [167], however, observed no significant correlation between serum uric acid and triglyceride in 295 executives participating in a periodic health evaluation program, from whom were excluded those who had clinical or electrocardiographic evidence for coronary artery disease or who were receiving drug therapy for diabetes, hypertension, gout, or hypercholesterolemia. Benedek's [39] findings in healthy men and women without gout were similar. It would therefore appear that while a relation between uric acid and triglycerides exists in gout, this relation does not hold for normouricemic subjects. The question arises whether relations that exist across the entire range of values are as relevant as those within the upper ranges that pertain to most subjects with a given disease.

ATHEROSCLEROSIS AND HYPERURICEMIA

A widely quoted paper by Traut et al [684] purported to show urates in the walls of arteries. No chemical evidence for this was presented. The identification was made on the basis of the shape of the crystal clefts, which more closely resembled the clefts seen from urate deposition than those from cholesterol crystals; around the clefts there was a granulomatous reaction with multinucleated giant cells, and no foamy macrophages were seen. Necropsy of their second patient with gout showed on the mitral valves chalky deposits that reacted positively with the murexide test. In 1897, Davis [135] stated that urate deposits on the heart valves had been found in rare cases of gout. While the interpretation of these observations is debatable, they certainly raise the question of the relation between hyperuricemia and atherosclerosis and the more remote possibility that urate crystals may actually form within vessel walls.

An early study by Kramer et al [390] was of 437 cases of peripheral vascular disorders including arteriosclerosis, arterial thrombosis, diabetes, and thrombophlebitis; 39 per cent of the patients had hyperuricemia. When those with arterial occlusive disease were graded clinically according to the severity of the occlusion, it was found that the percentage of those with hyperuricemia gradually increased, from 11.8 per cent in those with calcified vessels but no occlusions, to 28.2 per cent in those with severe occlusion. Another early contribution, by Gertler et al [240], was a study of 97 men who had experienced a myocardial infarction before the age of 40 years. One of the control groups consisted of 97 men individually matched to the coronary disease group in age, physique, occupation, racial origin, and economic status. While 24 per cent of the patients with myocardial infarction had serum uric acid levels exceeding 6 mg/100 ml, only 6 per cent of the controls had such high values. Examination of the purine intake of the two groups showed that the differences in uric acid levels could not be accounted for on this dietary basis. It is worth emphasizing that somatotype was not a factor contributing to the relation between serum uric acid and coronary artery disease. This study has been criticized for not containing such crucial data as the point in time after the myocardial infarction when serum uric acid was estimated, and the factors of treatment that might have influenced serum uric acid levels; but these detractions lose weight in the light of other findings that serial determinations of serum uric acid for several months after the acute episode of either myocardial or cerebral infarction did not show important falls in these levels [286, 542]. In the Framingham observations, 5,127 men and women aged 30–59 years on admission to the study, were followed for 14 years, and the incidence of coronary heart disease was assessed at the end of 10 years [281]. There was a significantly higher incidence of coronary heart disease in subjects with gouty arthritis; and within the general population, the incidence of coronary heart disease in those with serum uric acid levels over 7.0 mg/100 ml was twice that in the group with values lower than 4.0 mg/100 ml. Among the 5, 967 persons in the Tecumseh study were 94 men and 53 women in whom coronary heart disease developed; 17.0 per cent of the men and 20.8 per cent of the women with coronary heart disease were hyperuricemic [507].

Hyperuricemia was found by Hansen [286] in 41 (36 per cent) of 115 persons with acute cerebral infarction. All of the 34 controls admitted to the surgical and neurosurgical wards for treatment of traumatic injuries were normouricemic, eliminating stress as the cause for the hyperuricemia. Serial uric acid determination in 17 patients for as long as 2–16 months after the stroke showed persistent hyperuricemia in 10. Similarly, Pearce and Aziz [542] found hyperuricemia in 25 per cent of 60 consecutively admitted patients with stroke, excluding those with many of the general medical conditions known to induce hyperuricemia: hypertension, diabetes mellitus, and antihypertensive treatment. The hyperuricemia did not seem to be a transitory phenomenon. Serial estimations in 16 patients (the second value was obtained 3–9 months after the ictus) showed no significant pattern of change in the levels. Most recently, Viozzi et al [699] reported that the prevalence of arterial thrombosis in various sites was higher in patients with gout than in a general population.

Our observations showed that coronary artery disease developed in two of 124 young patients with asymptomatic hyperuricemia during a 4¼-year period but in none of the control group (Table 5-3) [204]. Computer-assisted studies of more than 10,000 patients in our clinic show that while the mean serum uric acid was 5.5 mg/100 ml in those considered to have no clinically significant abnormality, it was approximately 1 mg higher in those with peripheral arteriosclerosis (6.4 mg/100 ml), in those with cerebral vascular insufficiency (6.7 mg), and in those with thrombophlebitis (6.4 mg). Although only 2.6 per cent of the 10,000 patients had serum uric acid levels in excess of 8.5 mg, this percentage was more than doubled (to 6.4 per cent) in the 110 patients with peripheral arteriosclerosis.

A Canadian group of workers [506, 640] found that patients with gout had shortened partial thromboplastin times, increased platelet adhesiveness, diminished platelet survival time, and increased platelet turnover. In related work, which may have considerable bearing on whether or not hyperuricemia predisposes to arterial thrombosis, Kellermeyer and Breckenridge [372] showed that uric acid crystals could activate Hageman factor. Activated Hageman factor may initiate the clotting mechanism. Newland [514] examined the effect of uric acid on platelet aggregation induced by adenosine diphosphate (ADP) under the hypothesis that uric acid, being a metabolite of the adenine nucleotides, may influence the degradation of ADP. In rats given uric acid intravenously 1 minute before the injection of ADP, the mean serum uric acid level rose 50 per cent, and the incidence of pulmonary platelet thrombi rose significantly above that of control animals. In rats pretreated with warfarin for 2 days, the mean serum uric acid level was lower and the incidence of ADP-induced pulmonary platelet thrombi was less. These results suggest that one mode of action of warfarin is through uricuria and that its effect on platelet aggregation may be indirect.

Table 5-3. Consequences of Asymptomatic Hyperuricemia

	Hyperuricemic Subjects	Normouricemic Subjects	P
Total subjects	124	211	
Gout	3	1	NS
Renal stone	1	2	NS
Urinary tract infections*	6	15	NS
Hypertension	8†	0	< .01‡
Heart disease	2	0	NS‡§
Diabetes	4†	0	NS‡§
Thrombophlebitis	2	2	NS

* Two or more clinically apparent urinary tract infections in all cases except one normouricemic patient with acute pyelonephritis.

† In 2 patients, diabetes and hypertension developed concurrently.

‡ The combined occurrences of hypertension, heart disease, and diabetes were significantly higher in the hyperuricemic than in the normouricemic group (p < .01).

§ The combined occurrences of heart disease and diabetes were significantly higher in the hyperuricemic than in the normouricemic group (p < .05).

(Reproduced by permission from Fessel, et al: Arch Intern Med 132:44, 1973)

HYPERTENSION AND HYPERURICEMIA

Both Breckenridge [69] and Cannon et al [83] saw hyperuricemia in 27 per cent of untreated, nonazotemic hypertensive patients. The mechanism seemed to be from a diminished uric acid clearance and an increase in the miscible uric acid pool. Although lacticemia is quite frequent in hypertension, Cannon et al [83] saw no direct correlation between serum lactic acid and uric acid levels. In the patients studied by Breckenridge [69], there was a highly significant increase in cerebrovascular accidents and in the development of ischemic heart disease among those who had hyperuricemia, in contrast to those whose uric acid levels were normal. Because hypertension developed in 6.3 per cent of our patients with asymptomatic hyperuricemia during a $4\frac{1}{4}$-year follow-up period, it would seem that the hyperuricemia is not a mere epiphenomenon of hypertension (Table 5-3) [204].

RELATION BETWEEN URIC ACID AND CARBOHYDRATE METABOLISM

The confusing and often apparently conflicting literature relating uric acid and carbohydrate metabolism can be best understood on the basis of a uricuric effect of hyperglycemia. It is generally agreed that there is a high prevalence of impaired carbohydrate metabolism in gout, yet glucose infusions are uricuric, and groups of patients with clinical diabetes have a low mean serum uric acid [60, 141, 309, 477, 637]. Although, allegedly, clinical gout and clinical diabetes do not commonly coexist, coexistent gout and diabetes were studied in 29 patients by Bartels et al [32]. The diabetes followed the onset of gout in 25 of the patients, preceded gout in only two, and occurred simultaneously with the onset of gout in another two. In 15 of the 25 patients with preexisting gout, the authors believed there was a definite decrease in frequency of gout attacks after the onset of diabetes. These 15 patients were apparently not receiving uricuric therapy. De Coek [141] compared 32 diabetic men with 32 nondiabetic, age-matched controls. The diabetic group had significantly higher urate clearances than the controls and significantly lower serum uric acid levels. There was no significant difference between the creatinine clearances of the two groups. De Coek suggested that there might be impaired urate reabsorption in the diabetic patient on the basis of thickening of the tubular basement membranes. He found mean serum uric acid levels of 3.94 mg/100 ml in the diabetic group and 6.03 mg/100 ml in the control group. Similar but smaller differences between the mean serum uric acid of diabetic patients and that of the total population were seen in the Tecumseh Health Study [477]. In a survey of more than 10,000 male government employees, Herman et al [309] saw a significant inverse relation between diabetes and serum uric acid. Even those men with previously unknown diabetes had significantly lower uric acid levels, showing that these levels must be related to the disease diabetes rather than to its treatment.

Paradoxically, there is general agreement that groups of patients with clinical gout uniformly have a high prevalence of impaired carbohydrate tolerance. Boyle et al [67] found significantly higher fasting blood sugar levels in patients with gout than in weight-matched controls. Higher prevalences of carbohydrate intolerance in patients with gout than in normal persons were seen by Weiss et al [713], Herman et al [309], and Denis and Launay [143]. Between 7 per cent and 55 per cent of the subjects studied by Denis and Launay [143] would be termed diabetic, depending on the diagnostic criteria used for diabetes. Glucose intolerance of a degree sufficient to diagnose chemical diabetes was seen in about one-third of their patients. In our patients with asymptomatic hyperuricemia, diabetes developed in 3.2 per cent (Table 5-3) [204].

In contrast to reports that show chemical diabetes in both gout and asymptomatic hyperuricemia, there is some question whether clinical diabetes and clinical gout coexist less frequently than expected. Joslin et al [352], for example, reported coexistent gout in only one diabetic patient among 1,500, and no patient in the Tecumseh Health Study [477] had both gout and diabetes. Whitehouse and Cleary [718] found one case of gout among 100 diabetic patients, and others have seen clinical diabetes in as many as 10 per cent of patients with gout [334].

RELATION BETWEEN WEIGHT AND SERUM URIC ACID

Our patients with asymptomatic hyperuricemia had significantly greater values for weight, triceps skinfolds, and subscapular skinfolds, and a smaller value of ponderal index (height/weight $\frac{1}{3}$) than the control group [204]. In the Tecumseh Health Study [507], serum uric acid and relative weight were studied in 5,967 subjects. Relative weight was computed by a regression equation taking into account actual weight and biacromial and bicristal diameters. Hyperuricemia was found in 3.4 per cent of those whose relative weight was below or at the 20th percentile; in 5.7 per cent of those whose relative weight was from the 21st to the 79th percentile; and in 11.4 per cent of those whose relative weight was at or above the 80th percentile. Examining serum uric acid in 460 persons with various body weights, Křížek saw a practically linear relation between serum uric acid and weight, starting from 80 kg, with a highly significant correlation coefficient between serum uric acid and weight for both males and females [391]. Among the 213 people who had lost an average of 6.6 kg, the relation between the change in serum uric acid and the change in weight was not statistically significant. Although Benedek [39] saw a significant relation between ponderal index and serum uric acid in women, no such relation existed in men. In an early study of this problem, Gertler et al [240] found a significant correlation between serum uric acid and weight, ponderal index, and somatotype, yet their studies showed a significantly lower serum uric acid in physique-matched controls than in a group of patients with coronary heart disease.

Further evidence that body size is not the sole common determinant in the constellation of factors that includes hyperuricemia, diabetes, hyperlipidemia, and atherosclerosis was shown by Berkowitz [43], who found that 19 of 25 patients with gout had hypertriglyceridemia and that 74 per cent of the 19 had impaired carbohydrate tolerance. Likewise, 72 per cent of 25 patients with hypertriglyceridemia but no gout had impaired carbohydrate tolerance, but all of the six gouty patients with normal triglyceride levels had normal fasting blood sugar levels, and the mean weight of these six patients was identical with that of the 19 gouty patients with hypertriglyceridemia. In the studies of Wiedemann and coworkers [719], approximately half the gouty patients manifested type IV hyperlipoproteinemia that was unrelated to obesity or glucose intolerance.

Other evidence that weight is only one of multiple variables comes from population studies. Acheson and Florey [6] observed a strong association between serum uric acid and body weight in recruits to the armies of Argentina and the United States. Among Brazilian recruits, this association held only for those who weighed more than 135 pounds, and there was no such association among Colombian army recruits. In 80 male Australian aborigines, Emmerson et al [175] saw no significant correlations between serum uric acid and height, weight, or surface area; but among 138 females there was a significant regression of serum urate with weight. A subgroup of Polynesians, the Maori, are hyperuricemic, obese, diabetic, and atherosclerotic. Another subgroup, the Pukapukans, are hyperuricemic yet thin, nondiabetic, and nonatherosclerotic. Yet a third subgroup, the Hawaiians, tend to be obese, atherosclerotic, and diabetic but not hyperuricemic.

RELATION BETWEEN THE LIVER AND URIC ACID

A relation between the liver and gout has been postulated since earliest times. Wolfson et al [731], in 1949, made a thorough study of liver function in patients with gout, using the tests then available. They concluded that the liver is ordinarily both functionally and anatomically normal in gout unless there is a complicating disease process, and they observed an increased mean level of albumin in patients with gout who had no apparent hepatic or renal impairment. A population survey in New Haven, Connecticut, by Acheson and Chan [5] showed a weak but statistically significant correlation between both gamma and beta globulin levels and uric acid in women but not in men. Our own studies show that serum glutamic oxalacetic transaminase and other values obtained as tests of hepatocelluar function are normal in asymptomatic hyperuricemia, and confirm the significant elevation in mean serum albumin [204].

A study of liver function was made by Grahame et al [262] in 73 patients with gout, 16 patients with asymptomatic hyperuricemia not due to renal failure, and 30 control subjects. The mean sulfobromophthalein (BSP) retention in the patients with gout was 9.2 per cent (2–27 per cent); in the patients with asymptomatic hyperuricemia, 7.1 per cent (2–12 per cent), and in the control group, 3.5 per cent (0–10 per cent). The differences between the control group and the other two groups were statistically significant. The means for alkaline phosphatase in the three groups were, respectively, 9.5, 9.9, and 7.7 King-Armstrong units. These differences were also statistically significant. The authors induced hyperuricemia in five healthy subjects by feeding them RNA; there were no resultant changes of importance in responses to any of the liver function tests. The various abnormalities in response to the liver function tests of their patients remained even when the overweight subjects were excluded.

Sørenson [650] made an extensive review of the literature concerning the extrarenal excretion pathways of uric acid and conducted his own studies with ^{14}C-labeled uric acid. He estimated that the normal adult male excretes approximately 200 mg of uric acid per 24 hours in the digestive juices. In 10 subjects, the uric acid concentration in bile was 4.4 mg/100 ml (1.97–6.47 mg/100 ml). If approximately 1 liter of bile is produced per day, the average biliary excretion accounts for 50 mg/day.

Gouty patients are traditionally supposed to be heavy drinkers, and our studies extend this observation to patients with asymptomatic hyperuricemia [204]. Although Grahame et al [262] saw a correlation between raised BSP retention and regular alcohol consumption in their patients with gout, this was not of statistical significance. Of the gouty subjects with raised BSP retention, 64 per cent did not admit to regular drinking. It is possible that the acute rises of serum uric acid and occasional clinical gout induced by heavy drinking are caused by lacticemia resulting from the metabolism of ethanol [424].

POPULATION STUDIES: HEREDITY VERSUS ENVIRONMENT

Ethnic studies of serum uric acid distribution are important to the present subject because they shed light on the relative influences on uric acid levels of genetic versus environmental factors and show the concentrations in which associated conditions occur in groups of subjects relatively homogeneous for racial and social factors. The genetic analysis is directly relevant because if idiopathic hyperuricemia is primarily genetically determined, so presumably might also be its associated conditions, and the same argument would apply if environmental factors were found to be primary. This knowledge is obviously important in advising hyperuricemic patients regarding prophylactic measures against associated conditions discussed in this chapter.

An early study by Hauge and Harvald [296] showed that mean serum uric acid levels in the siblings of gouty patients were significantly higher than in controls, but the siblings' values fitted a normal distribution curve, making untenable the previously advanced hypothesis of a dominant inheritance. These observations were confirmed by O'Brien et al [526] in their studies of Blackfoot and Pima Indians. Other authors have found a bimodal distribution curve for serum uric acid values in the general population, but Finn et al [207] ascribed this to technical factors and showed that uric acid is normally distributed in the general population. Our own findings confirm this.

A population study in England reported by Popert and Hewitt [558] included 100 relatives of those hyperuricemic subjects identified by the study. None of the hyperuricemic persons had had gout. Their 100 relatives had a normal distribution of serum uric acid values. When Popert and Hewitt analyzed another English community, they found three hyperuricemic persons among 18 relatives of hyperuricemic subjects. Hauge and Harvald [296] had observed significantly more urinary calculi in relatives of persons with gout than in controls, and Duncan and Dixon [163] had reported a heavy aggregation of renal disease and toxemia of pregnancy in the siblings of a patient with primary gout. In light of their findings, Popert and Hewitt [558] considered that a distinction should be drawn between simple familial hyperuricemia and the familial hyperuricemia of gouty families.

The observation by Jensen et al [343] that the variance of uric acid was significantly greater in dizygotic than in monozygotic twins is clear evidence that genotype exerts a significant effect on normal serum uric acid levels. There is also an environmental influence, because when all twins of each type were considered, uric acid variance was greater among those twins who lived apart than among those who lived together. This evidence for both genetic and environmental influence on uric acid levels was confirmed in similar studies in twins by Boyle et al [66].

Hauge and Harvald [296] found no evidence for a genetic linkage between the predisposition to hyperuricemia and the blood groups ABO, Rhesus, MNS, P, Lewis, or Duffy and Kell. Saha and Banerjee [597] confirmed these findings for the ABO and Rhesus blood groups in Indians. Acheson and Florey [6], however, observed significantly higher than average serum uric acid levels in young Colombian men of blood-group B and significantly lower than average serum uric acid levels in young Brazilian men of blood-group AB. No such relationships were seen in men from Argentina or the United States. Acheson and Florey considered it unlikely that they had identified a genetic linkage but wondered if the red blood cell, a source of purines, might be catabolized differently in different circumstances. Flatz [209] saw significantly lower mean serum uric acid levels in young Thai men with blood-group A. Although those with blood-group B had the highest mean serum uric acid levels, the differences did not reach statistical significance. We did not find different mean serum uric acid levels according to the various ABO blood groups [204], but confirmed the observation of Acheson and Florey [6] and that of Flatz [209], that hyperuricemic patients include fewer individuals with blood-group A and significantly more with blood-group B than a contrast population.

Studies of indigenous Pacific populations have given much information about the relative roles of genetic and environmental factors on the genesis of hyperuricemia and about the constellation of conditions associated with hyperuricemia. Observations in New Zealand initiated by Rose [587] have shown hyperuricemia in a number of the Polynesian subgroups (Maori, Pukapukans, and Rarotongans) [561]. Whereas the historical evidence is convincing that gout was rare in the Maori before the twentieth century, Lennane et al [410] found that gout is now much more prevalent in the Maori people than in those of European stock. The Maori and Rarotongan peoples are hyperuricemic and gouty and have high prevalence rates for ischemic heart disease, hypertension, diabetes, and obesity. The Pukapukan people are hyperuricemic with a strong tendency to gout but have low prevalence rates for ischemic heart disease, hypertension, diabetes, and obesity [561]. One's immediate reaction to ascribe these interesting findings to genetic factors is modified by the observation of Evans et al [183] that the Pukapukans live in the Northern Cook Islands under a subsistence level economy on a diet composed of coconut, taro (related to the sweet potato), and fish and that they only uncommonly use alcohol. The Rarotongans, on the other hand, live in the Southern Cook Islands where they have ready access to a varied diet including canned goods, and almost half of them were classified as either moderate or heavy drinkers. Evans et al [183] showed a stepwise increase of mean serum uric acid with increasing alcohol consumption.

Further evidence for the interaction of environmental and genetic factors, with environmental ones perhaps playing the active role and genetic ones a passive or permissive role, comes from studies of Filipino people. Whereas the mean serum uric acid levels of Filipinos living in the Philippine Islands and the prevalence of gout in the Philippines are the same as of Caucasians in the United States, the mean level of serum uric acid in Filipinos living in Hawaii and Seattle is higher than in Caucasians. Healey et al [302] suggested that in the Filipinos the ability of the renal tubules to increase uric acid secretion in response to an increased plasma urate load might be defective.

O'Brien et al [526] calculated a "heritability factor" that reflects the correlation of parents' phenotypic values with those of their offspring. For a known genetic trait in Pima Indians, an abnormally short middle phalanx of the fifth finger, they estimated the heritability factor at about 70 per cent, but for uric acid levels the heritability factor was only 23.8 per cent in the Blackfoot and 21.6 per cent in the Pima. They concluded that the uric acid level is largely determined by environmental rather than genetic factors.

On serum uric acid levels, these population studies appear to show a weak genetic influence and a stronger environmental influence. In some populations they confirm a remarkable tendency for hyperuricemia, gout, hypertension, atherosclerosis, diabetes, and obesity to occur together in a constellation.

PHOSPHORIBOSYL TRANSFERASE (PRT) DEFICIENCY

Any discussion of hyperuricemia would be incomplete without mention of hypoxanthine-guanine phosphoribosyl transferase (HGPRT) deficiency as a

CHAPTER 6

Synopsis of Clinical Immunology

Although a comprehension of immunological principles is essential to an understanding of modern investigations into the pathogenesis of connective tissue diseases, such understanding is becoming increasingly difficult for the clinician because of the explosive growth of knowledge in this field. In this chapter, I shall give a simplified overview of the physiology of immunity as it is understood at the time of writing, in 1974. The chapter is mainly a verbal explanation of Figure 6-1.

It is customary to divide immune reactions into those that are cell-mediated and those that are antibody-mediated. It is also usual to consider the thymus-derived lymphocytes (T lymphocytes) and the bone marrow-derived lymphocytes (B lymphocytes) as central respectively to each of these branches of the immune response.

Antigen is processed by macrophages, whether tissue histiocytes or blood monocytes. B lymphocytes, in response to the presence of this processed antigen and assisted by T lymphocytes by an uncertain mechanism, transform into plasma cells, which, in their turn, produce immunoglobulins. Immunoglobulin G or M reacts with the antigen to form antigen-antibody complexes. Immunoglobulin E attaches to membrane receptors on basophils, causing release of histamine and of platelet activating factor; the latter induces the release of other vasoactive amines from the platelet. The antigen-antibody complex causes activation of prekallikrein in the plasma to active kallikrein, which has both direct chemotactic properties and the capacity to activate plasma kininogen, resulting in the formation of kinins. Kinins induce the typical inflammatory response of pain, vasodilatation, and increased capillary permeability.

The antigen-antibody complex also induces the activation of the first component of complement. Figure 6-1 shows complement, for the sake of simplicity, unattached to cells; but *in vivo* it would be attached either to cells or to the antigen-antibody complex. The first component of complement has three subunits, labeled respectively C1q, C1r, and C1s. The second element of complement in the complement cascade is labeled C4, for historic reasons. This is activated by the first component of complement to form C14; C2 then enters the sequence. A byproduct at this point in the sequence of complement activation is the formation of C-kinin, which has the general properties of kinins already alluded to. An offshoot of the entry into the sequence, of the third and fifth components of complement is the formation of anaphylatoxin. Anaphylatoxin causes liberation of histamine; when injected into animals, it may cause urticaria and, even, a syndrome resembling anaphylactic shock.

It is important to note that the complement cascade may be initiated at the level of the third component of complement, bypassing the prior sequence, by

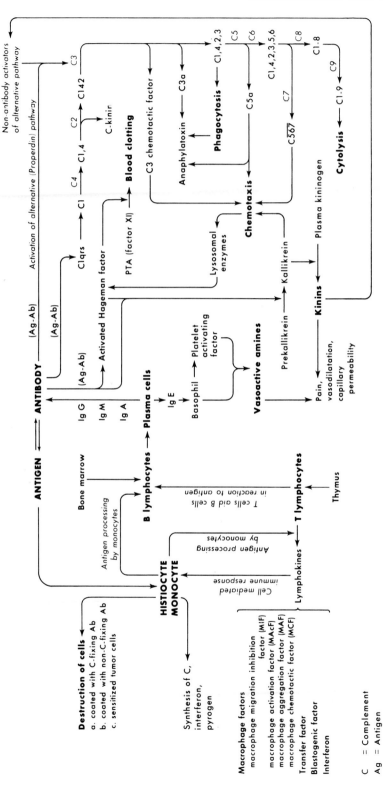

Fig. 6-1. The physiology of immunity.

means of the so-called "alternative" or properdin pathway. This alternative pathway may be activated by the antigen-antibody complex.

The compound, C1423, has the property of promoting phagocytosis. The byproduct, C5a, not only has anaphylatoxic properties, but most importantly, promotes chemotaxis (as does active kallikrein).

Next in the sequence of the complement cascade is the introduction of the sixth and seventh components of complement with an important byproduct, the so-called "trimolecular complex", C567; the latter, too, is chemotactic. After the insertion of C8 and C9 into the sequence, the end product, C1-9, is formed; this is responsible for cytolysis by an unknown mechanism.

Thus, at various points of the reaction sequence, the complement system may mediate such features of the inflammatory response as enhanced phagocytosis, increased vascular permeability, and chemotaxis.

Turning now to the cell-mediated immunity, it will be noted from Figure 6-1 that the histiocyte or monocyte is central to this reaction: not only is this the final effector cell for this form of immunity; it may initiate cell-mediated immunity by processing the antigen and presenting it to the T lymphocyte. In response to the presence of appropriate antigen, the T lymphocyte produces lymphokines, which in general are factors that localize and amplify the histiocytic response. Approximately a dozen lymphokines have been isolated, the most important being blastogenic factor, transfer factor, and migration inhibition factor (MIF). Blastogenic factor hastens the self-reproduction of sensitized T lymphocytes so that a clone of sensitized T lymphocytes is rapidly produced. Transfer factor induces sensitivity to the offending antigen in previously uncommitted T lymphocytes. Between them, transfer factor and blastogenic factor form an important amplification mechanism to bring more histiocytes to the scene of inflammation. MIF prevents the histiocytes from wandering from the site of the inflammatory response. The histiocyte typifies cell-mediated immunity: it causes destruction of cells coated with complement-fixing antibody; it may also cause destruction of cells coated with noncomplement-fixing antibody, as in autoimmune hemolytic anemia.

The antigen-antibody complex influences the opposing systems of blood clotting and fibrinolysis. It activates Hageman factor (Factor XII). Factor XII causes activation of plasma thromboplastin antecedent (Factor XI) which, in its turn, initiates the coagulation sequence that terminates in the formation of fibrin. At the same time, Factor XII catalyzes the conversion of plasminogen to plasmin, permitting fibrinolysis; for simplicity, this is not depicted in Figure 6-1. A further important function of Factor XII is to activate kininogenase, which mediates the formation of kinin. Note that not only antigen-antibody complexes, but also plasmin, can amplify the complement cascade by activating the alternative pathway.

THE ROLE OF PROSTAGLANDINS

The prostaglandins are implicated in the inflammatory and immune reactions, but their precise roles have not been fully delineated. Although the prostaglandins are found throughout the plant and animal kingdom, and are present in virtually every tissue of the human body, their name derives from the original observation that pharmacologic effects, of which prostaglandins were eventually recognized as the cause, could be obtained with semen and prostatic extracts. The basic 20-carbon skeleton of the prostaglandins has been named prostanoic acid (Fig. 6-2).

Four series of natural prostaglandins have so far been described, designated by the letters E, F, A, and B. The two major compounds, prostaglandins E and F, were so named because prostaglandin E is more soluble in *e*ther; whereas prostaglandin F is more soluble in *p*hosphate buffer ("phosphate" is spelled in Swedish with an F). Prostaglandins A and B are produced by dehydration of a prostaglandin E molecule.

Lichtenstein and coworkers [421] found that prostaglandins inhibited the release of histamine, as induced by antigen and mediated by IgE, from human leukocytes. Testing a series of prostaglandins, they found that compounds E_1 and E_2 were most efficient in this respect. They observed that prostaglandins similarly inhibited cytolysis of mouse cells by sensitized lymphocytes. Prostaglandins caused an increase of cyclic AMP in the human leukocytes and in mouse lymphocytes, an observation that supports the hypothesis that the level of cellular cyclic AMP regulates the expression of humoral and of cell-mediated hypersensitivity.

Zurier and Ballas [743] saw suppression of experimental adjuvant arthritis in rats that had been treated with prostaglandin E_1. Prostaglandin E_1 has been found to increase the formation of corticosteroids by perfused rat adrenal glands; to reduce lysosomal enzyme release from leukocytes, and to prevent phytohemagglutinin-induced transformation of lymphocytes. These experiments showing inhibition of the immune and inflammatory responses by prostaglandin E run counter to others that showed a possible mediation of the inflammatory response by prostaglandin E: inflammatory exudates contain prostaglandin E; the latter has chemotactic activity for leukocytes and increases vascular permeability more powerfully than does bradykinin, histamine, or serotonin [358]; in tissue culture, larger amounts of prostaglandins were produced by synovium from patients with rheumatoid arthritis than by synovium from patients with osteoarthritis [581]; and prostaglandins E_1 and $F_{2\alpha}$ caused increased collagen biosynthesis [56]. Thus, although the role of the prostaglandins in regulation of the inflammatory response is complex and incompletely unraveled, these compounds are clearly relevant, and the clinician should be familiar with them. It is of related interest that aspirin and indomethacin block production of prostaglandins [384, 638], and it has been suggested that this may be the mechanism underlying their therapeutic actions. Furthermore, prostaglandins E_1 and E_2 in-

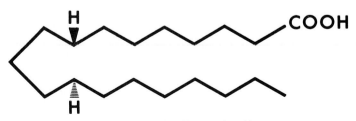

Fig. 6-2. Prostanoic acid.

duced resorption of bone in tissue culture to a degree comparable to that from parathormone [379]. Since prostaglandins are released by rheumatoid synovium in tissue culture [581], it is possible that these substances are also involved in causation of the characteristic juxta-articular osteoporosis of rheumatoid arthritis.

The following measurements for assessing the immune response mechanism are commonly available to the clinician. *Humoral antibody responses*: immunoglobulin levels; individual complement components, C1q, C3, C4; total hemolytic complement (CH50); percentage of circulating B lymphocytes (see below). *Cell-mediated immunity*: presence of delayed hypersensitivity to such antigens as PPD, mumps, candida, and trichophyton; development of contact allergy to dinitrochlorobenzene; nonspecific blast response by lymphocytes to mitogens such as phytohemagglutinin or pokeweed; production of lymphokines such as MIF; number of circulating T cells (see below).

The B and T lymphocytes may be distinguished by cytoplasmic membrane markers. B cell markers include membrane-associated immunoglobulins, detectable by direct immunofluorescence with fluorescein-labeled anti-immunoglobulin sera. In addition, the spontaneous formation of rosettes by sheep erythrocytes under specific conditions appears to be a characteristic property of the B and T lymphocytes. Unsensitized sheep erythrocytes adhere to T cells and form rosettes; sheep erythrocytes sensitized by antibody and the first four components of complement specifically bind to B lymphocytes and form rosettes. This is the basis of the so-called "rosette test" for distinguishing T cells from B cells. In mice, T lymphocytes bear a specific membrane antigen, theta; recently an antiserum has been made against a similar membrane antigen to human T lymphocytes, which may in the future form the basis for rapid identification of T cells.

CHAPTER 7

Angiitic Reactions

The angiitic reaction is central to the so-called "collagen diseases." The lesion is basic in periarteritis nodosa, microscopic polyarteritis, and systemic lupus erythematosus, is probably a forerunner to the formation of the rheumatoid granuloma, is prominent in dermatomyositis, especially in the childhood variety, and appears in progressive systemic sclerosis, particularly when the kidneys are affected. Midway between the pure angiitic reaction and the pure granulomatous reaction are 1) the lesion of Wegener's granulomatosis, where there is a granuloma contiguous to the angiitis, and 2) giant cell arteritis, where there is a granuloma within the wall of the artery. It is no wonder that the term, "collagen-*vascular* disease" is sometimes used. However, of all aspects of the collagen diseases, the classification of angiitis is the most difficult to approach because its histopathology is somewhat monotonous from case to case (cf. muscle reactions, Chapter 11; and granulomatous reactions, Chapter 8); its clinical manifestations offer but little nosologic help, and its known causes are diverse.

CLASSIFICATION OF ANGIITIS

A classification that is based upon the *size* and *location* of the affected vessel is unsatisfactory for the most part. Zeek [739] devised a classification based partly upon size of vessel involved: according to this, periarteritis nodosa affects larger vessels and spares pulmonary vessels, while hypersensitivity angiitis affects arterioles, venules, and capillaries, including those of the lungs. A major objection to this classification is its implication that hypersensitivity is known to be etiologic in the one but not in the other; whereas, in fact, immune mechanisms are probably involved in many cases of both sorts yet are not known with certainty to be involved in all cases of either sort. Further problems with this separation into periarteritis nodosa and hypersensitivity angiitis are discussed during the course of this chapter: at this point it will be mentioned only that Rose [588] saw no differences between cases with and those without lung involvement with respect to the incidence of polyarteritis in other organs or with respect to the accompanying clinical manifestations; that, although Moskowitz and coworkers [494] saw some differences in clinical findings and histopathology between groups with and without lung involvement, there was considerable overlap among the two groups, and finally, that neither Rose's [588] nor Frohnert and Sheps' [228] analysis demonstrated any prognostic value to the separation of those cases of periarteritis with pulmonary involvement from those without.

With further regard to classification according to *location* of involved vessels, some evidence suggests that in certain cases the lesions are completely or almost completely confined to the skin (although abdominal angiograms should be obtained to ascertain this in future cases). But, contrariwise, many patients with systemic angiitis have cutaneous involvement as well. In the special instance of giant cell arteritis, on the other hand, classification according to location does have utility because of the predilection of this form of the illness for the superficial temporal, ophthalmic, and posterior ciliary arteries, and the aortic arch.

With regard to classifying angiitis on the basis of the *size* of involved vessels, giant cell arteritis commonly affects medium-sized or larger vessels, but may occasionally affect arterioles; and although periarteritis nodosa is classically said to be a disease of medium-sized arteries, as such it is rare and almost always affects small-sized arteries. No particular vessel, whether artery, venule, or capillary, is the sole primary site of histopathologic change in any variety of angiitis.

A classification of angiitis that is based on the *histopathologic appearances* is, likewise, unsatisfactory because of the limited number of histologic reactions that occur in the vessel wall. Giant cell arteritis gives the impression of a specific histopathological reaction; but giant cells may be sparse, and these are themselves unspecific, being seen also, for example, in atheroma, lues, and Takayasu's disease. Further, in classic cases of giant cell arteritis, small vessels may show necrotizing arteritis without granulomata.

Whether or not there is fibrinoid material; whether there is intramural or perivascular infiltrate; whether the infiltrate is lymphocytic or polymorphonuclear neutrophilic; and, if the infiltrate is neutrophilic, whether it is leukocytoclastic with nuclear dust—these are basic yet confusing issues related to the classification and definition of angiitis. Immunofluorescence has shown that fibrinoid material contains, and may even be entirely composed of, fibrin. Such studies have also shown that fibrinoid substance, as defined by the immunofluorescent demonstration of fibrin in the vessel wall, may be present even when not seen by tinctorial staining: this vitiates the requirement that the definition of vasculitis must include the demonstration of fibrinoid material by tinctorial staining procedures; on the other hand, the presence of fibrinoid substance certainly implies vasculitis. More vexing yet is the question, whether perivascular infiltration alone, without intramural infiltration by inflammatory cells and without fibrinoid necrosis of the wall, is adequate to justify the label "vasculitis." Certainly, in many cases of widespread systemic vasculitis, areas of perivasculitis alone may be seen. Overall, however, one so often sees perivascular cuffing by inflammatory cells without intramural infiltrate or fibrinoid material [703], especially in the skin, that it is utilitarian to reject mere perivascular cuffing as a criterion for the label "vasculitis," recognizing that one may thereby miss the diagnosis in a few cases.

Aside from the granulomatous form, the main types of vasculitis are lymphocytic and neutrophilic. The import of seeing a purely lymphocytic reaction, rather than a purely neutrophilic one (sometimes termed "leukocytoclastic" because of the neutrophilic cell fragmentation that may be seen), is severalfold. Lymphocytic vasculitis is usually self-limited, is seen especially in certain drug eruptions and in reactions to insect bites, and seems likely to represent a cell-mediated immune reaction. Whether this is a true vasculitis, or the vascular wall is merely a pathway to the site of reaction in the tissues, is debatable. This histopathological reaction may be seen in erythema multiforme, erythema nodosum, and nodular vasculitis, all of which are probably clinical manifestations of delayed hypersensitivity or cell-mediated immunity. Neutrophilic vasculitis, on the other hand, is probably due to immune complex deposition (see below), i.e., humoral immunity. The presence of polymorphonuclear leukocytes in the wall of the vessel usually signifies vasculitis, but not always, because tissue inflammation requires that leukocytes pass from the blood to the tissues via the vessel wall.

A singular feature of neutrophilic vasculitis is the persistence of the polymorphonuclear reaction however long the angiitis may last: even after 21 years of recurrent angiitis, the cell type was polymorphonuclear [360]. This is unlike any other inflammatory reaction, where the morphological representation of chronicity is the mononuclear cell. It must imply either that the inciting factor for this form of vasculitis is ongoing, or that the chemotactic factor induced by the inciting agent is specific for polymorphonuclear cells and ineffective on mononuclear cells.

A classification of angiitis based upon its *known causes* is most logical (See Table 7-1). Unfortunately, in the majority of cases the etiologic factor is unknown. Nevertheless, hypersensitivity is probably the cause in most patients: there was an unmistakable drug reaction at the onset of illness in 26 of 72 cases analyzed by McCombs [455]. Students of angiitis will note that one is forced in Table 7-1 to borrow from Zeek's [739] classification because she constructed her groupings from an artificial blend of histopathological and clinical criteria. Aside from the special case of giant cell arteritis with its prognostic implications, there is little pragmatic value to any classification that is not based upon causation.

MODELS AND CAUSES OF ANGIITIC REACTIONS

At the present stage of our knowledge, immune complex deposition disease is the best available model to explain the allergic, the rheumatic, and the idiopathic groups of neutrophilic angiitis. It is therefore in order to review briefly our current understanding of how immune complex deposition produces the

Table 7-1.   Causes of Angiitic Reactions

Infection: septic embolism; syphilis; rickettsia; mycoplasma; fungus; virus

Trauma

Allergy: hypersensitivity reactions to drugs; deposition of immune complexes that contain viruses or bacterial antigens; insect bites

Raised hydrostatic pressure: malignant hypertension

Drug abuse: especially amphetamines

Atheroembolism

Idiopathic: periarteritis nodosa; rheumatoid arthritis; systemic lupus erythematosus; scleroderma; polymyositis; giant cell arteritis; Takayasu's disease.

finale that is manifested as angiitis. Certain animal models of angiitis seem likely to represent direct infection of vessels. A brief description of these will also be given; however, it currently seems dubious that this mechanism accounts for the angiitis of collagen diseases. The model of stress as causing angiitis, studied exhaustively by Selye, will not be outlined (vide Chapter 2 for calciphylaxis); its relevance to human medicine has never been clearly assigned. The following description of immune complex disease in experimental animals and man derives in part from the superb review by Cochrane and Koffler [113], to which the interested reader is directed for encyclopedic detail and bibliography.

Experimental **acute** *immune complex disease* occurs during the phase of immune-elimination after a single intravenous injection of a foreign protein. By means of fluorescence microscopy, the antigen, host γ-globulin, and C3 are detected at the very onset of injury in the vicinity of the internal elastic lamina of the artery. It is of great interest, however, that these are so rapidly removed that they are no longer detectable one or two days after the onset of arteritis. Neutrophils are clearly crucial for the development of this arteritis because it is completely inhibited if neutrophils are eliminated when the immune complexes enter the circulation. Complement depletion also inhibits the development of arteritis, presumably because it entails loss of chemotactic factors for neutrophils. Interesting and unexplained is the fact that glomerulitis develops even after neutrophils and C3 are eliminated.

Experimental **chronic** *immune complex disease* is somewhat different from the acute disorder. If rabbits are injected daily with heterologous serum protein antigens, those animals that have a strong antibody response develop chronic membranous glomerulonephritis within about 5 weeks. The amount of antigen that is injected intravenously is critical: the dose must be manipulated so as to obtain a temporary excess antigenemia after each injection in order to permit the formation of soluble immune complexes, which circulate in the presence of excess antigen. This chronic experimental disorder differs from the acute form in that glomerulonephritis rather than arteritis develops; moreover, no endocarditis occurs in the chronic disease.

The deposition of immune complexes depends upon an involved series of events. Hydrodynamic forces play a role. For example, in acute complex disease of rabbits, aortic lesions occur mostly at its bifurcation and at the origins of the coronary arteries; the intensity of the lesions in serum sickness increases when there is hypertension. It is also interesting that necrotizing arteritis (but with minimal cellular infiltrate) in the kidneys and elsewhere is seen in malignant hypertension. Increased vascular permeability occurs, probably related to the release of vasoactive amines as described below; the large, macromolecular immune complexes are then deposited along the vascular basement membranes. Because deposition of the immune complexes within the vessel wall depends on increased vascular permeability, the release of vasoactive amines from platelets is an important mechanism in the whole process. Vasoactive amines are released from platelets under the following conditions: 1) when immune complexes are in contact with the platelets in the presence of either complement or neutrophils; 2) when the antigen is particulate—this requires the presence of complement components 1, 4, 2, and 3; 3) when a platelet activating factor is released by IgE-sensitized basophils in the presence of antigen.

Other causes of angiitic reactions include infection of vessels, trauma, hypertension and, possibly, states of decreased fibrinolysis.

A model of polyarteritis in turkeys presumably involves *direct infection* of the vessels by *Mycoplasma gallisepticum* [676]. This is an interesting model for two additional reasons. First, the histopathology commences with a granulomatous reaction in the vessel wall, the later lesion being plasmacytic and lymphocytic. Second, the organism can be cultured only from the acute, not from the chronic arteritic lesion [111]. Finally, the distribution of the lesions is principally and often exclusively within the arteries of the brain, reminding one of a) the peculiar predilection of giant cell arteritis in humans for certain cerebral arteries, and b) the rare disease in humans, granulomatous angiitis of the central nervous system [386].

The interpretation of other experimental models of angiitis that involve infection is less clearcut because the mechanisms may be mixed. For example, spontaneous polyarteritis in certain animals could be from immune complex deposition, as is most likely in mice tolerant to lymphocytic choriomeningitis virus; or from direct infection, as it might be in the mice with a lymphocytic vasculitis studied by Wigley and coworkers [721]; or from a combination of immune complex deposition and direct infection of the vessel.

Rickettsial diseases in man, e.g., typhus, are characterized by panarteritis with fibrinoid degeneration and cellular infiltrate of the vessel wall. Organisms are rarely demonstrable and the lesion probably results from a combination of direct infection and immunological damage.

Direct trauma to a vessel may induce angiitis. An important example in man is atheroembolism. One of seven patients with diffuse atheroembolism studied by Anderson and Richards [17] had necrotizing angiitis with fibrinoid necrosis and cellular infiltrate, distinguishable from periarteritis nodosa only in those sections that happened to demonstrate the intraluminal cholesterol crystals. Reaction to the chemical was clearly involved, but trauma from impacted microcrystals may have played a role in causation of this angiitic process. In five of their seven patients the erythrocyte sedimentation rate was substantially elevated (up to 120 mm/hr), and six of the seven had eosinophilia (up to 11 per cent); the differential diagnosis from periarteritis nodosa was often difficult.

Necrotizing angiitis may be widespread in *malignant hypertension*: the walls of the afferent arterioles in the kidney have fibrinoid necrosis with little cellular infiltrate; but arterial lesions in other organs may be indistinguishable from periarteritis nodosa, so that Knowles and coworkers [383] considered hypertension an important mechanism in the pathogenesis of polyarteritis, even labelling these cases secondary periarteritis nodosa—a term that is not used today. Whether the interesting observation of polyarteritis in addicts who inject themselves intravenously with methamphetamine [109] is related to the angiitis of hypertension or depends upon hepatitis-B infection and consequent immune complex disease is uncertain. The likelihood that it is unrelated to hepatitis is increased by the experimental observations in monkeys that chronic intravenous injections of methamphetamine induced cerebral vascular spasm, shown angiographically, and microaneurysms and perivascular cuffing of arterioles by inflammatory cells, shown at autopsy [595].

Decreased fibrinolytic activity of the blood has been observed by Cunliffe and his coworkers [126, 127] in three patients with chronic vasculitis. The clinical condition improved after treatment with medicines that increased fibrinolysis. Cunliffe considered that the decreased fibrinolytic activity was the result rather than the cause of the local thrombosis [127].

CLINICAL ASPECTS OF ANGIITIC REACTIONS

The original descriptions of periarteritis nodosa in the nineteenth century emphasized the involvement of medium-sized arteries; the weakness of the vessel wall caused aneurysms to form, and nodules were often palpable in the superficial vessels. Yet, in their review of the cases reported up to 1939, Harris and coworkers [289] found that cutaneous nodules appeared in only 16 per cent. Periarteritis nodosa was apparently quite rare; by 1939 only 101 cases had been reported in the English literature [289]. Palpable aneurysms on superficial arteries are still rare: I have seen only one patient with this finding in the past 10 years. Yet microscopic polyarteritis of various causes is quite common. It seems likely that periarteritis nodosa as originally described, and the usual case of microscopic polyarteritis as seen today are merely variants of the same process which formerly was recognized only when it was sufficiently advanced to affect larger-sized vessels. My patient with periarteritis nodosa herself drew attention to the palpable nodule on a superficial temporal artery, biopsy of which showed panarteritis and a local aneurysm (Fig. 7-1): subsequent muscle biopsy showed necrotizing angiitis of arterioles (Fig. 7-2) characteristic of microscopic polyarteritis in any patient. It is preferable not to separate periarteritis nodosa from polyarteritis of smaller vessels, i.e., microscopic polyarteritis: regrettably, the term periarteritis nodosa is deeply rooted in medical terminology.

The symptoms, signs, and laboratory findings in any particular patient with polyarteritis depend upon the extent of organ involvement. Fever and tachycardia are common; disorders of peripheral nerves, usually a mixed motor and sensory polyneuropathy but occasionally classic mononeuropathy multiplex, are important clues to the diagnosis. An interesting pointer is leukocytosis, present in 75 per cent of the 175 patients reviewed by Nuzum and Nuzum [525]: the explanation for this frequent laboratory finding is unknown. Eosinophilia is widely recognized, but affects only one case in five [289]. Abnormalities of urinary sediment should be diligently sought in suspected cases: the number of red blood cells or cellular and granular casts may be few, and they may appear in showers, so that microscopy should be performed on many samples before concluding that the kidneys are spared.

Diagnosis of polyarteritis. Biopsy of skin and muscle showed polyarteritis in only 37 per cent of patients in whom the condition was demonstrated by other means [703]. This matches Nuzum's observation, in 175 patients collected from the literature, that skin and skeletal muscle were involved in only 20 to 40 per cent of patients [525]; on the other hand, abdominal viscera were frequently involved—the kidneys in 85 per cent, the liver in 66 per cent, the gastrointestinal tract in 51 per cent, the pancreas in 35 per cent, and the spleen in 34 per cent of cases. For this reason, the abdominal arteriogram, which evaluates several

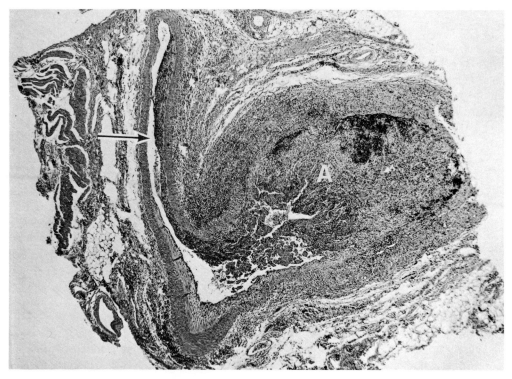

Fig. 7-1. Periarteritis nodosa in temporal artery. Arrow points to normal lumen of vessel; diffuse inflammatory reaction present in media and adventitia, with aneurysm formation (A). Hematoxylin and eosin, ×44. Same case as in Fig. 7-2.

organs simultaneously, is one of the most valuable investigative techniques. According to Bron and Gajaraj [73], pioneers in this field, the frequency of abdominal visceral aneurysms in polyarteritis approaches 60 per cent. Figure 7-3 shows numerous small aneurysms scattered throughout the liver; in the original x-ray, several aneurysms are demonstrated within the territory of the superior mesenteric artery, as well as within the kidneys. In a case reported by Capps and Klein [87], renal aneurysms were demonstrated angiographically; yet there were no red blood cells in the urine. Although angiographic findings in a number of other collagen diseases include vascular irregularities, narrowings, and complete obstructions (see, e.g., Fig. 1-7), multiple aneurysms are seen only in polyarteritis. An advantage of the angiographic demonstration of aneurysms is that it enables one to follow the course of the disease in a way unavailable by other means. For example, Robins and Bookstein [580] saw three cases in which renal aneurysms disappeared after treatment.

GOODPASTURE'S SYNDROME

Case 7-1. A 59-year-old man had been known to have mild emphysema for some years before a productive cough with blood-tinged sputum suddenly developed. He was considered to have acute bronchitis, but dyspnea persisted and iron-deficiency anemia with a hematocrit reading of 28 per cent was soon observed. The dyspnea and hemoptysis became more severe, and gross hematuria appeared. The arterial oxygen tension was 51 mm Hg during treatment with oxygen via face mask, then fell to only 34 mm Hg. Serum creatinine level was 1.6 mg/100 ml. The chest x-ray showed diffuse alveolar infiltrates (Fig. 7-4). He died from cardiopulmonary arrest about a month after the initial hemoptysis. Microscopic sections from lungs (Fig. 7-5) and kidneys showed findings consistent with Goodpasture's syndrome: immunofluorescence microscopic studies were not made.

Goodpasture's syndrome—lung hemorrhage and glomerulonephritis—is relevant to the present discussion because, although the major mechanism for production of the lung and renal lesions is not immune complex deposition, a number of patients show widespread polyarteritic lesions at autopsy. Dyspnea and hemoptysis are the major pulmonary features; hemosiderin-laden macrophages are seen in the sputum; the chest x-ray appearance represents blood in alveoli, a so-called "alveolar infiltrate," which often changes rapidly. Autopsy shows the alveolar hemorrhage and hemosiderin-containing macrophages (Fig. 7-5); in some cases, necrotizing and inflammatory changes are seen in the alveolar septa. Hematuria may be microscopic or macroscopic; proteinuria is usually slight but may be heavy. In the early stages of the disease, renal biopsy shows focal glomerulonephritis. At autopsy, the renal findings are those of severe,

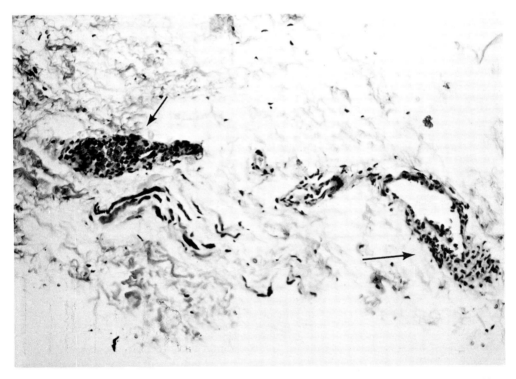

Fig. 7-2. Muscle biopsy showing acute arteriolitis (arrows). Hematoxylin and eosin, ×150. Same case as in Fig. 7-1.

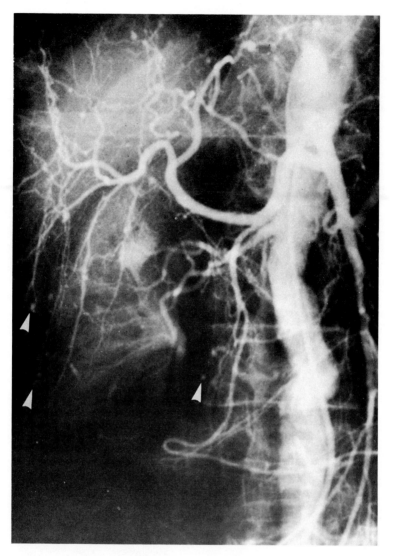

Fig. 7-3. Abdominal arteriogram in polyarteritis. Numerous tiny aneurysms (e.g., at arrows), especially in hepatic circulation.

widespread glomerular damage with focal necrotizing lesions in the tufts, and diffuse proliferative changes.

An antibody directed toward antigenic determinants that are shared by lung and kidney tissues is one of the mechanisms underlying Goodpasture's syndrome. The glomerular lesion is caused by an antibody directed against glomerular basement membrane [411], and in typical cases immunofluorescent staining for IgG shows linear deposition of antibody along the glomerular basement membrane. This is in contradistinction to the granular deposits of fluorescent antibody against IgG seen in immune complex deposition nephritis, such as that in systemic lupus erythematosus. Many reports indicate that the pattern of deposition of C3 on the glomerular basement membrane is also linear; but

Germuth and coworkers [239] saw a granular pattern in three cases of Goodpasture's syndrome, an observation that raises new questions about the mechanism for the renal lesion.

The mechanism for the pulmonary lesion is also considered to be immunological. Antibody eluted from the lungs of a patient with Goodpasture's syndrome was found to fix to glomerular basement membrane [385], and it is considered that there are some shared antigens in the lungs and kidney. Respiratory infection frequently precedes Goodpasture's syndrome: a well-studied case was closely associated with influenza A2 virus infection [725]; and hemoptysis usually antedates glomerulonephritis. This suggests that the lung is the initial site of damage; antibodies are consequently produced that damage both lung and kidney, causing release of more antigen which, in turn, induces further antibody formation. Bilateral nephrectomy has, however, been followed by cessation of lung hemorrhage in some patients [438], supporting the possibility that the kidney is the initial site of stimulus for antibody formation.

Beirne and Brennan [36] obtained occupational histories from eight patients with Goodpasture's syndrome and found that six of them had had extensive exposure to hydrocarbon solvents, e.g., degreasing and paint-removing solvents, and fuel oils. Frequently these solvents were heated and the patients had been ex-

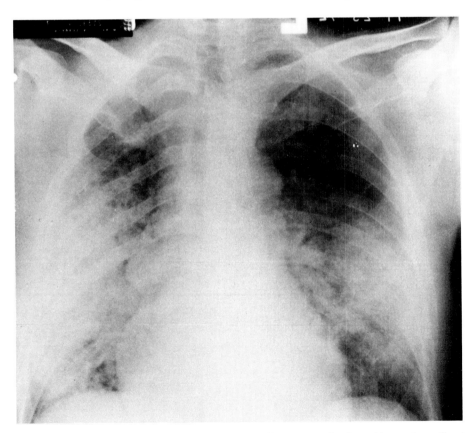

Fig. 7-4. Case 7-1. Goodpasture's syndrome. Chest x-ray showing widespread, confluent alveolar infiltrate.

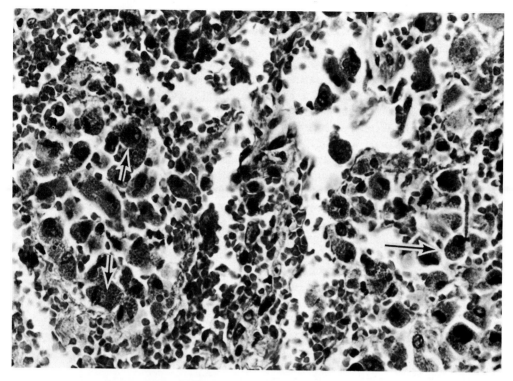

Fig. 7-5. Goodpasture's syndrome; numerous macrophages laden with hemosiderin (e.g., arrows) are within the alveoli.

posed to their vapor or fine mist. The reader is referred to the chapters on systemic lupus erythematosus reactions, muscle reactions, and sclerodermatous reactions for other examples of environmental chemicals associated with connective tissue diseases. A more systematic investigation than has so far been made, into the noninfectious environmental agents that are associated with the connective tissue diseases, might be productive.

The chaotic nosological situation relative to angiitic reactions is illustrated by those cases of Goodpasture's syndrome with systemic arteritis which are inseparable from microscopic polyarteritis except by the presence of linearly deposited immunoglobulins at the glomerular basement membrane. The finding of Germuth and coworkers [239] that C3 deposition may be granular even though IgG deposition is linear adds further confusion. It is probable that the various angiitides share mechanisms and histopathological reactions. It is worth reiterating the suggestion made at the beginning of this chapter, that angiitic reactions be classified only on the basis of known cause.

CHAPTER 8

The Problem of Granulomatosis in Rheumatology

Granulomatous reactions form an important part of the histopathologic picture in rheumatic diseases. A granuloma is defined as a focal accumulation of macrophages. The lesions in granulomatous disease may be pure granulomata, epithelioid granulomata, tuberculoid granulomata, or necrotizing granulomata; but the histologic and cytologic distinctions give little help in determining the specific etiologic agent. Clinically and anatomically, all granulomatous inflammatory diseases are fundamentally alike, though they are produced by specific agents of very wide variety [211].

Patients with diffuse granulomatosis of a chronic sort frequently have prominent accompanying rheumatic symptoms. When the histopathology includes necrotizing arteritis, the label *Wegener's granulomatosis* is applied and the clinician rests comfortably, having made the correct diagnosis. More frequently, there is no accompanying arteritis and the problem of diagnosis becomes intense. There are many known causes of diffuse granulomatous reactions. First, they may be associated with systemic infections by nonpyogenic organisms, such as syphilis, tuberculosis, leprosy, leptospirosis, and brucellosis. Second, they may be associated with protozoan infections, such as trypanosomiasis and toxoplasmosis. Next, they may be due to fungal infections, such as coccidioidomycosis and histoplasmosis. Finally, granulomatous reactions may result from Helminth infestation, either nematodal or cestodal. In the work-up of a case of chronic granulomatosis, all of the above known etiologic factors must be considered. After they have been excluded, the label *idiopathic* is applied. Within this idiopathic group are found Crohn's disease, Wegener's granulomatosis, and allergic granulomatosis; it would, also, be proper to add rheumatoid granulomatosis to this group.

It is likely that cell-mediated immunity is involved in the pathogenesis of all cases of granulomatosis. Germuth [238] has shown that a single injection of bovine serum albumin into rabbits may lead to typical generalized granulomatosis, indistinguishable from any other sort, including even the presence of the intermediate epithelioid cell form. An interesting series of studies by Warren and his coworkers (551, 708) concerned the granulomata that may be induced experimentally by means of schistosome eggs. Typical granulomata formed around these intravenously injected ova; an augmented and accelerated reaction appeared in animals previously given sensitizing injections of the eggs; the sensitization was specific for these eggs, and was transferable to uninfected mice by means of lymph node or spleen cells taken from infected mice. Suppression of circulating antibody by means of x-irradiation had no effect on the granuloma formation; it was greatly inhibited by thymectomy.

The model of granulomatous inflammation using intravenously injected schistosome eggs obviously involves complex antigens. Similar findings have been made using simple antigens. Kasdon and Schlossman [365] sensitized guinea pigs to human serum albumin (HSA) and subsequently challenged the animals with intravenous injections of HSA covalently linked to Sepharose® beads (2 per cent agarose gel in the form of beads from 60 to 300 μm in diameter). Granulomata developed around the pulmonary arteries. Of great rheumatological interest was the presence of severe, *focally necrotizing,* but mainly *granulomatous arteritis.* Unanue and Benacerraf [688] used as antigen keyhole limpet hemocyanin that was conjugated to dinitrophenyl hapten; this antigen was then linked to polyacrylamide beads. When injected intravenously, these coated polyacrylamide beads induced severe granulomata in the lungs of immune guinea pigs. Granulomatous reactivity was passively transferred into normal animals by lymph node cells but not by serum antibody from sensitized guinea pigs.

Studies in leprosy show the balance that exists between tissue reactions dependent upon humoral and cell-mediated immunity, and illuminate the situation that probably exists in rheumatic diseases. In patients with leprosy there exists a continuous spectrum of clinical, immunological, bacteriological, and histological features between the tuberculoid form at one extreme and the lepromatous form at the other, with some patients having overlapping features of both of these types [577]. In the tuberculoid form, response to the lepromin skin test is positive, there is a marked lymphocytic reaction in the granuloma, and no bacilli are seen within the reactive tissue. In the lepromatous type, response to the lepromin skin test is negative, the granuloma contains scanty or no lymphocytes, and bacilli are superabundantly present within the lesion. Lepromatous leprosy is serious and progressive; whereas the tuberculoid form is more benign and often selflimiting. There is substantial evidence that the position of a patient within the clinical spectrum of leprosy is related to his capacity to mount a cell-mediated immune response to *Mycobacterium leprae.* Thus, patients with tuberculoid leprosy, who have many leprosy bacilli in their tissue lesions, have a high degree of cell-mediated immunity that is reflected by infiltration of their lesions with numerous lymphocytes; in contrast, patients with lepromatous leprosy, whose tissue lesions are massively infected by bacilli, have severe depression of the cell-mediated immune response and few lymphocytes in the tissue lesions. *In vitro* studies have confirmed this: responses of lymphocytes to phytohemagglutinin, purified protein derivative (PPD), streptolysin O, and antigens of *M. leprae* were significantly depressed in patients with lepromatous leprosy but were normal in patients with tuberculoid leprosy [77].

An interesting reaction, the so-called "erythema nodosum leprosum" (ENL), occurs only in patients with the lepromatous or near-lepromatous form of the disease. This is characterized by crops of tender, erythematous papules, and fever; it affects as many as 50 per cent of patients by the end of their first year of chemotherapy. The lesions show intense perivascular polymorphonuclear leukocytic infiltration. Sometimes there are systemic manifestations similar to those found in chronic serum sickness: arthritis, iritis, orchitis, peripheral neuritis, lymphadenopathy, and proteinuria. A high percentage of lepromatous patients with active ENL had factors in their sera that precipitated with the C1q component of complement, suggesting the presence of circulating immune complexes [489]. In this form of leprosy one sees the situation described by Talal in New Zealand black mice [669]: these animals, which have a high prevalence of spontaneous systemic lupus erythematosus, have depressed cellular immunity with enhanced humoral immunity. Perhaps, then, it is not surprising that a high prevalence of LE cell phenomenon and antinuclear antibody formation has been reported [59] in patients with leprosy. Clinical systemic lupus erythematosus, however, is uncommon in association with leprosy.

The functional capacities of lymphocytes in leprosy and other granulomatous diseases have been analyzed. In lepromatous leprosy, the absolute and relative numbers of B lymphocytes in the blood are greatly increased, while the T lymphocytes are decreased [169, 232]. In contrast, there were normal numbers of B lymphocytes in the circulating blood of a patient with the tuberculoid form of leprosy, the granulomata of which contain more lymphocytes than do the granulomata of the lepromatous form [232]. In sarcoidosis, higher than normal mean levels of circulating B lymphocytes have been found [537]. Patients with active systemic lupus erythematosus, and with rheumatoid arthritis accompanied by vasculitis, also had higher numbers of circulating B lymphocytes [740]. Patients with rheumatoid arthritis without vasculitis had values comparable to those of healthy controls [740]. In patients with untreated Hodgkin's disease, the percentage of circulating B lymphocytes was either normal or low, but rose after therapy [117, 185].

In the present context, granulomatous reactions derive interest both from their rheumatic manifestations and from the light they shed upon the possible pathogenetic and nosologic relationships of the collagen diseases. The literature contains case reports of lymphoma with associated systemic rheumatic disease, drug-induced pseudolymphoma with associated polyarteritis or systemic lupus, and granulomatous angiitis that was associated in man with herpes zoster and that is caused in turkeys by *Mycoplasma gallisepticum*. The following case histories illustrate several interesting points, especially the overlapping clinical features of granulomatoses and the difficulty of reaching an etiologic diagnosis.

Case 8-1. In a white women aged 40, a papule approximately ⅝-inch in diameter appeared on the forearm; the regional axillary lymph nodes were enlarged. Results of all tests were normal. Although the nodule regressed somewhat, biopsy was performed. The most striking finding was the presence in the dermis of small granulomata composed of large, eosinophilic cells with indistinct borders, which formed small, irregularly rounded groups surrounded by lymphocytes and plasma cells. Although these granulomata were occasionally found in relation to small blood vessels, there was no evidence of vasculitis. There was no caseation. No organisma were revealed by special stains.

The patient remained well until approximately 3 years later, when she was seen for repair of a rectovaginal fistula which had recently appeared. Microscopic sections of tissue removed from the fistulous tract showed a number of small, noncaseous granulomata; the cytoplasm of the giant cells contained no identifiable foreign material. Again, no organisms were seen on sections stained for acid-fast organisms and fungi.

During the following year, she complained of pain in the neck, shoulders, elbows, wrists, fingers, hips, and knees together with almost incapacitatingly severe morning stiffness. Aside from pain that was induced in many joints by motion, no abnormality was found on physical examination. Results of the following laboratory studies were either negative or within normal limits: hematocrit, white cell count, erythrocyte sedimentation rate, serum calcium, phosphorus, alkaline phosphatase, bilirubin, creatinine, uric acid, potassium, sodium, chloride, bicarbonate, creatine phosphokinase, SGOT, lactic dehydrogenase; antinuclear antibody, rheumatoid factor, urinalysis, and chest x-ray. Cryoglobulins were absent from the serum. Biopsy of bone marrow, liver, and muscle showed no abnormality and no granulomata. Intermediate PPD skin test elicited a positive reaction. Reactions were negative to skin testing and complement fixation tests with coccidiodin, blastomycin, and histoplasmin. Cultures of material from muscle and bone marrow biopsies were negative for tubercle bacillus and fungi. During the next 6 months, the patient required as much as 75 grains of aspirin daily to control muscle stiffness and joint pain, and there were definite effusions into each wrist and one knee. Abdominal pain and a palpable abdominal mass led to barium enema examination, which demonstrated a large colonic mass. At laparotomy, a large mass was resected from the descending colon. Histopathologic examination of the resected material showed numerous noncaseating granulomata in the wall of the colon as well as in the pericolonic lymph nodes; i.e., the patient had granulomatous colitis. The material was cultured for tubercle bacillus and fungi, with negative results.

All of the patient's rheumatic complaints ceased abruptly after 2 days of preoperative bowel prophylaxis with neomycin, and these complaints did not recur during the next 5 years. Almost exactly 1 year after the colectomy, hemiparesthesiae developed over the entire left side. She stated that 8 years previously she had had similar paresthesiae in all four limbs, with associated diplopia, and urgency of both micturition and defecation and that a neurologist had diagnosed multiple sclerosis; no details of that illness are available. Physical examination at this final hospital admission revealed analgesia in the C_5 distribution of the left arm, impairment of vibratory sense in the upper and lower limb on the left, and pyramidal tract signs on the left side. Stereognosis was impaired in the left hand. The cerebrospinal fluid was normal with respect to cell count, glucose and total protein levels; the globulin percentage of total serum protein was at the upper limit of normal, 13.3 per cent. A neurologist consultant considered that the findings were suggestive of multiple sclerosis. During the next month, bilateral impairment of posterior column functions developed. There was gradual improvement; but the patient was lost to follow-up a few months later.

In this woman who had granulomata of skin and rectovaginal wall, polyarthralgia and myalgia were the dominant symptoms for 18 months until severe granulomatous colitis supervened. After surgical resection of the involved colon, her rheumatic symptoms dramatically cleared: the patient herself related the improvement to the preoperative bowel preparation with neomycin. An associated neurological disorder was consistent with multiple sclerosis.

Case 8-2. A black man was first seen at age 42 with a one-year history of typical palindromic rheumatism. Aside from mild aortic regurgitation, a tiny effusion in the left knee, and a subcutaneous nodule over the left olecranon process, findings on physical examination were within normal limits. The nodule disappeared before it could be removed for examination. Laboratory findings included negative serologic tests for syphilis, negative reactions for rheumatoid factor and antinuclear antibodies, normal level of blood uric acid, and erythrocyte sedimentation rate of 56 mm/hr.

Four months later he had severe periumbilical pain, and appendectomy was performed. Histopathologic examination revealed noncaseating granulomata within the wall of the appendix; special stains for organisms, including acid-fast organisms, showed none. At this time, soft, enlarged lymph glands were noted in the left axilla. Reaction was positive to skin testing with intermediate strength PPD and negative to coccidioidin and histoplasmin. Chest x-ray showed no evidence of parenchymal lung disease or lymph node enlargement. Biopsy of axillary lymph nodes showed noncaseating granulomata. Cultures of these nodes were negative for both tubercle bacillus and fungi. X-rays of hands, feet, and sacroiliac joints showed no abnormalities.

About 9 months after these events, the patient complained of pleuritic chest pain. Chest x-ray showed pleural thickening and bilateral basilar infiltrates of the lungs. Attempt at pleural biopsy was unsuccessful. Liver biopsy showed noncaseating granulomata. Several sputum samples and the liver biopsy material were cultured for tubercle bacillus and fungi with negative results.

This patient's first cousin, a 53-year-old woman, was seen subsequently with complaints of pain in the shoulders, elbows, wrists, metacarpophalangeal and proximal interphalangeal joints of her fingers, hips, knees, and ankles. Morning stiffness lasted about 20 minutes. She had experienced Raynaud's phenomenon with the phases of pallor, cyanosis, and rubor. Review of her record revealed that she had had regional enterocolitis for 15 years. Several tests for rheumatoid factor in her blood were negative; two of four tests for antinuclear antibodies were positive; LE cell preparations were negative.

Case 8-2 underscores the difficulty of making a precise nosologic diagnosis in a case of noninfectious granulomatous disease. James [338] has offered two minimal criteria for the diagnosis of sarcoid: the presence of a suggestive clinicoradiologic picture with evidence of generalized involvement, and histologic proof of sarcoid. Although, as indicated in Case 8-6 (below), palindromic rheumatism may be an occasional accompaniment of sarcoidosis, it is nevertheless rarely so. Similarly, appendiceal involvement is uncommon. One cannot maintain, therefore, that this patient had a suggestive clinical picture. There was no evidence of sarcoidosis on the x-rays of hands and feet, and the acute pleuritis and basilar infiltrates seen on chest x-ray were atypical for sarcoid. Thus, although the histopathological picture was consistent with sarcoidosis, he had neither clinical nor radiologic evidence of the disease. How, then, is his case to be classified? Had the small-bowel x-rays given evidence of Crohn's disease, one might be satisfied to call it an example of that condition; just as, in the preceding case, the colonic lesion permitted the diagnosis of granulomatous colitis. Haslock and Wright [294] have reviewed the musculoskeletal complications of Crohn's disease. Although they did not find patients with palindromic rheumatism, active synovitis was seen in approximately 20 per cent of their patients. In Crohn's disease, the synovitis is mostly of a nonspecific sort; Lindström, Wramsby, and Östberg [426] reported a rare case in which they found actual granulomata in the synovium cells.

The next case is similarly difficult to classify: inflammatory polyarthritis, hepatosplenomegaly, generalized lymphadenopathy, pericarditis, low-grade fever, macrocytosis, posterior column and spinothalamic column disorder of the spinal cord, and abnormal urinary sediment were all features of her illness.

Case 8-3. In a white woman, inflammatory polyarthritis with swelling and redness of several joints first appeared at age 41 years, in 1953, when the observation of hepatomegaly prompted exploratory laparotomy. A large abdominal lymph node was removed, together with a sample of liver. The lymph node was found to contain a noncaseating granuloma, but the liver was histopathologically normal. Three years later, generalized peripheral lymphadenopathy and fever first appeared, both thereafter recurrent. During the next few years her main complaints derived from the inflammatory polyarthritis. In 1963, at age 51, acroparesthesiae led to the findings of impaired senses of vibration, touch, pinprick, and cold in all four limbs. The patient was mildly anemic, with prominent macrocytosis in the peripheral blood. The bone marrow appeared normal, as was response to the Schilling test for vitamin B_{12} absorption. At this time, up to 10 granular casts per high power field were seen in the urine.

In early 1964, pericarditis developed; a few months later the voice became hoarse and the vocal cords were edematous. Concurrently, a fine papular rash appeared on the trunk and arms, and the spleen was enlarged. Biopsy of the liver, a lymph node, and skin revealed noncaseating granulomata in each. During the next year, biopsy of the liver and bone marrow revealed noncaseating granulomata. Result of a Tine test was borderline, at 0.5 cm. Skin test reactions to first-strength PPD, coccidioidin, and histoplasmin were negative. Serum globulin and calcium levels were within normal limits. On repeated hematologic studies during this lengthy illness, rheumatoid factor was absent and several LE cell preparations were negative. Aside from some mild thickening at the apices of each lung, the findings on repeated chest roentgenograms remained with normal limits. X-rays of hands and feet gave evidence neither of rheumatoid arthritis nor of sarcoidosis.

From 1965 onward, the arthritis and general malaise were severe and she was treated with large doses of prednisone and isoniazid. She became more and more anorectic and cachectic, and eventually died of cardiac arrest. Autopsy revealed generalized arteriosclerosis, chronic fibrous pericarditis, and interstitial pulmonary fibrosis. There was no evidence at autopsy of granulomatosis or arteritis.

A chronic granulomatous disease during which many specimens were cultured for organisms with negative results had prominent rheumatic accompaniments. Although there was a posterior column disorder and macrocytic anemia was present, the bone marrow contained no megaloblasts, and vitamin B_{12} absorption was normal.

Case 8-4. A woman born in the Philippines came to the United States at age 32. At age 35, she complained of dysuria, urinary frequency, fever, and a loss of 20 pounds; she had been treated with a sulfonamide drug for presumptive pyelonephritis. About one month later, an infiltrate was seen in the upper lobe of the left lung on a routine chest film. Aside from a low-grade fever at this time, the physical findings were unremarkable. A hematocrit reading was 34 per cent; 3–5 red blood cells and 10–15 white blood cells per high power field were seen in the urine. A roentgenogram of the chest now showed an infiltrate at the apex of the right lung and in the mid and upper lung fields on the left. The skin test reaction was positive to intermediate strength PPD, and negative to histoplasmin and coccidioidin. Many samples of sputum and urine, cultured for tubercle bacillus and other organisms, yielded no growth.

The diagnosis of probable pulmonary tuberculosis was made and treatment with isoniazid and para-aminosalicylic acid was begun. Nevertheless, daily spikes of fever, to as high as 41.1 C (106 F), persisted and several episodes of spontaneous thrombophlebitis occurred in all four limbs. Prednisone, 45 mg daily, was started empirically and the patient began to feel better.

During the first, lengthy hospitalization, a number of other studies were of interest. On several occasions, marked hyperglobulinemia was observed, between 5.3 and 6.5 gm/100 ml; electrophoresis showed γ globulin to be 36.5 per cent of the total serum proteins. Sulfobromophthalein retention was 34 per cent at 45 minutes; liver biopsy showed many areas of cloudy swelling but no granulomata. Bone marrow aspiration and scalene node biopsy were, likewise, unrevealing. Findings on excretory urography were normal.

Her second admission to the hospital was occasioned by the appearance of a new in-filtrate in the upper lobe of the left lung, seen on chest x-ray about one year after the original admission. On this occasion, her blood pressure was 160/110. Results of many further laboratory studies were negative; these included cultures of sputum and gastric washings for tubercle bacilli, and LE cell preparations.

After a short while, the antituberculosis medicine and prednisone were stopped. During the next five years her main problem related to persistent hypertension, for which she was treated with thiazides.

At age 41, she suddenly felt pain in the right ear, and was found to have serous otitis media. A few days later, facial weakness and severe conductive hearing loss occurred on the right. The right mastoid process was tender and radiolucent. The area was explored surgically. A large mass completely filled the mastoid region. Histopathological exami-nation of this lesion showed many plasma cells on a background of fibrosis.

Little transpired for the next $2\frac{1}{2}$ years; she then had sudden pain, complete external ophthalmoplegia, and blindness of the right eye. X-rays revealed a retro-orbital mass. Laboratory tests results at this time included total serum proteins of 7.2 gm/100 ml, 20.9 per cent of which were γ globulins; normal eosinophil count; negative reaction to Coombs' test, and to tests for antinuclear antibodies and cryoglobulins.

She was treated with large doses of prednisone, and with isoniazid. Slowly, some function returned in the external ocular muscles, but the affected eye remained totally blind, with optic atrophy. During the next 2 years her main problem was hypertension.

Although the histopathology in this case is not entirely characteristic, it is most consistent with Wegener's granulomatosis; one would be more confident in this diagnosis had necrotizing arteritis been seen in the tissue removed from the mastoid process. A remarkably similar case was reported by Cassan, Divertie, and others [93]: bilateral orbital pseudotumors with cavitary pulmonary lesions. Their patient, also, had a prolonged—15-year—survival. Ocular or orbital in-volvement in Wegener's granulomatosis is not rare; Straatsma [662], reviewing 44 cases of this disease, found that there had been ocular or orbital involvement in 19, and that 7 of these 19 patients had had proptosis. Prolonged survival in this usually rapidly fatal disease was reported by Carrington and Liebow [90] in cases that they designated as representing limited forms of angiitis and granulo-matosis.

It is well known that arthritis may appear in sarcoidosis. Siltzbach and Duberstein [632] encountered joint manifestations in 38 (12 per cent) among 311 patients with a tissue-confirmed diagnosis of sarcoidosis, observed over a 20-year span. The most common type was an acute, transient polyarthritis that appeared at the outset of sarcoidosis and was commonly associated with erythema nodosum. It is of interest that both synovial effusions and radiological articular changes are distinctly uncommon in the arthritis of sarcoidosis [47, 632]. Nevertheless, one must consider sarcoidosis in the differential diagnosis of acute polyarthritis, as was demonstrated by the following experience.

Case 8-5. A 23-year-old black woman had noted pain and swelling in the left ankle for one month and mild pain in the right ankle for one week. Physical examination showed swelling and warmth of the left ankle, which was extremely painful to the touch; the right ankle was clinically normal. The erythrocyte sedimentation rate was 83 mm/hr (Westergren); all other laboratory tests were unrevealing. Synovial fluid and cervical cul-tures were negative for gonorrhea. Response to a skin test for tuberculosis was negative. With the presumptive diagnosis of acute gonococcal arthritis, penicillin was given intravenously. There was initial improvement, but even after 7 days there were residual symptoms in the ankle. When the patient was seen a month later, her only symptom was drenching night sweats. Physical examination showed no residue of the arthritis but superficial lymphadenopathy was observed for the first time. The diagnosis of sarcoidosis was now entertained: erythrocyte sedimentation rate was still elevated, at 45 mm/hr; serum globulin level was slightly higher than normal, but serum calcium level was normal. Three weeks later, peripheral facial nerve palsy occurred suddenly. Biopsy of a scalene node showed the appearances characteristic of sarcoidosis.

Palindromic rheumatism is a condition characterized by recurrent arthritis of brief duration, which usually affects one joint at a time for hours or days and affects a different joint when it next occurs. The intervals between episodes gradually lessen and the numbers of joints affected in the attack gradually increase. Many cases eventuate, usually after many years, in fixed rheumatoid arthritis. In the following case, typical palindromic rheumatism was a manifestation of sarcoid arthritis.

Case 8-6. A 28-year-old black man had had histopathologically proved sarcoidosis 4 years previously, after a respiratory illness that was accompanied by bilateral hilar and superficial lymphadenopathy. Despite continuous prednisone therapy since that time, he had experienced episodic arthritis for the last couple of years. For the most part the arthritis was transitory, lasting 3 or 4 days and affecting only one joint at a time. During an attack the joints were warm but not red. Physical examination revealed enlargement of superficial lymph nodes, including those of each epitrochlear group, a tiny effusion in one knee, and pain with pressure in a few of the proximal interphalangeal joints. X-rays of the hands and feet (Fig. 8-1) showed distortion of the trabecular pattern in some of the phalanges, compatible with sarcoid of bone.

SYMPTOMATOLOGIC OVERLAP

In chronic granulomatosis of known cause, the symptoms are widespread because almost no organ or tissue is spared the lesions. Even in the idiopathic varieties, the manifestations may be extremely diffuse, as is well known in sarcoidosis and Wegener's granulomatosis. However, it is important to note that there may be a very considerable clinical overlap between conditions in which the granulomatosis is confined to or mainly concentrated in a single organ system. Crohn's disease, for example, may have an important associated polyarthritis [294], most commonly of a nonspecific inflammatory sort according to both synovianalysis and biopsy [649]; only very rarely has a granulomatous reaction been seen in the synovium itself [426]. A similar nonspecific inflammatory polyarthritis of the rehumatoid type is seen in ulcerative colitis [81]. The arthritis seen in sarcoidosis may be either granulomatous or nongranulomatous of a nonspecific sort; even in chronic beryllium disease there may be an associated nonspecific arthralgia [661]. Cutaneous polyarteritis may be seen in Crohn's disease [170] and ulcerative colitis [397]. Kurlander and Kirsner [395] have described the associations among systemic lupus erythematosus, ulcerative colitis, and right-sided colitis, and between discoid lupus and granulomatous ileocolitis. Our own group of 64 patients with systemic lupus erythematosus (See Chapter 10) in-

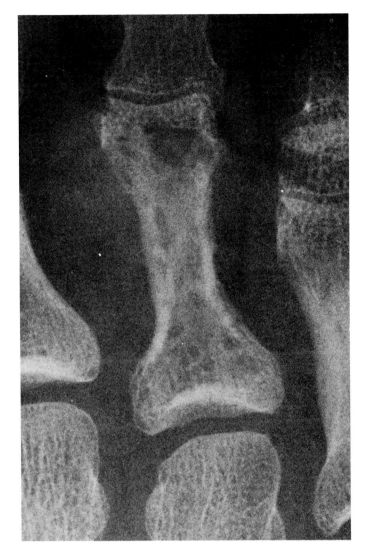

Fig. 8-1.   Case 8-6.   Sarcoidosis causing lytic lesions in proximal phalanx of toe.

cludes one with associated ulcerative colitis, and a patient with pure discoid lupus who has granulomata in the skin biopsy specimen. Granuloma formation in systemic lupus erythematosus is uncommon but has been reported occasionally [557, 672]. An interesting patient reported by Wasserman, Krosnick, and Tumen [709] had ulcerative colitis with associated allergic granulomatosis; in addition, there was enlargement of peritracheal and hilar lymph nodes.

An extraordinary case demonstrating this clinicopathologic overlap in Whipple's disease was reported by Rodarte and coworkers [582]: a man had joint pain, and a nodule over the left olecranon. Biopsy of the nodule showed changes consistent with rheumatoid arthritis. One year later, generalized lymphadenopathy appeared; biopsy of a lymph node revealed noncaseating granulomata. Six months after this, pleural thickening led to biopsy of pleura and lung: the removed material was sterile on culture for bacteria. Skin tests for tuberculosis and histoplasmosis were negative. Yet nine months later, there was further joint pain and another nodule, this time over the right olecranon. After an illness of about three years, diarrhea and vomiting occurred together with a petechial rash, generalized edema, anemia, bilateral knee effusions, myocarditis, and evidence of a circulating anticoagulant. He died. Autopsy revealed that histiocytes containing the PAS-positive, sickle-shaped particles characteristic of Whipple's disease were preset in the jejunum, mesenteric lymph nodes, liver, spleen, lung, pleura, pericardium, and heart. The biopsy specimens were re-examined. No evidence of sickle-shaped particles could be found in them.

The early clinical manifestations of this man's illness were consistent with rheumatoid arthritis. They were also consistent, both clinically and histologically, with sarcoidosis. It seems likely that these sarcoid and rheumatoid reactions were early manifestations of the Whipple's disease. It is remarkable, yet certainly apposite to the present discussion, that biopsy of the subcutaneous nodule at the olecranon revealed changes of rheumatoid arthritis.

The picture that emerges from the literature and from the above case histories is of a very marked overlap in clinical manifestations among the various sorts of idiopathic granulomatoses. There would seem to be no good reason why we should distinguish rigidly as separate disease entities, those clinical patterns in which the idiopathic granulomata are confined to or mainly concentrated in a single organ. It is merely convenient and descriptive to speak of idiopathic granulomatous uveitis, sarcoidosis, Crohn's disease, granulomatous colitis, or idiopathic granulomatous hepatitis; each diagnostic label only indicates the dominant organ affected. This problem is well illustrated by the first three cases described above and was recognized by James [338], who emphasized the many causes of a sarcoid reaction and stated that the diagnosis of sarcoidosis requires a suggestive clinical and radiological picture, together with histological proof. The histological picture of sarcoidosis is, however, entirely nonspecific; so that, pragmatically, the diagnosis of sarcoidosis rests upon the clinical and radiological picture in the presence of an idiopathic granulomatous reaction. If in Cases 8-2 and 8-3 the typical radiological features had been present in the lungs, one would not hesitate to label those patients as having sarcoidosis; but in the absence of such radiologic evidence, that label remains moot. If, on the other hand, Case 8-3 had shown evidence of necrotizing arteritis, then in the presence of pericarditis, myocarditis, pleuritis, and prominent inflammatory polyarthritis, one would be justified in giving to her disease the label of Wegener's granulomatosis. Yet, in some cases of Wegener's granulomatosis and allergic granulomatosis, the vascular lesions may be very slight, as in Case 8-4. Two of the 13 patients reported by Churg and Strauss [108] in their original paper describing allergic granulomatosis had either minimal or no arteritis. In discussing the concept of limited forms of Wegener's granulomatosis, Cassan, Coles, and Harrison [92] postulated a continuum between isolated angiitis on the one hand and granulomatosis on the other, and indicated the possibility of great overlap. In their prospective study of seven patients who had granulomatous hepatitis of unknown cause, Guckian and Perry [270] noted that there seemed to be more than a chance relationship between granulomatous diseases, abnormal immune globulins, autoimmune diseases, and various malignant neoplastic diseases. They

speculated that the excessive antigenic stimulus which produced the granulomatous disease and hypergammaglobulinemia might also cause aberrant immunologic responses or even exhaustion of immunologically competent cells,
failure to reject self-antibody clones and neoplastic cell lines, and consequent
autoimmune disease and malignant neoplasia.

The second case reported by Guckian and Perry [270] serves admirably to
summarize this chapter. A 44-year-old black woman had fever and lymphadenopathy in 1956, generalized migratory arthritis and nodular lesions on the legs
and arms in 1959, and granulomatous hepatitis proved by biopsy in January
1963. Serologic reaction for syphilis and skin reaction for tuberculosis were both
positive. Culture of the liver biopsy specimen was negative for tubercle bacillus.
In February 1963 she had carcinoma of the cervix. In April 1963 the polyarthralgia and subcutaneous nodules recurred. In September 1966 there were
further nodules on the legs, and lymphadenopathy. Biopsy of the lesions on the
legs showed a pattern consistent with erythema induratum, but acid-fast bacteria
could not be identified. Biopsy of a superficial lymph node showed partial replacement with granulomatous inflammation, without true caseous necrosis.
Ziehl-Neelson stain revealed acid-fast bacilli, but cultures for mycobacteria were
sterile. A kidney biopsy specimen showed necrotizing arteriolitis and focal
glomerulitis. Two LE cell preparations were strongly positive. Clearly, rheumatic
disease and chronic granulomatous disease overlap so closely both in their
clinical manifestations and in their underlying pathophysiology that it is spu-
rious, even if convenient, to separate them nosologically.

CHAPTER 9

Rheumatoid Reactions

DIAGNOSIS

Rheumatoid arthritis in its typical form is easy to diagnose. The patient, often a woman, has had an inflammatory polyarthritis for many weeks or months. The small joints of the hands are characteristically involved, excluding, however, the terminal interphalangeal joints; the large joints of the limbs, especially wrists and shoulders, ankles and knees, are often affected. No synovial joint of the body is immune, even such small ones as the atlanto-odontoid or the crico-arytenoid. The symptom of severe morning stiffness, and the findings of subcutaneous nodules at the elbows, erosions of the joints seen on x-rays, and rheumatoid factor in the serum complete the picture. It is necessary to exclude other causes of chronic inflammatory polyarthritis, e.g., ankylosing spondylitis, systemic lupus erythematosus, periarteritis nodosa, polymyositis, scleroderma, rheumatic fever, chronic gout, chronic infectious arthritis, Reiter's syndrome, sarcoidosis, and hypertrophic pulmonary osteoarthropathy. Indeed, it cannot be sufficiently emphasized that the diagnosis, "rheumatoid arthritis," like that of any other connective tissue disease, requires not only the characteristic clinical picture but also the exclusion of any other cause of such a clinical picture. It is superfluous to list the entire gamut of diseases that must be excluded before diagnosing rheumatoid arthritis: many of them are considered within the body of this book. Lists of criteria for the diagnosis of rheumatoid arthritis have been proposed, but it must be stressed that these lists themselves are derived from the knowledge of experienced clinicians and cannot substitute for a careful assessment of the overall clinical picture. The American Rheumatism Association (ARA) criteria [585] require that five or more of the following be present for the diagnosis of definite rheumatoid arthritis: morning stiffness; joint tenderness or pain on motion; soft tissue swelling of one joint; soft tissue swelling of a second joint within 3 months of the first; soft tissue swelling of symmetrical joints, excluding distal interphalangeal joints; subcutaneous nodules; appropriate x-ray changes, and rheumatoid factor in the serum. The so-called "New York criteria" [40] require the following: 1) a history of an episode of three painful limb joints; 2) the occurrence of swelling, limitation of motion, subluxation, or ankylosis of three limb joints that must include a hand, wrist, or foot, and symmetry of one joint pair and must exclude distal interphalangeal joints, the fifth proximal interphalangeal joints, the first metatarsophalangeal joints, and the hips; 3) erosive changes seen in x-rays of the joints, and 4) rheumatoid factors in the serum.

PREVALENCE

The prevalence of rheumatoid arthritis in the population has been variously estimated to be between 0.5 per cent and almost 4.0 per cent [401, 402, 531].

Our own studies show that the prevalence of rheumatoid arthritis in San Francisco is approximately 1 per cent of the adult population. This figure is based upon 924 patients for whom the diagnosis, "rheumatoid arthritis," was entered into the computer when they were seen in our clinic between the years 1966 and 1973; during those years the average number of Kaiser Foundation Health Plan members in San Francisco was 121,000. No attempt was made to ascertain whether the diagnosis of rheumatoid arthritis for these 924 patients accorded with the criteria of the American Rheumatism Association; nor was the task undertaken to remove those patients, possibly 10 per cent of the 924, who lived outside the geographic boundaries of San Francisco. Counterbalancing this, on the other hand, is the fact that for a large number of patients the diagnosis was undoubtedly not entered into the computer because their disease was inactive on the occasion of their visit to the clinic for other reasons. If we accept, as an approximation, the prevalence of rheumatoid arthritis as 924 cases in the population of 121,000, the prevalence rate is 1 case per 131. Since the disease is overwhelmingly one of adults, and 77.6 per cent of the Kaiser Foundation Health Plan membership in San Francisco is 15 or more years old, the prevalence may be adjusted to one case in 102, or 1 per cent of the adult population.

OUTCOME OF RHEUMATOID ARTHRITIS

The importance of these figures on prevalence is twofold. First, they give some idea of the magnitude of the public health problem posed by the disease. Second, the prevalence figure of 1 percent provides a yardstick against which one may measure the likelihood of devastation from this disease. If one carefully observes a crowd of people, it is obvious that 1 per cent of its members are not crippled by rheumatoid arthritis. Indeed, upon casual inspection away from the examining room, one is often hard pressed to observe the presence of rheumatoid arthritis. One of the first questions asked by a patient who has been informed that she has rheumatoid arthritis concerns what the future holds for her. In popular belief, rheumatoid arthritis is a crippling disease that sooner or later condemns the sufferer to a wheelchair. The patient must be reassured that 1 per cent of the population is not in a wheelchair because of rheumatoid arthritis. In fact, away from a university arthritis clinic, rheumatoid arthritis is seen to be generally not a crippling disease. In the overwhelming majority of cases, the patient is able to function at a moderately satisfactory level.

In estimating prognosis, one must separate early cases from later, well-established ones, because the outlook for each of these groups is entirely different. The outcomes of early rheumatoid arthritis were studied by Otten and Boerma [532] in 141 patients for whom the diagnosis of rheumatoid arthritis was made on clinical grounds and in whom the duration of the disease was less then 6 months. There were 106 patients whose symptoms had been present for between 1 and 3 months: after 1 year only 46 patients, after 2 years only 34 patients, and after 3 years only 22 patients had any continuing indication of joint disease.

Thirty-seven (35 per cent) of these 106 patients had a positive response to tests for rheumatoid factor within 3 months of onset of their condition. Recovery from joint symptoms occurred after 1 year in 71 per cent of those without rheumatoid factor, and in only 30 per cent of those whose serum contained rheumatoid factor. Once recovery had taken place, no relapses were observed in the seronegative patients during a 3-year follow-up period; but relapses did occur in the seropositive group. On the other hand, even in some patients whose tests for rheumatoid factor remained positive over a 5-year period of observation, complete remission was observed. In 35 patients, the disease had been present between 4 and 6 months at first observation. Among these, 11 of the 22 whose sera did not contain rheumatoid factor recovered during the first year of observation, but no patient whose serum contained rheumatoid factor was so fortunate.

Another important study of outcomes of early rheumatoid arthritis was made by Wawrzynska-Pagowska and coworkers [711]. They examined patients whose joint pain and swelling had been present for at least 3 months, and for whom the diagnosis of rheumatoid arthritis was based on at least four of the ARA criteria, except that they excluded patients who had radiological abnormalities in the affected joints or in the hands or feet. They followed 202 adult patients for between 2 and 6 years: 37 had probable rheumatoid arthritis; the remainder had either definite or classic rheumatoid arthritis according to the ARA criteria. After 2 years the patients were restudied, and categorized as follows: 1) 41 patients (25 per cent) in whom all previous signs and symptoms had completely disappeared, 2) 124 patients (61.4 per cent) in whom erosions had developed, and 3) 21 patients (10.4 per cent) in whom a certain diagnosis could not be established at the 2-year follow-up examination. After 4 to 6 years of follow-up, 51.4 per cent of the group that had been labeled originally as having probable rheumatoid arthritis were in complete remission; only 18.3 per cent of those originally considered to have definite rheumatoid arthritis, and 2 per cent of those originally classified as having classic rheumatoid arthritis were so fortunate.

In a more prolonged observation, Short and Bauer [625] studied 300 unselected patients who had been admitted to the medical wards of the Massachusetts General Hospital between the years 1930 and 1936 with the diagnosis of rheumatoid arthritis. The average duration of follow-up was 9½ years (range, 6 months to 16 years). At the follow-up examination, 15.2 per cent were in remission, 38.0 per cent were moderately or slightly improved, 12.8 per cent were considered to have had no change, and 34.0 per cent were worse.

In their study of the population of Sudbury, a small town in Massachusetts, O'Sullivan and Cathcart [531] observed, as had others in different population surveys, that there is a large group of patients who appear normal on physical examination but who have a past history of a polyarthritis compatible with an earlier diagnosis of rheumatoid arthritis. Their data showed that only half of the persons with verified rheumatoid arthritis had evidence of any limitation, and those with a characteristic past history who lacked current verification had no residual disabilities. They concluded that the true proportion of persons progressing to physical impairment must be less than one-sixth of all persons with present or past evidence of rheumatoid arthritis, and suggested that rheumatoid arthritis exists most frequently as a benign, nondeforming condition.

Ragan and Farrington [564] concluded that those features seen on first examination which suggest the future development of sustained disease include the following: 1) lengthy duration of active disease, 2) the presence of severe disease, and 3) the presence of rheumatoid factor in the serum. Constitutional features such as severe stiffness, fever, or anemia seemed unimportant for outcome.

As a general rule, those patients who are seen within 1 year of onset have a strong chance of complete remission some time during the next 2 to 3 years, particularly if rheumatoid factor is absent from their serum. There is a good chance of improvement or remission in approximately half of all patients with established disease.

ACUTE RHEUMATOID ARTHRITIS

At its onset, rheumatoid arthritis may mimic gout. Four patients among the 100 studied by Jacoby, Jayson, and Cosh [337] had had episodes of pain in the first metatarsophalangeal joint 8 months to 4 years before the onset of the disease; and in two patients, both men, it was sufficiently acute to suggest gout but their serum uric acid levels were normal. Even after the disease has become well established, there may be episodes reminiscent of acute gouty arthritis.

Case 9-1. A woman aged 43 had had episodic pain and swelling in the ankles and anterior portion of the feet for several months. Attacks of pain, intense redness, and swelling in the region of the first metatarsophalangeal joints, lasting 2 days at a time, had occurred once or twice monthly. More recently, an episode of swelling and bright redness in the right wrist had occurred; it had lasted for several hours only, and was much better by the next day. She had experienced occasional pain in other joints, including the shoulders, elbow, and both hips. Morning stiffness had recently appeared. Physical examination showed swelling in the affected wrist and in the metatarsophalangeal joints. There were no subcutaneous nodules. X-rays showed a striking degree of erosion, with a punched-out quality, affecting particularly the first metatarsophalangeal joint (Fig. 9-1). Rheumatoid factor was present in her serum. Serum uric acid level was normal. Within 1 year she had typical, generalized rheumatoid polyarthritis.

SUBCUTANEOUS NODULES AND THE SPECTRUM OF RHEUMATOID DISEASE

Subcutaneous nodules that are histopathologically indistinguishable from those seen in rheumatoid arthritis may occur in the *absence* of any other manifestations of rheumatoid disease. Mesara, Brody, and Oberman [472] followed 12 patients who had subcutaneous nodules and no other demonstrable evidence of rheumatoid arthritis or rheumatic fever for between 1 and 17 years. Although the nodules recurred or persisted in half of the patients, rheumatoid arthritis developed in none of the 12. The nodules were indistinguishable from those seen in rheumatoid arthritis or rheumatic fever. A similar case history follows.

Case 9-2. A 28-year-old woman gave a history of having had a subcutaneous nodule on the volar aspect of each of three fingers for the previous 5 years. She had never had

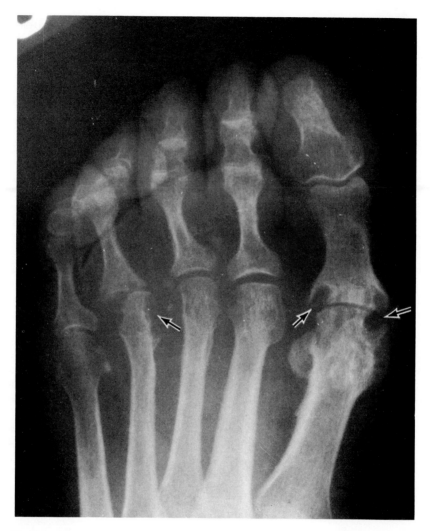

Fig. 9-1. Case 9-1. Early rheumatoid arthritis simulating gout both clinically and radiologically. Punched-out lesions at first and third metatarsophalangeal joints (arrows).

arthritis, but had noted morning stiffness of the fingers, lasting approximately 1 hour. Exposure to sunshine induced urticaria; there was no other significant symptom. The only finding of note on physical examination was a small subcutaneous nodule at the volar aspect of the terminal interphalangeal joint of an index finger. Results of tests for erythrocyte sedimentation rate, C-reactive protein, rheumatoid factor, and antinuclear antibody were negative or within normal limits. Two nodules that had been removed during the previous 2 years were histopathologically typical for rheumatoid nodules. No further symptoms developed during the subsequent 2 years.

In the next case, the rheumatoid arthritis was more in evidence, yet still not prominent.

Case 9-3. Polyarthralgia first appeared in a woman at age 24. There were no other significant symptoms, and all laboratory studies gave completely normal results at that time. During the next year, the polyarthralgia persisted and no joint was observed to be swollen. About 1 year after onset, definite swelling developed in several proximal inter-phalangeal joints of the fingers, and a soft tumor was seen underneath one of the metatarsophalangeal joints. The tumor was excised and found to be a typical rheumatoid nodule. About 6 months later, she awoke one morning with severe pain over the dorsum of one foot, which was red and swollen. She was thought by one observer to have acute gout, but the serum uric acid level was normal. When she was seen 5 days after this epi-sode, there was obvious tenosynovitis affecting the tendons of extensor digitorum longus. Thereafter, the synovitis became an insignificant problem but numerous subcutaneous nodules developed in both feet. Several of these were excised and were histopathologically typical for rheumatoid nodules. Interestingly, x-rays of the hands and feet showed no erosive changes at the joints. Rheumatoid factor appeared in modest titer, 1:3,200 (FII hemagglutination).

It is always somewhat surprising to find nodules in the absence of clinical arthritis or in patients with relatively mild arthritic manifestations because, as al-ready mentioned, experience has shown that subcutaneous nodules accompany the more severe forms of rheumatoid disease. This experience has been con-firmed by Gordon, Stein, and Broder [259], who analyzed 127 hospitalized patients with definite or classic rheumatoid arthritis: 76 per cent had one or more extra-articular features including nodules, pulmonary fibrosis, digital vasculitis, skin ulceration, lymphadenopathy, noncompressive neuropathy, splenomegaly, episcleritis, or pericarditis. Subcutaneous nodules were the most common extra-articular feature, occurring in 53 per cent of this group of patients with severe rheumatoid arthritis. This study confirmed that extra-articular features confer a poor prognosis on patients with rheumatoid arthritis. In the total group of patients, the mortality rate at 5 years was surprisingly high—20 per cent; the rate was twice as high in the group with extra-articular features as in those without such features. The following patient had many interesting extra-articular fea-tures, including innumerable subcutaneous nodules, but disproportionately mild arthritic manifestations.

Case 9-4. When first seen at age 54, this man had had subcutaneous nodules for 10 years. They were, presently, scattered over his hands (Fig. 9-2), olecrana, tendo-Achilles, and feet. He had experienced polyarthralgia for 8 years. Although x-rays showed erosive changes at many metacarpophalangeal joints, there had been virtually no joint swelling, and there were no joint deformities. For a couple of years, he had experienced numbness and tingling in the tips of all fingers and in each great toe. The only significant findings on physical examination were the uncountable subcutaneous nodules and mild swelling at some of the metacarpophalangeal joints.

A nodule was removed and showed the histopathological findings typical of a rheumatoid nodule. Rheumatoid factor (by FII hemagglutination method) was present in a titer of 1:200,000. Serum IgM level was raised, at 335 mg/100 ml. Antinuclear anti-bodies were absent. X-ray of the chest showed no abnormalities.

During the next year, the acroparesthesiae worsened, and although sensation and deep tendon reflexes had been normal originally, pinprick sensation was now impaired in the tips of the right first through fourth fingers and left first, third, and fourth fingers, in the entire right great toe, and in the medial half of the left great toe. The deep tendon re-flexes at the knees and ankles became severely depressed.

Drenching night sweats occurred and he lost 5 pounds. All tests for pulmonary tuber-culosis were negative, but chest x-ray showed interstitial fibrosis for the first time (Fig. 9-3).

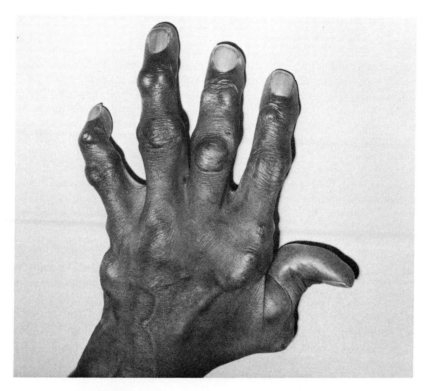

Fig. 9-2. Case 9-4. Rheumatoid nodules situated over most of the prominences of the hand.

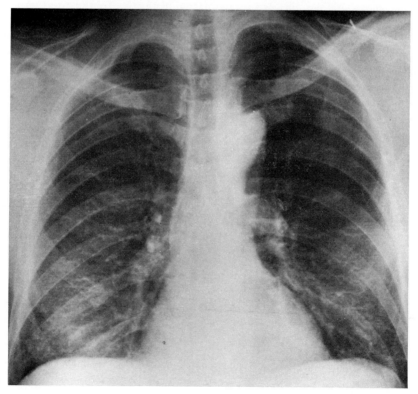

Fig. 9-3. Case 9-4. Rheumatoid arthritis, with early pulmonary fibrosis.

Cyclophosphamide therapy was started. After a year, staphylococcal infection of a nodule occurred, and cyclophosphamide was stopped. By now the sensory disturbances had ceased, and the deep tendon reflexes at knees and ankles had increased.

The nodules underwent interesting changes during treatment with cyclophosphamide. The old nodules tended to shrink in size and to soften in their centers, and several of them discharged cheesy material. But concomitantly, many new nodules appeared elsewhere.

The titer of rheumatoid factor fell to 1:12,000. During the next 18 months, while cyclophosphamide was not given, more new nodules appeared; the interstitial pulmonary fibrosis and accompanying nonproductive cough worsened, and spontaneous epididymo-orchitis occurred. When the patient was last seen, new nodules were continuing to form, and sensation to pinprick was again decreased in the fingertips of one hand.

Two other informative cases will be mentiond briefly.

Case 9-5.   At a time when her peripheral rheumatoid arthritis was quite active, a 60-year-old woman noted considerable enlargement of subcutaneous nodules which had been present at the elbows and, simultaneously, had symptoms of acute congestive heart failure. Her arterial oxygen concentration at this time was only 58 mm Hg. The chest x-ray (Fig. 9-4) showed interstitial pulmonary fibrosis with areas of plate-like atelectasis. Her condition gradually improved in response to combined diuretic and cyclophosphamide therapy.

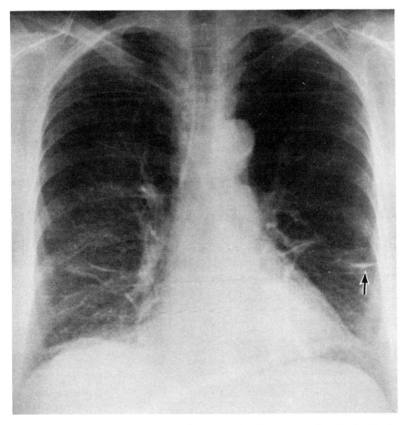

Fig. 9-4.   Case 9-5.   Discoid atelectasis (arrow) in chest x-ray of patient with rheumatoid disease.

A similar situation occurred in the next patient.

Case 9-6. A 65-year-old woman had chronic rheumatoid arthritis. Concomitantly with a sudden acute exacerbation of her peripheral arthritis and increase in size of subcutaneous nodules, high fever and dyspnea developed. Chest x-ray showed moderately severe interstitial fibrosis (Fig. 9-5). Test for rheumatoid factor was positive at a titer of 1:5,120. All of her symptoms improved markedly under the influence of 60 mg prednisone daily; a noteworthy, but fortunately transient, side effect of the therapy was an acute schizophrenic reaction.

Involvement of the lungs by rheumatoid arthritis may take a number of forms. Interstitial pneumonitis or fibrosis are the most common. Pleuritis with effusion sometimes occurs.

Case 9-7. A 72-year-old man whose chest x-ray (Fig. 9-6) showed a large pleural effusion had had active rheumatoid arthritis, lasting approximately 10 years, about 25 years previously; for the last 15 years, the arthritis had been inactive. The effusion had been ushered in by an episode of pleurisy about one month before. Physical examination revealed chronic deforming changes of rheumatoid arthritis in the fingers, wrists, and toes but no clinical sign of active synovitis. There were subcutaneous nodules at one elbow and over one foot. Reactions to skin tests with PPD, histoplasmin, and coccidioidin were

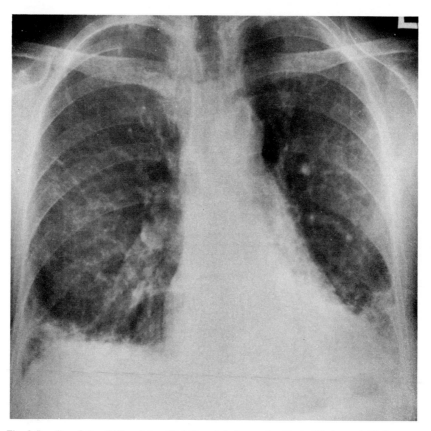

Fig. 9-5. Case 9-6. Diffuse interstitial fibrosis in lungs of patient with rheumatoid disease.

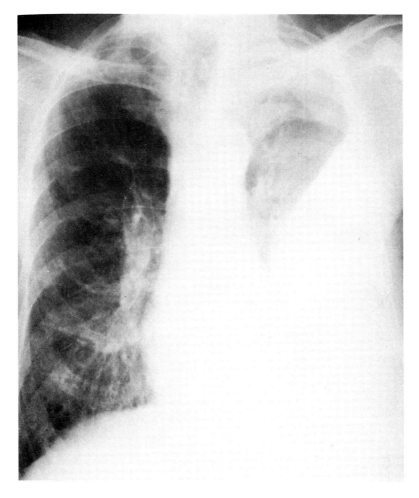

Fig. 9-6.   Case 9-7.   Pleural effusion caused by rheumatoid arthritis.

negative. The pleural fluid contained no neoplastic cells; its white blood cell content was 110,000/cu mm, 94 per cent polymorphonuclear leukocytes; its total protein level was 3.7 g/100 ml; lactic dehydrogenase was 25,917 I.U.; glucose, 2 mg/100 ml. Rheumatoid factor was present in the pleural fluid. Cytological study of the pleural fluid (Fig. 9-7) revealed some of the features described below. Biopsy of the pleural membrane showed nonspecific, subacute inflammation, without evidence of arteritis, rheumatoid nodule, or tuberculosis.

A characteristic cytological picture in the fluid of rheumatoid pleural effusion was described by Nosanchuk and Naylor [521] and confirmed by Boddington and coworkers [58]. The stained films show abundant necrotic leukocytes and a background of amorphous material, which is variable in its staining characteristics, mostly basophilic but sometimes eosinophilic. Fluorescent antibody studies have shown that this material probably contains various immunoglobulins. There are both polymorphonuclear leukocytes and many mononuclear cells; bare nuclei are common, sometimes losing their chro-

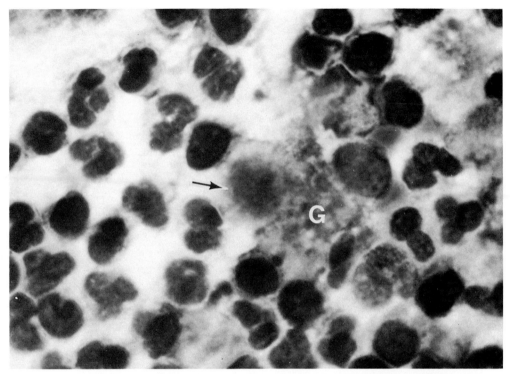

Fig. 9-7. Case 9-7. Rheumatoid pleural effusion. Cell-button of centrifuged pleural fluid. Poly-morphonuclear cells have swollen nuclei. There is a diffuse background of amorphous granular ma-terial, G, showing a tendency to round-off (arrow) but not forming the discrete hematoxylin bodies seen in systemic lupus erythematosus (see, also, Fig. 15-1).

matin pattern and becoming hyaline. Macrophages produce bizarre giant epithe-lioid forms, some of them multinucleate or with a large, irregular nucleus. These epithelioid cells often take on a highly characteristic tadpole shape, with a pointed tail. Boddington and coworkers [58] stated that in an experience of 2,800 pleural effusions they had never observed these findings except in rheumatoid arthritis.

Pleurisy or pleural effusion occurs in 2 or 3 per cent of patients with rheumatoid arthritis. In some, histologic examination of the pleural membranes has shown granulomatous inflammation identical with the changes in the subcutaneous rheumatoid nodules, but often only nonspecific pleuritis, as in Case 9-7. One of the most characteristic, virtually pathognomonic, features of the pleural effusion is its exceptionally low level of glucose. According to Lillington and coworkers [425], a low glucose level in pleural fluid that is nonpurulent, negative for bacteria on smear and culture and for malignant cells on cytologic examination almost invariably indicates that the effusion is due to rheumatoid pleuritis unless pleural biopsy reveals tuberculosis. Data from the literature plus their own experience indicated that the glucose content of the fluid is less than 30 mg/100 ml in about 80 per cent of rheumatoid effusions. Men seem to be over-represented among the patients with rheumatoid pleural effusions; 14 of the 17 patients reported by Lillington and coworkers were men. The low levels of glucose in these effusions are apparently due to its impaired transport from the blood to the pleural fluid across the inflamed pleural membrane: raising the blood glucose level did not raise the pleural fluid glucose in patients with rheumatoid pleural effusion; whereas it did so in patients with pleural effusion from other causes [89, 152]. The fluid from effusions due to coincidental lung diseases in patients with rheumatoid arthritis may not have the characteristics described above.

Case 9-8. A 55-year-old woman was crippled with rheumatoid arthritis. She had undergone extensive corrective surgery to her joints and many subcutaneous nodules were present. A transient pleural effusion was caused by a large pulmonary embolism: the fluid contained 4,600 leukocytes per cu mm (30 per cent polymorphonuclears, 70 per cent lymphocytes); total protein, 5.0 g/100 ml; glucose, 130 mg/100 ml. Cytological study showed only hyperplasia of mesothelial cells.

Large nodules due to rheumatoid disease may appear in the lungs in two circumstances. First, typical rheumatoid nodules may appear and actually cavitate [517]. Secondly, large nodules may appear in so-called "Caplan's syndrome" [86]. Caplan's syndrome is interesting in that it seems to be a modification of the pneumoconiotic reaction in patients with rheumatoid arthritis.

The more common disorder of the pulmonary parenchyma in rheumatoid arthritis is diffuse interstitial fibrosis. Patterson, Harville, and Pierce [538] studied 702 patients with rheumatoid arthritis and discovered eight with diffuse pulmonary fibrosis of no obvious cause. Most of their patients had moderately severe rheumatoid disease and over half had subcutaneous nodules. At autopsy, in one patient the lung showed a chronic inflammatory cellular infiltrate with lymphocytes and plasma cells in the alveolar septa, and numerous nodules, some with central areas of fibrinoid necrosis.

Tomasi, Fudenberg, and Finby [680] found rheumatoid factor in the serum of 11 of 18 patients with idiopathic pulmonary fibrosis; conversely, nine of 14 patients who had rheumatoid arthritis with high serum titers of rheumatoid factor showed x-ray evidence of pulmonary disease. In most of the patients with high titers of rheumatoid factor, circulating intermediate complexes were seen on ultracentrifugal analysis. The authors postulated that the lungs filtered out these complexes, which had pathogenic significance in relation to the pulmonary fibrosis. Ward and Stalker [707] studied 19 patients with chronic interstitial pulmonary fibrosis, excluding those with clinical rheumatoid arthritis. The sheep cell agglutination test for rheumatoid factor was consistently positive in five of the patients, and positive at some time during the course of the observations in another six.

The most common extra-articular features other than subcutaneous nodules and pulmonary fibrosis are digital vasculitis, skin ulceration, lymphadenopathy, noncompressive neuropathy, splenomegaly, and episcleritis, all of which occur in approximately similar prevalence. Pericarditis is frequently seen at autopsy, but seldom causes clinical manifestations. Although peripheral neuropathy is quite common, involvement of the central nervous system is exceptional [533].

Patients with extra-articular manifestations of rheumatoid arthritis, representing the most severe form of this disease, have provided opportunities to understand the underlying pathogenesis of rheumatoid arthritis. Current research has followed two converging pathways: 1) the possible participation of an infectious agent, 2) the immune reactions that underlie the synovitis and extra-articular manifestations.

In the first half of the twentieth century, students of rheumatoid arthritis suspected that it was infectious in origin. This idea is being re-examined. Early test systems for rheumatoid factor used streptococcal agglutination because it was considered that streptococcus might be the offending infectious agent. Sclater [608] found that infection had occurred within the 2 months preceding onset of rheumatoid arthritis in 72 (18.5 per cent) of 388 patients. Barland [30], reviewing the possible relationships between an infectious agent and the immune reactions of rheumatoid synovitis, considered that there were two possible relations: either a nonarthrotropic infectious agent was trapped in an antigenically active form that persisted in joint tissues; or an arthrotropic infectious agent was present in a latent or defective state in the synovial membrane or articular cartilage, producing intracellular viral antigen, extracellular virus coat antigens, cellular neoantigens, or antigenically altered intracellular or extracellular products.

Many attempts have been made to grow known bacteria or viruses from the synovial fluid or the synovial membrane of rheumatoid joints. Although some claims for success have been made, for the most part these remain unconfirmed. In general, it is held that no organism has yet been identified. The concept that immune factors are important to the pathogenesis of rheumatoid disease is upheld by the tendency of two features to occur with high frequency in patients with extra-articular manifestations of rheumatoid arthritis: high titers of rheumatoid factor in the serum, and necrotizing vasculitis in the tissue lesions. Mongan and coworkers [486] showed that necrotizing vasculitis occurred exclusively among their patients who were seropositive for rheumatoid factor and did not occur in those who were seronegative. They also found that serum complement activity, which is generally normal in rheumatoid arthritis, was significantly lower in the patients with vasculitis. Hunder and McDuffie [326] studied 16 patients with classic rheumatoid arthritis whose serum complement values were lower than normal. There was a high prevalence of extra-articular manifestations. Most noteworthy was the frequency of bacterial infection during the period of observation. There was some evidence, i.e., anticomplementary serum factors, of circulating immune complexes. They held that the findings of high titers of rheumatoid factor, decreased complement levels, and anticomplementary serum factors in their patients might all have developed in response to chronic immunization, and that immune complexes were the ultimate cause of the clinical manifestations. Zvaifler [744] considered that the role of IgM rheumatoid factors in joint inflammation is to enhance phagocytosis of immune complexes, leading to the release of lysosomal enzymes. Possible mechanisms whereby IgM rheumatoid factor might improve the interaction of immune complexes with phagocytic cells include 1) conversion of soluble complexes into larger, more particulate, and less soluble ones, and 2) conversion of noncomplement-fixing complexes into complement-fixing ones, allowing the complexes to bind to the leukocyte membrane at the C3 receptor. This fixation of complement by the complexes induces depletion of complement from the joint fluid in rheumatoid arthritis. In Hedberg's extensive studies [304, Appendix Tables I–VII] normal levels of total hemolytic complement (CH50) in joint fluid, i.e., >300 units/ml, were seen in 15 of 17 patients with degenerative joint disease, meniscus lesions, trauma, or loose bodies in the knee joints; and low levels of total hemolytic complement, i.e., <300 units/ml, were seen in 26 of 27 adults who had rheumatoid arthritis with nodules, in 33 of 49 adults with seropositive rheumatoid arthritis, in six of 12 adults with seronegative rheumatoid arthritis, in all of seven juveniles with seropositive rheumatoid arthritis, in one of five juveniles with seronegative rheumatoid arthritis, in three of 14 patients with psoriatic arthritis, and in all of 10 patients with systemic lupus erythematosus. Although the above observations are of great theoretical interest, our own studies of synovial fluid C3 complement level show that measurements of this component of complement are not helpful clinically in distinguishing between rheumatoid arthritis, and osteoarthritis or acute traumatic synovitis (Table 9-1). It is not clear why results from measurement of CH50 should be so different from those of C3; but the results shown in Table 9-1 are important because C3 levels are assayed in most hospital laboratories; whereas CH50 levels are not so easily obtainable. Bunch and coworkers [78] related synovial fluid CH50 levels to total protein in the fluid; lowest ratios were seen in the classic or definite cases of rheumatoid arthritis, and intermediate values in the probable cases. However, 39 per cent of the patients with classic or definite rheumatoid arthritis, and 81 per cent of those with probable rheumatoid arthritis, had values overlapping those of the controls.

The typical histopathological features of rheumatoid arthritis are the granulomatous synovitis of joints and tendon sheaths, and the rheumatoid nodule in the subcutaneous tissue and viscera. Most authorities are content to accept both the synovitis and the subcutaneous nodules as granulomata, since they contain aggregates of histiocytes. Unexplained, is why the histiocytes in the subcutaneous nodules palisade around central foci of necrosis. Sokoloff and Bunim [642] examined a number of subcutaneous nodules very early in the course of their development, and saw conspicuous inflammatory changes in the small arteries. Concomitantly, some of their patients had arteritis in muscle biopsy specimens. An interesting example was their patient number 7, who had active rheumatoid arthritis but no reported evidence of peripheral neuropathy or cutaneous ulceration. During the course of hospital therapy, a subcutaneous nodule developed and was removed when only 7 days old; 2 weeks later, biopsy of the gastrocnemius muscle was performed. Each of these biopsy specimens was found to contain small arteries with active inflammatory changes in their walls. Sokoloff and Bunim raised a number of questions in 1957 which remain unanswered today. Why are the vascular lesions not found consistently in rheumatoid arthritis? What is the histological relationship of rheumatoid arteritis to polyarteritis nodosa? What is the pathologic significance of polyarteritis nodosa in rheumatoid arthritis? What relationship do the perivascular infiltrates of lymphocytes in the striated muscles in rheumatoid arthritis bear to rheumatoid arteritis? One also wonders what factors determine that one immunologically mediated disease should appear, i.e., rheumatoid arthritis, rather than another, e.g., polyarteritis nodosa or systemic lupus erythematosus? Although some patients have so-called "overlap syndromes" or mixed connective tissue diseases, such overlap is the exception rather than the rule; the clinical picture of the

Table 9-1.   Synovial Fluid and Serum C3 and C4 Levels in
Rheumatic Diseases

	Synovial Fluid		Serum*	
	C3	C4	C3	C4
Rheumatoid arthritis	27	2	99	26
	28	4	126	34
	30		105	
	30		90	
	33	9	108	
	36	21	84	45
	36			
	37			
	42		102	
	45		27	
	45			
	53		113	
	54		132	
	54		96	
	58		150	
	60		126	
	66			
Juvenile rheumatoid arthritis	24	6		
	24	4	135	
	28 }†			
	42			
	32	18		
	36 }†			
	36			
Psoriatic arthritis	42		108	
	42			
Systemic lupus erythematosus	9	3		
	28			
Rheumatic fever	66	26	156	
Osteoarthritis	21			
	23	14		
	23			
	28	11	110	56
	33			
	35	11		
	36			
	40	8		
	40	18	106	48
	42	11		
	44	23		
	45	16		
	90		123	

Table 9-1—Continued

	Synovial Fluid		Serum*	
	C3	C4	C3	C4
Traumatic effusion	16			
	18	20		
	21	4		
	23			
	23 †			
	30			
	31	9		
	35			
Post-traumatic prepatellar bur-sitis	21	14		

* Normal serum levels: C3 > 90 mg/100 ml; C4 > 25 mg/100 ml.

† Bracketed values were obtained from the same patient on different occasions.

disease as it develops at the onset of illness, be it rheumatoid arthritis, systemic lupus erythematosus, polyarteritis, scleroderma, or polymyositis, tends to remain constant throughout the course of that illness rather than to become blurred by an overlap with a nosological neighbor.

The percentage of patients with rheumatoid arthritis who are found to have LE cells varies markedly from series to series according, probably, to the test method used. If large numbers of patients with rheumatoid arthritis are tested, the LE cell will be found in approximately 5 per cent. Goldfine and coworkers [249] studied the clinical significance of the LE cell phenomenon in rheumatoid arthritis. They found that the presence or absence of LE cells made no difference to the degree of joint inflammation, the duration of arthritis, the presence of subcutaneous nodules, or the occurrence of systemic involvement of any sort. Their data gave no support to the concept that rheumatoid arthritis with LE cells is either an entity distinct from rheumatoid arthritis or a variant of systemic lupus erythematosus.

The nosological question, whether rheumatoid arthritis and polyarteritis truly represent different disease entities or are merely polar expressions of the same underlying disease, is unlikely to be resolved until we have better understanding of the pathogenic mechanisms involved. From the clinical viewpoint, the separation is usually easy: either the patient has established peripheral rheumatoid arthritis with ensuing extra-articular manifestations that include necrotizing vasculitis; or the patient has typical polyarteritis with relatively trivial synovitis. As usual, it is the overlapping cases that are not only puzzling, but also nosologically instructive.

Case 9-9. A 36-year-old woman had been investigated 6 years earlier because of productive cough and dyspnea, and found to have severe pulmonary fibrosis and hypergammaglobulinemia. For the last 9 months, she had suffered from inflammatory polyarthritis, small papules along the free margins of the nose, and intracutaneous papules over both olecrana. For 2 or 3 months she had experienced painful paresthesiae in the hands and feet, and livedo reticularis on the legs.

Physical examination showed some pain with full motion in several joints, but no joint effusions or deformities. The skin showed livedo reticularis over the legs and feet, and intracutaneous small nodules at the nasal margins and over the olecrana. There was definite impairment of pinprick and cold sensations in the feet and in the distribution of the right ulnar nerve; the ankle jerks were absent. Pertinent laboratory findings included 15 per cent eosinophils in the peripheral blood; 26 per cent γ-globulins in the serum protein, as determined by electrophoresis; positive response to test for rheumatoid factor, negative to test for antinuclear antibodies; erosive changes in several interphalangeal joints seen in x-rays of the hands, and diffuse interstitial fibrosis seen in radiographs of both lungs (Fig. 9-8). Muscle biopsy showed evidence of inflammatory arteritis. Biopsy of one of the intracutaneous nodules showed changes typical for either granuloma annulare or rheumatoid arthritis (Fig. 9-9) (see below).

About a month later, acute median nerve palsy developed. The patient received chlorambucil without any corticosteroid, and made a slow but almost complete recovery from her neuropathic and cutaneous lesions. Subsequently, her main difficulty has been the inflammatory polyarthritis.

A point of parenthetic interest in the above case is the occurrence of intracutaneous nodules. These are quite rare in adult rheumatoid arthritis, but are seen occasionally in the juvenile form of the illness (Fig. 9-10). Some fine points

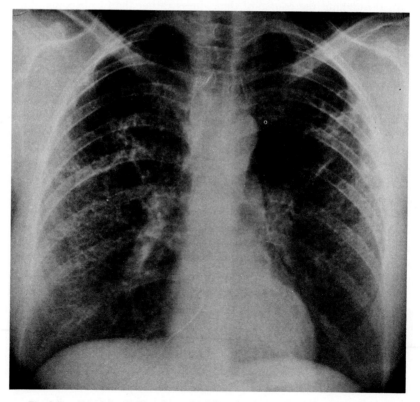

Fig. 9-8.   Case 9-9.   Diffuse interstitial fibrosis of lungs in rheumatoid arthritis.

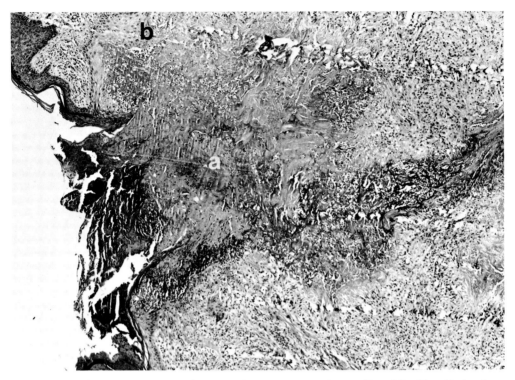

Fig. 9-9. Case 9-9. Histopathology of intracutaneous rheumatoid nodule. Necrobiosis of collagen (a) with surrounding histiocytes (b).

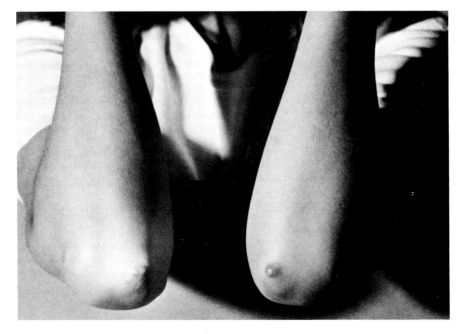

Fig. 9-10. Intracutaneous nodules at the elbows in a patient with juvenile rheumatoid arthritis.

of histologic distinction between the cutaneous lesion of granuloma annulare and the intracutaneous rheumatoid nodule have been reviewed by Bowers [65]. In rheumatoid arthritis, the nodules are usually larger than in granuloma annulare, and the degenerated collagen is more homogeneous and less fragmented in appearance. In granuloma annulare, the cellular infiltrate is more pleomorphic, with eosinophils, many lymphocytes, and occasional plasma cells and neutrophils; whereas the rheumatoid nodule contains mainly histiocytes and fibroblasts.

An example of predominantly extra-articular rheumatoid disease follows:

Case 9-10. A 40-year-old woman had a 3-year history of Raynaud's phenomenon with subungual hemorrhages, polyarthralgia, trigger fingers, flexor and extensor tenosynovitis at the wrist (Fig. 9-11), prepatellar bursitis (Fig. 1-1), and subcutaneous nodules in various sites including the elbows. The enlarged prepatellar bursae contained nodules. Although antinuclear factor and rheumatoid factor (sought by latex agglutination, FII hemagglutination, and anti-Ripley techniques) were absent from her serum, biopsy of one of the subcutaneous nodules at the elbow showed the histological appearances of a rheumatoid nodule. No erosions were seen in x-rays of the hands.

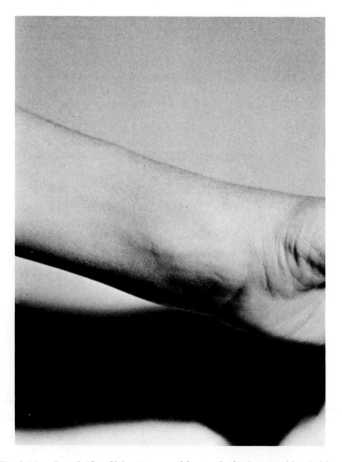

Fig. 9-11.   Case 9-10.   Volar tenosynovitis at wrist in rheumatoid arthritis.

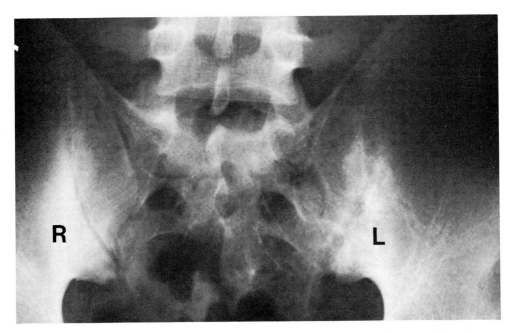

Fig. 9-14. Patient with ankylosing spondylitis. A (above), anteroposterior x-ray of sacroiliac joints: the left side is abnormal, with erosions and sclerosis of both sacral and iliac sides of the joint. The right side appears normal. B (page 140), oblique view of right sacroiliac joint. C (page 141), oblique x-ray of abnormal left sacroiliac joint.

Thompson [678], account for approximately 1 per cent of all patients with the disease.

It should be noted that sacroiliitis is a reaction that is seen not only in ankylosing spondylitis, but also in psoriatic arthropathy, Reiter's syndrome, juvenile rheumatoid arthritis, brucellosis, fluorosis, and in paraplegics. Sometimes confusing to the clinician is the condition known as osteitis condensans ilii, in which the radiological appearances consist of osteosclerotic lesions occurring on the iliac side of the joint. Rarely, the sacrum may also be involved [678]. The joint margins remain intact. The changes may be either unilateral or bilateral. Osteitis condensans ilii occurs predominantly in females, and commonly starts after pregnancy. It is apparently not histologically a true osteitis and Thompson [678] indicated that sacroiliac osteosclerosis would be a preferable term. Thompson considered that the condition could cause back pain; but other authorities hold a contrary opinion. It is interesting in this regard that among nine women with acute anterior uveitis who were positive for HL-A27 (see also p. 238), two had osteitis condensans ilii [71].

Psoriatic arthritis differs in several ways from rheumatoid arthritis: the sex ratio of affected individuals is approximately equal; there is a predilection for the terminal interphalangeal joints; so-called "sausage digits" occur, in which the inflammatory reaction from the involved interphalangeal joint extends both proximally and distally to the subcutaneous tissues of the contiguous phalanges; there may be arthritis mutilans, with telescoping digits caused by severe osteolysis; sacroiliitis appears in 10 to 20 per cent of patients, and subcutaneous

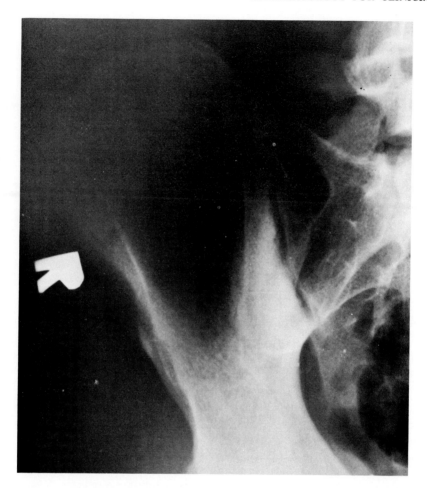

Fig. 9-14. B.

nodules and rheumatoid factor are usually absent. According to Moll and Wright [483], asymmetrical involvement of a few terminal interphalangeal joints, proximal interphalangeal joints, or metatarsophalangeal joints, sometimes only one of these, is the most typical clinical pattern of psoriatic arthritis, occurring in more than 70 per cent of patients. The radiological picture of psoriatic arthritis not only is characterized by the distribution of involved joints, but is said to show much more severe osteolysis than is seen in rheumatoid arthritis. Severe erosive changes may appear with great rapidity (Fig. 9-15), although such rapid changes are seen occasionally in patients with rheumatoid arthritis who have no psoriasis (Fig. 9-16). So far as skin involvement by psoriasis is concerned, it is worth emphasizing the need to search carefully for lesions unsuspected by the patient; for example, in the scalp, in the umbilicus, and in the natal cleft. The nails repay careful inspection; they may show pitting, transverse ridging, onycholysis, hyperkeratosis, and yellow discoloration.

   In *Reiter's syndrome* as in psoriatic arthritis, sausage digits occur; other features of Reiter's syndrome include chronic psoriasiform lesions of the skin and nails, and keratoderma blenorrhagica especially of the soles and palms which is very similar in appearance to pustular psoriasis affecting these areas. Histopathologically, too, the changes in the synovium of psoriatic arthritis and Reiter's syndrome are indistinguishable both from one another and from those seen in rheumatoid arthritis; the skin lesions of psoriasis and Reiter's syndrome are also identical [552]. Other clinical features of Reiter's syndrome, besides the polyarthritis, urethritis, and conjunctivitis, include uveitis, diarrhea, lesions of the oral mucosa, balanitis, hemorrhagic cystitis, prostatitis, and cardiac lesions [712].

A potentially clarifying observation which at this time raises more questions about nosologic interrelationships than it answers is the association between

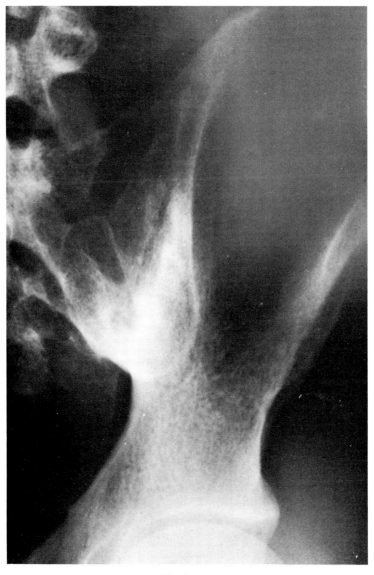

Fig. 9-14. C.

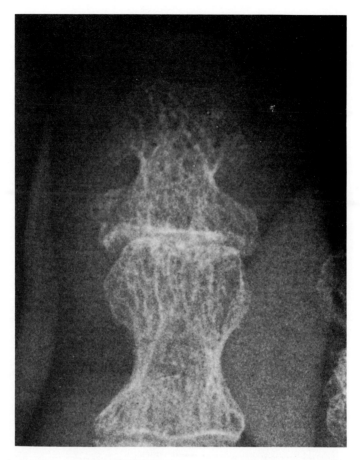

Fig. 9-15. Distal interphalangeal joint of second toe, right foot, of a patient with psoriatic arthritis. A (above), 6/20/73. B, 9/25/73. Note large lytic lesions, that have appeared at the lateral and medial aspects of the joint during the three months between x-rays.

certain histocompatibility antigens and some of the diseases under discussion [457]. This topic is considered in more detail in Chapter 15. A strong association exists between possession of HL-A antigen W27 and both ankylosing spondylitis and Reiter's syndrome [10, 16, 70, 72, 491, 603, 732]. The same histocompatibilty antigen, HL-A W27, is associated with psoriatic spondylitis [464] and with juvenile rheumatoid arthritis, although not with adult-onset rheumatoid arthritis [563], and with acute anterior uveitis [71, 173]. Other HL-A antigens, 13 and W17, are present in high frequency in patients having psoriasis without spondylitis [457]. Thus, in several of the conditions in which rheumatoid reactions occur and in which sacroiliitis and anterior uveitis are common, there is an additional unifying factor of an increased frequency of HL-A W27 antigens, and this increased frequency is not seen in idiopathic rheumatoid arthritis.

Further illustrating the fact that rheumatoid joint reactions occur in diseases that are separable on other grounds from idiopathic rheumatoid arthritis are the peripheral polyarthritis sometimes seen in patients with ankylosing spondylitis, the inflammatory polyarthritis seen in certain nonrheumatoid granulomatous diseases (See Chapter 8), and an acute polyarthritis that may appear in a specific granulomatous disease, i.e., leprosy accompanied by erythema nodosum leprosum; this may be indistinguishable from rheumatoid arthritis, even to the extent of a positive response to test for rheumatoid factor [364].

Other observations that unify some of the illnesses in which a rheumatoid reaction appears are: 1) the high prevalence rates of ankylosing spondylitis in Crohn's disease (7 per cent) [293, 294] and ulcerative colitis (3 per cent) [4]; 2) conversely, the prevalence of inflammatory bowel disease in ankylosing spondylitis (17 per cent) [341]; 3) Morris and coworkers [492] studied 31 patients with inflammatory bowel disease and observed that 6 of 8 patients with associated spondylitis had the HL-A W27 antigen; whereas none of the 23 patients who had either peripheral arthritis or no arthritis had this antigen. This suggests that different pathogenic mechanisms may underlie the spondylitis and peripheral arthritis of inflammatory bowel disease; and 4) a family reported by Good [255] in which three brothers had respectively, ankylosing spondylitis, Reiter's syndrome, and Reiter's syndrome followed by rheumatoid arthritis.

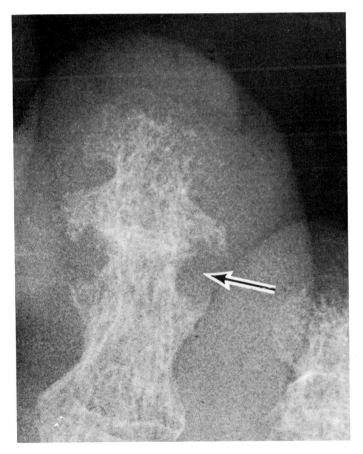

Fig. 9-15. B.

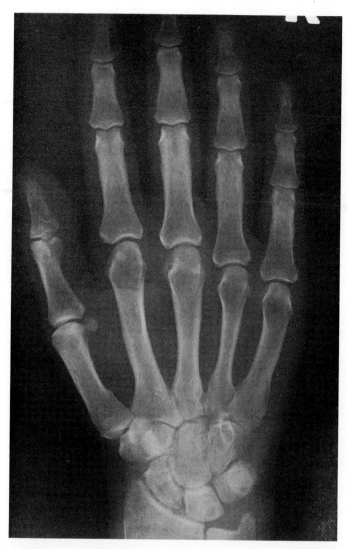

Fig. 9-16.   Early rheumatoid arthritis. A (above), July 1971: sparse, faint subchondral erosions in carpus. B, same hand, February 1973: note numerous subchondral and cortical erosions, especially at arrows.

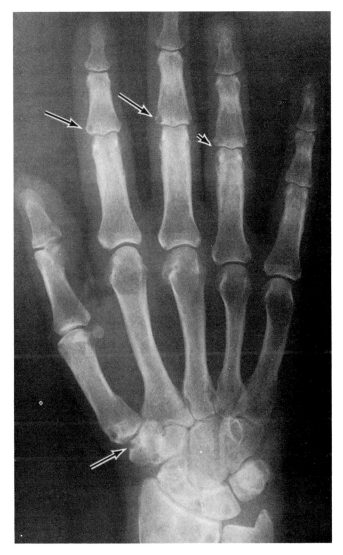

Fig. 9-16. B.

This chapter will be concluded by reiterating what was stated at its beginning. The label *rheumatoid arthritis* implies an idiopathic rheumatoid reaction.
Before applying this label, the clinician must undertake a process of excluding a
variety of conditions that may cause or be associated with chronic inflammatory
polyarthritis: psoriasis, Reiter's syndrome, ankylosing spondylitis, systemic connective tissue diseases, gout, Crohn's disease, ulcerative colitis, sarcoidosis,
amyloidosis, Behçet's syndrome are a few of them. The process of exclusion is
difficult because some of these latter disorders include associated manifestations
that overlap broadly with those of rheumatoid arthritis itself.

CHAPTER 10

Lupus Erythematosus Reactions

Lupus erythematosus (LE) may be a reaction to drugs or to known viral infection, but most frequently has no recognized cause. This chapter will pay most attention to idiopathic systemic lupus erythematosus (SLE); the merit of emphasizing LE as a reaction is that it draws attention to antecedent causation.

PREVALENCE AND OUTCOMES

It is obvious in a busy community rheumatological practice that SLE is common and most often benign. Recent estimates of the 10-year survival rate have been 59 per cent [181] or higher [404]. Two population surveys of the incidence and prevalence of SLE reported from the United States gave estimates of prevalence of 1 case in 12,300 in New York City [628] and 1 case in 2,400 in Rochester, Minnesota [516].

Our own studies show that the prevalence of definite SLE, according to American Rheumatism Association (ARA) criteria [115], in San Francisco is 1 case in 1,969 persons, approximately 20 per cent higher than the highest previous estimate; that the prevalence in black women aged 15 to 64 years is 1 case in 245; and that the disease is usually benign, with a 10-year survival rate exceeding 90 per cent. For inclusion in our study, a patient had to be a member of the Kaiser Foundation Health Plan (KFHP) and resident in the city and county of San Francisco between July 1965 and June 1973. An important feature of this study is that The Permanente Medical Group gives total medical care to the KFHP members; complete medical records of this care are available, in some instances extending back for 20 years.

Only the records of patients diagnosed by an internist as having possible or definite SLE, or by a dermatologist as having discoid LE, were scrutinized. Patients with the lupus syndrome induced by drugs or associated with chronic active hepatitis were carefully excluded from the analysis, as were those whose major diagnosis was clearly rheumatoid arthritis, Felty's syndrome, scleroderma, or polyarteritis. The years of study were those between July 1965 and June 1973.

The ARA preliminary criteria for the classification of SLE [115] were used. Cases were classified as "definite" if any four of the 14 preliminary criteria were present serially or simultaneously during any period of observation. Those cases that did not meet the criteria for diagnosis of definite SLE were allotted to one of three further groups: those in which three criteria were present, those with only two criteria, and those with only one criterion. The 14 proposed criteria include 21 items as follows: 1) facial erythema or butterfly rash, 2) discoid lupus, 3) Raynaud's phenomenon with at least a two-phase color reaction, 4) alopecia,

5) sun-sensitivity, 6) oral or nasopharyngeal ulceration, 7) arthritis without deformity, 8) LE cells, 9) chronic false-positive reaction to tests for syphilis present for at least 6 months, 10) profuse proteinuria (>3.5 g/day), 11) cellular casts, 12) pleuritis or pericarditis, 13) psychosis or convulsions, and 14) hemolytic anemia, leukopenia (white blood cell count <4,000/cu mm on two or more occasions), or thrombocytopenia. The only minor deviation in this study from the ARA criteria was the use in our laboratory of the fluorescent treponema antibody-absorbed test, instead of *Treponema pallidum* immobilization or Reiter's test, for the diagnosis of chronic false-positive tests for syphilis.

The incidence of new cases diagnosed on the basis of the ARA criteria as being definite SLE, in the 8-year period July 1965–June 1973, was 74. The mean KFHP membership resident in San Francisco city and county during this period was 121,444. Thus, the annual incidence of SLE was 7.2 cases per 100,000.

The prevalence of SLE is 1 case per 1,969 population. This calculation is based on the 64 cases of definite SLE (in 57 women and 7 men) in persons known to be alive, members of KFHP, and resident in the city and county of San Francisco in June 1973, and on the known KFHP membership in San Francisco of 126,000 in March 1973 (Table 10-1). This figure is a conservative estimate, because in June 1973 there were an additional nine patients for whom a reasonable working diagnosis was SLE. These nine patients were: 1) a black woman with polyarthralgia, recurrent oral ulcers, pleurisy, and positive test for antinuclear antibodies (ANA), 2) a black woman with polyarthritis, pleuritis, positive LE cell preparations, clinical and laboratory evidence of polymyositis, and leukocyte counts of 3,600/cu mm in May 1973 and 2,300/cu mm in October 1973, 3) a

Table 10-1. Demographic Data: Membership of Kaiser Foundation Health Plan Resident in the City and County of San Francisco

Total resident members in March of successive years:		
	1965	113,000
	1966	115,000
	1967	118,000
	1968	122,000
	1969	126,000
	1970	123,000
	1971	125,000
	1972	125,000
	1973	126,000
Mean of above years		121,444
Age composition of resident members, March 1973:		
	0–14	22.4%
	15–44	45.4%
	45–64	23.6%
	≥64	8.6%
Skin color of resident members, June 1971:		
	White	81%
	Black	9%
	Other	9%

(Reproduced by permission from Fessel, W. J.: Arch Int Med, 134: 1027–1035, 1974.)

black man with diffuse proliferative nephritis seen on renal biopsy, and three positive LE cell preparations, 4) a Chinese man with polyarthritis, positive LE cell preparation, and hemolytic anemia, 5) a Chinese woman with nephrotic syndrome, membranous glomerulonephritis, epimembranous electron-dense deposits and virus-like particles in endothelial cells seen on renal biopsy, leukocyte count <4,000/cu mm on three occasions, and positive ANA, 6) a white woman with polyarthritis, psychotic episodes, focal proliferative nephritis seen on biopsy, and positive ANA, 7) a white woman with severe, generalized discoid LE, psychotic episodes, recurrent thrombophlebitis, cerebral artery thrombosis, positive LE cell preparations, and intermittent hypocomplementemia, 8) a white woman with polyarthritis, discoid LE, alopecia, conversion of ANA from negative to positive, and hematoxylin bodies and rosettes in the LE cell preparation, and 9) a white woman with sun-sensitivity, polyarthritis, epilepsy of late onset, and positive ANA in titer of 1:200. If these nine cases with a working diagnosis of SLE were included in the assessment of prevalence, the figure would be 1:1,726.

The prevalence in black persons. There was a striking over-representation of black persons among the 64 patients with definite SLE known to be alive and resident in the city and county of San Francisco in June 1973 (Table 10-2). Nineteen (29.7 per cent) of the 64 patients were black, and 16 of the black patients were women. Nine per cent, or 11,340 of the KFHP members in the city and county of San Francisco are black (Table 10-1); 50 per cent of these, or 5,670, are female. This gives a prevalence of 16 cases of SLE per 5,670; 2.8 per 1,000, or 1:354 of the total black female population. Since the range of ages of these 16 black women was 16 to 62 years, and 69 per cent of the KFHP population in the city and county of San Francisco is between 15 and 64 years of age, we may adjust the prevalence of SLE in black women aged 15 to 64 years to 16 cases per 3,912, 4.1 per 1,000, or 1:245.

Table 10-2 shows the prevalence rates per 10,000 for four groups of patients: those with four or more diagnostic criteria, i.e., definite SLE; those with three diagnostic criteria, those with two, and those with only one diagnostic criterion. These prevalence rates are based upon both KFHP membership and residence in

Table 10-2. Skin Colors, Males, and Prevalences* According to Numbers of Diagnostic Criteria† Present

Diagnostic Criteria No.	Patients No.	Skin Color				Male %	Prevalence per 10,000
		White %	Black %	Other %	Unknown %		
≥4	64	54.7	29.7	15.6	0	10.9	5.1
3	14	50.0	28.6	21.4	0	14.3	1.1
2	9	44.4	11.1	44.4	0	22.2	0.7
1	20	55.0	30.0	10.0	5	30.0	1.6

* Prevalence in first 6 months of 1973.

† Diagnostic criteria are the 14 "preliminary ARA criteria" for diagnosis of SLE [115].

(Reproduced by permission from Fessel, W. J.: Arch Int Med, 134: 1027–1035, 1974.)

the city and county of San Francisco during January to June 1973 for patients in all groups. All of the patients with one criterion alone have discoid LE except for the Chinese woman mentioned above as having a working diagnosis of SLE with positive ANA, nephrotic syndrome, consistent appearances on renal biopsy, and leukopenia. Two striking observations (Table 10-2) are that 1) in all groups, not just the patients with definite SLE, the black population is grossly over-represented, and 2) accompanying a decreasing number of diagnostic criteria is a stepwise increase in the percentage of male patients, starting with 10.9 per cent among those with four or more diagnostic criteria and reaching 30.0 per cent among those with only one diagnostic criterion; however, these gender differences are not statistically significant ($x^2 = 4.44$, df = 3).

It is not clear why SLE is now so common, whereas formerly it was considered so rare. Heightened awareness of the diagnosis and widespread availability of testing for antinuclear antibodies evidently contribute to the frequency with which the disease is recognized. Whatever the reasons, however, it is plain that SLE has replaced acute rheumatic fever as the gravest rheumatic disease that is encountered on the hospital wards and in the clinic. Moreover, the prevalence of SLE in this San Francisco population, 51 per 100,000, is remarkably similar to the 52.9 cases of acute rheumatic fever per 100,000 found by Collins [120] in the National Health Survey and the Supplementary Communicable Disease Study made in 1935 to 1936 in the United States.

That a heightened awareness of the possibility of this diagnosis is partly, at least, responsible for an apparent increase in prevalence is illustrated by the following patient.

Case 10-1. A 61-year-old woman had received medical care at this clinic for the last 4 years, mainly because of vague abdominal symptoms that defied accurate diagnosis. At the time of a routine Multiphasic Health Checkup, it was noted that the leukocyte count was 3,900/cu mm, and that the year before it had been 4,400/cu mm. This observation led to questions directed toward the possibility of SLE. For the first time during her treatment at this clinic, she stated that she had been sun-sensitive throughout life, with blistering after the slightest exposure to sunlight; for the past 4 or 5 years she had had polyarthralgia without swelling, affecting wrists, metatarsophalangeal joints, and ankles, and had had recurrent oral ulcers; during the previous year her hair had started to fall excessively despite her daily ingestion of 3 gr of thyroid extract. Both parents and two sisters were said to have rheumatoid arthritis. Physical examination revealed only a generalized alopecia. Repeat leukocyte count was 4,400/ cu mm; antinuclear antibodies were present in the serum.

MORTALITY RATE

The mortality rate for patients with SLE in the San Francisco KFHP population was low. Only five (6.75 per cent) of the patients with definite SLE newly diagnosed between July 1965 and June 1973 died during the 8-year period, an annual mortality rate of 0.84 per cent. The projected 10-year survival rate thus exceeds 90 per cent. The prolonged course of the disease as it exists in the community is further exemplified by the fact that for the 11 patients who died

between July 1965 and June 1973 (including six whose definite diagnosis ante-
dated June 1965), the mean survival period after the appearance of the fourth
diagnostic criterion was 5.2 years (range, 0–14.08 years).

ORDER OF APPEARANCE OF DIAGNOSTIC CRITERIA

The first of the ARA criteria to appear was arthritis in 34.5 per cent of all
patients; discoid LE in 10.7 per cent, sun sensitivity in 6.0 per cent; all of the
other criteria accounted for fewer than 5 per cent of the first-appearing diagnostic manifestations. In 10 (15.6 per cent of the 64 patients), more than one criterion appeared simultaneously as the initial diagnostic sign.

The interval between the appearance of the first and the fourth definitely
diagnostic criterion was extremely variable. The mean interval was 5.7 years, the
standard deviation 7.4 years, the range 0–34 years. In 11 of the 64 patients, an
interval of 10 or more years elapsed between the appearances of the first and the
fourth diagnostic signs; in four of these, the interval was 20 or more. In these 11
patients, the initial manifestation was arthritis in five, chronic false positive
reaction to tests for syphilis in two, psychosis in two, discoid LE and sun
sensitivity each in one.

Table 10-3 shows the frequency with which each of the 14 ARA criteria appeared as one of the initial four. Arthritis was among the first four criteria to appear in all but three of the 64 patients (95.3 per cent); hematologic abnormalities

**Table 10-3. Frequency of Occurrence of
the 14 Criteria for Diagnosis of SLE* Among
First 4 Manifestations, in 64 Patients**

Criterion	%
Arthritis	95.3
Hematologic	54.7
LE cells	46.9
Discoid LE	37.5
Serositis	34.4
Alopecia	32.8
Sun sensitivity	26.6
Facial erythema	18.8
Raynaud's phenomenon	15.6
Psychosis/epilepsy	12.5
Chronic biologically false positive test for syphilis	12.5
Cellular casts in urine	10.9
Oral ulcers	7.8
Proteinuria >3.5 g/4 hr	3.1

* The listed criteria are abbreviations for
those proposed by the American Rheumatism
Association for the diagnosis of SLE [115].

(Reproduced by permission from Fessel,
W. J.: Arch Int Med, 134: 1027–1035, 1974.)

Table 10-4. Differences Between Black and Nonblack Patients
in Occurrence of first 4 Criteria* for the Diagnosis of SLE

	Black N = 19		Nonblack N = 45		
	No.	%	No.	%	Probability†
Hematologic‡	16	84.2	19	42.2	<0.01
Facial erythema	0		12	26.7	<0.05
Pleurisy/pericarditis	11	57.8	11	24.4	<0.05
Epilepsy/psychosis	0		8	17.8	N.S.

* First 4 of the ARA proposed criteria for diagnosis of SLE to appear in the given patient.
† χ^2 test used to analyze significance of differences across rows.
‡ Platelet count <100,000, or hemolytic anemia, or leukocyte count <4,000/cu mm on two occasions.
(Reproduced by permission from Fessel, W. J.: Arch Int Med, 134: 1027–1035, 1974.)

in 54.7 per cent, LE cells in 46.9 per cent, discoid LE in 37.5 per cent, serositis in 34.4 per cent, alopecia in 32.8 per cent. Thus, six of the 14 ARA criteria affected two-thirds of the patients early in the disease.

There were interesting differences between black and nonblack patients with respect to the occurrence of certain of the diagnostic criteria among their first four manifestations (Table 10-4). Serositis and hematologic abnormalities were significantly more common as initial criteria in black patients; facial erythema, not surprisingly, was not observed in black persons. Of main interest is the fact that epilepsy or psychosis did not occur as a first manifestation in black persons; possibly because of small numbers, this difference from nonblack patients did not reach statistical significance.

INVOLVEMENT OF SPECIFIC SYSTEMS

Renal involvement. Prevalence of renal involvement, as shown by abnormalities [27] on the renal biopsy specimen, was seven (10.9 per cent) among the 64 patients who were alive in June 1973. Three others had casts or proteinuria in an occasional urine sample, insufficient to justify renal biopsy; the mean survival period in these three patients from the time of first appearance of cellular casts in the urine was 73 months (range, 42–125 months). Three patients had focal proliferative nephritis seen on renal biopsy; their mean survival period to date from the time of biopsy is 54 months (range, 9–92 months). In only four (6.25 per cent) of the 64 patients has diffuse proliferative nephritis been seen on renal biopsy. These four patients are alive for a mean period of 45.5 months (range, 5–90 months) since biopsy.

There are no precise figures in the literature with which to compare the above experience of prevalence and mortality from renal disease in SLE, because all other reported groups of patients are highly ˙selected ones. Baldwin and coworkers [27] reported on 52 patients with abnormal renal biopsy findings. They did not consider patients on whom renal biopsy was not performed for one or another reason; and the patients with abnormal renal findings were among those with SLE seen in a large rheumatology clinic in New York, a group that is probably not representative of SLE as it exists in the community. Among these 52 patients, 25 were alive at follow-up; 12 of these had survived five or more years since biopsy. The least lethal forms of lupus nephritis were the focal proliferative and the membranous; there were 14 patients with each of these forms, and nine in each of the subgroups were alive at follow-up. Most lethal was diffuse proliferative glomerulonephritis; only seven among 24 patients with this form were still alive at the point of follow-up.

It is standard practice to study the renal biopsy specimen by electronmicroscopy, but even severe abnormalities seen on this examination are not necessarily ominous. Dujovne and coworkers [162] studied the distribution and character of the glomerular deposits in SLE in 40 renal biopsy specimens from 24 patients. The most important site of electron-dense aggregates was the subendothelial space, where such aggregates were seen only in the most active disease. Subendothelial deposits tended to decrease in prominence or to disappear following therapy, and in one patient a recrudescence of severe lupus nephritis was accompanied by the appearance of extensive subendothelial deposits. Subepithelial deposits, on the other hand, even when extensive, underwent relatively few changes with time and, once present, tended to persist. The study indicated that glomerular deposits should not by themselves be interpreted as evidence of active disease unless they are subendothelial or present in massive amounts after treatment. In general, the clinical course of patients with subepithelial deposits was benign.

In the present series, the incidence of renal involvement as found by biopsy or autopsy was low, only ten (13.5 per cent) of the 74 patients in whom the diagnosis of definite SLE was first made between July 1965 and June 1973 (Table 10-5). Four of the ten had focal proliferative nephritis; six had diffuse proliferative nephritis. Five of these 74 patients died during this period: one, with diffuse proliferative nephritis, died from acute necrotizing alveolitis and respiratory failure; one with focal proliferative nephritis died from uncontrollable lupus crisis, and one patient had had a few granular casts in her urine on several occasions during the 12½ years preceding her death from chronic interstitial pulmonary fibrosis and acute pulmonary embolism. Thus, in only two (2.7 per cent) of 74 patients freshly diagnosed as having SLE in the 8-year period did renal disease contribute, and then only indirectly, to death.

Previous estimates of the incidence of lupus nephritis and of its prognostic implications have been based on groups of patients who were unrepresentative of the community experience for three possible reasons: 1) the diagnosis of SLE may have been overlooked in mild cases, 2) patients with SLE are usually referred to large clinics or university hospitals when they have severe disease that is difficult to manage, and 3) reports based upon the findings at renal biopsy of necessity comprise those from patients, already members of a skewed group, with worst disease, because ethical considerations preclude biopsy where the condition is mild. Nevertheless, Heptinstall [307], who reviewed the literature in 1966, emphasized that while clinical renal involvement in five reported series varied from 56 per cent to 70 per cent, and although the kidney was found to be affected in approximately 80 per cent of cases coming to autopsy, lupus nephritis was determined as the cause of death in only 16 (21.6 per cent) of 74 patients.

On the basis of light microscopy, Baldwin and coworkers [27] observed the following clinicopathological correlations among 52 patients with lupus nephritis: in 14 with focal proliferative nephritis, where lesions involve only portions of some glomeruli, only five died and in none of these was the blood urea nitrogen elevated at the time of death; among 24 patients with diffuse proliferative nephritis, where all or nearly all glomeruli are involved in the inflammatory process, 17 died but renal failure was the cause of death in only nine; and among 14 patients with membranous lupus nephritis, in which there is uniform thickening of peripheral capillary loops with little or no hypercellularity, five patients died but only three of uremia. Thus, in this highly selected group of patients with lupus nephritis, only 12 of the 27 deaths were due to renal disease.

Rather similar observations were made by Zweiman and coworkers [746], who performed renal biopsy in 40 patients irrespective of the presence or absence of kidney disease. Twenty-five of the renal specimens showed changes of lupus nephritis; five of these were from patients who had no clinical evidence of renal involvement. Among 15 patients whose kidney tissue showed minor abnormalities or normal features, three died; among 24 patients with lupus nephritis, seven died but only four from renal causes. Thus, renal death occurred in only four of 39 patients. Hospitalized patients with SLE were the source of material for this study; even so, a few were not subjected to biopsy. Apparently, biopsy was not considered for patients who were not in hospital. This is one of the few reported studies in which an attempt was made to perform biopsy in all patients; nevertheless, the skewed nature of the patient sample is reflected in the high death rate, 10 (25.6 per cent) among 39 patients, followed for a mean of only 30 months.

The experience of Nanra and Kincaid-Smith [511] with 'the outcome of lupus nephritis is closest to ours. They studied 72 patients with lupus nephritis, of whom 63 (87.5 per cent) had the diffuse proliferative form. Although 13 (18.1 per

Table 10-5. Incidence of Renal Involvement in 74 Patients with SLE First Diagnosed* Between July 1965 and June 1973

Patients	Total	Urinary Casts Only	Focal Proliferative Glomerulitis†	Diffuse Proliferative Glomerulonephritis†
Living	64	3	3	4
Moved	5‡	0	1	0
Dead	5	1	0	2
All	74	4	4	6

* I.e., the fourth of the ARA criteria [115] to be observed in this patient appeared during this period.

† Classification of Baldwin and coworkers [27] was used.

‡ These 5 patients had either moved from San Francisco or left the Health Plan before 1973, so are not included in the computation of prevalence.

cent) of their patients died during the mean follow-up period of 4.4 years (range, 1 month to 7 years), only two deaths were from renal failure.

Lung involvement. Pulmonary dysfunction is very frequent in SLE. In their pulmonary function studies on 28 patients, Huang and coworkers [319] saw a restrictive pattern of respiration even in those patients who had no history of pleural involvement, no previous or present respiratory symptoms, and whose chest x-rays showed no abnormality. For the group, the mean forced vital capacity and the mean total lung capacity were, respectively, 62 per cent and 75 per cent of the predicted normal values; and in 16 patients for whom the diffusing capacity was estimated, the mean was only 65 per cent of the predicted value.

The abnormalities seen most commonly in the chest x-ray of patients with SLE are diffuse interstitial fibrosis and areas of plate-like atelectasis, some examples of which are illustrated (Fig. 10-1).

Eisenberg and coworkers [174] estimated the prevalence of diffuse interstitial pulmonary disease as not more than 3 per cent in their outpatients with SLE. This is confirmed in our group of 64 living patients, among whom only two (3.1 per cent) have diffuse interstitial disease; one other has discoid atelectasis alone, one has had recurrent pulmonary emboli, one associated lymphoma in the lung, and two have had chronic interstitial infectious pneumonitis (*Pneumocystis carinii* and miliary tuberculosis). Pleural involvement by SLE, on the other hand, was common, affecting 15 (23.4 per cent) of the 64 patients as one of the four

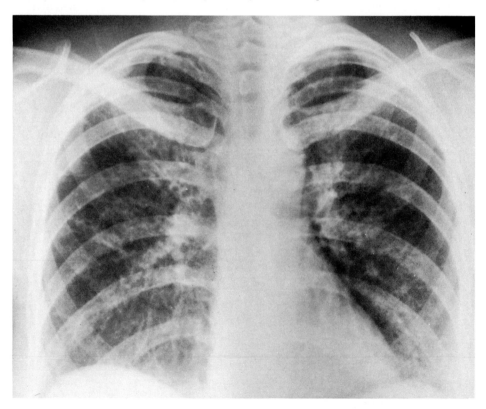

Fig. 10-1.   Systemic lupus erythematosus. A (above), diffuse micronodular interstitial infiltrate of lung (Case 10-9). B, discoid atelectasis at left lung base.

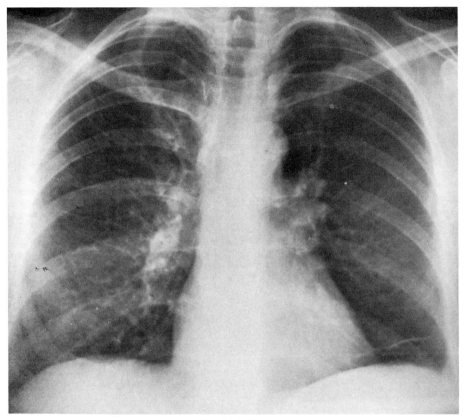

Fig. 10-1. B.

initial manifestations. Although pleuritic pain may be extremely severe and difficult to control by medication, patients with this complaint often have no pleural
effusion. When pleural fluid is present, it has a normal glucose value, it may
contain LE cells, and the levels of various components of complement may be
low [327].

Two of our patients with lung disease are of particular interest because they
demonstrate the ever-present need to consider all possibilities besides SLE as the
cause of the patient's difficulties:

Case 10-2. A Chinese woman aged 50 had had recurrent polyarthritis since 1962,
positive LE cell preparations first observed in 1963, an episode of psychotic behavior in
1966, and white blood cell counts as low as 1,100/cu mm. There was a family history of
active pulmonary tuberculosis and the patient had been known to have a positive reaction
to the PPD skin test for many years, although she had never shown evidence of active
pulmonary tuberculosis. The polyarthritis had necessitated prednisone in various doses for
the previous 7 years. Prophylaxis with isoniazid, 300 mg daily, together with pyridoxine,
50 mg daily, was started in June, 1971. She was admitted to the hospital in 1973 because
of increasing weakness and painful acroparesthesiae that had arisen during the previous 2
months. Physical examination showed marked weakness of the muscles of shoulder girdle
and hip, minimal weakness of the anterior tibial muscles, absence of deep tendon reflexes
at the ankles, and impairment of pinprick sensation in both feet. Chest x-ray revealed a

diffuse micronodular pattern throughout all lung fields; it was recognized in retrospect that this pattern had been present since 1971 (Fig. 10-2). The recent onset of myopathy and neuropathy was considered to represent evidence of activity of the underlying SLE; it seemed possible that the radiological abnormalities in the lungs likewise represented involvement by lupus. Review of a sequence of roentgenograms taken since she had started prednisone and isoniazid therapies showed a striking fluctuation in the miliary nodular infiltrate so that, at one point in time, the lung fields had become virtually clear. Liver biopsy showed numerous caseating granulomata, with Langhans' giant cells. *Mycobacterium tuberculosis,* resistant to isoniazid, grew from cultures of sputum, liver, and bone marrow.

Case 10-3. A 17-year-old black girl whose SLE had been present for the previous 3 years had experienced polyarthritis, pericarditis, and pleuritis, and had diffuse proliferative glomerulonephritis seen on biopsy. LE cell preparations were positive. She had been treated with a combination of prednisone and azathioprine since the diagnosis of nephritis 3 years earlier. Her most recent admission to the hospital was occasioned by progressive anemia, and symptoms and signs of a new polyneuropathy. Chest x-ray at the time of hospital admission is shown in Figure 10-3A with, for contrast, the chest x-ray from 2 months previously (Fig. 10-3B). The earlier film shows only mild changes suggestive of diffuse interstitial fibrosis. The later one shows more progressive diffuse interstitial fibrosis, as well as alterations consistent with plate-like atelectasis. It was considered that the latter were consistent with SLE affecting the lungs. The patient's vital capacity fell to only 800 ml/min, and she was short of breath at rest. For this reason, and because she had been treated with a combination of prednisone and azathioprine for 3

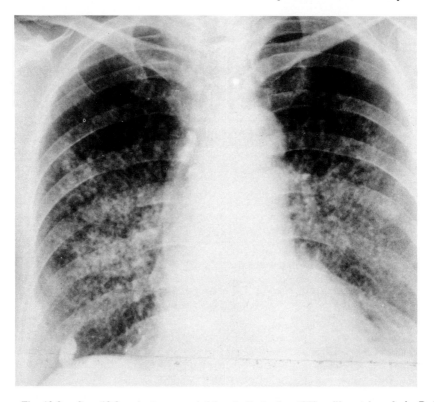

Fig. 10-2.   Case 10-2.   chest x-rays. A (above), September 1973: miliary tuberculosis. B, September 1971: faint miliary mottling is evident. C, June 1972: virtual clearing of miliary mottling.

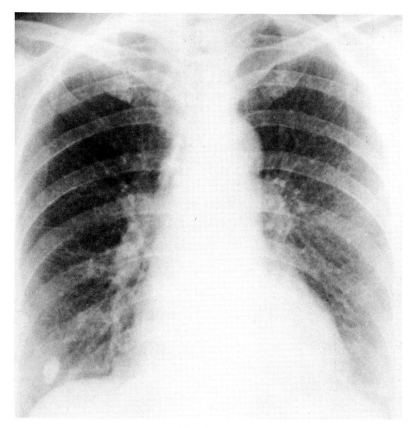

Fig. 10-2. B.

years, thoracotomy and lung biopsy were performed. Examination of the lung tissue revealed *Pneumocystis carinii* infection.

The first of these two cases is of importance because it shows that isoniazid does not provide total security against the supervention of active tuberculosis. In conjunction with the observation that the reaction to the PPD skin test is depressed in patients with SLE [280], it serves as a warning that tuberculosis may reactivate in patients being treated for SLE. The second case is of importance in demonstrating the well-known fact that infection with *P. carinii* may supervene in patients receiving immunosuppressive therapy, and as a reminder that the radiological appearances of this infection may be indistinguishable from those usually attributed to lupus lung disease.

Whitcomb and coworkers [717] were able to trace the development of interstitial fibrosis in a patient with proved *P. carinii* pneumonia, treated with pentamidine. Most patients in whom *P. carinii* pneumonia develops have some immunological defect, either intrinsic or induced; but it is interesting that among 194 patients with histologically confirmed *P. carinii* as the cause of their pneumonia, only five had SLE as their basic disease, and the several collagen diseases accounted for only nine (4.6 per cent) of all the cases [706]. Dyspnea and a nonproductive cough were the most common symptoms; physical findings were

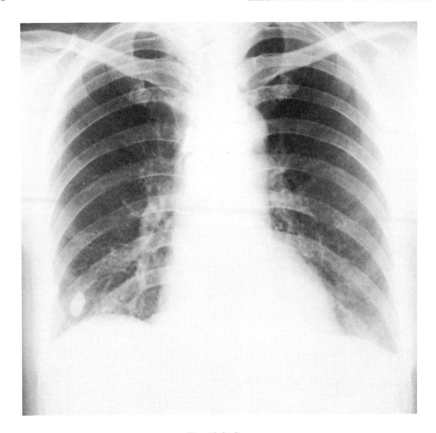

Fig. 10-2. C.

minimal or absent in this series of patients. It is noteworthy that *P. carinii* pneumonia affects males twice as often as females in the United States [706], and that in European cases a very high rate of spontaneous recovery from pneumocystis pneumonitis has been reported [231]. Is SLE associated with a low rate of *P. carinii* pneumonitis by virtue of the dominance of female patients with this condition; or does the female dominance permit a higher rate of spontaneous recovery than is otherwise anticipated in patients with this infection?

Prolonged fever. Prolonged high fever as an isolated symptom of SLE is uncommon and, when it occurs, may present a perplexing problem of differential diagnosis.

Case 10-4. A 63-year-old man had fevers up to 40.6° C (105° F) over a 6-week period. He had had polyarthritis of an inflammatory sort within the last 5 years, partial gastrectomy for duodenal ulcer, and positive response to serologic test for syphilis. During his hospitalization for the fever, several small exudates appeared in his optic fundus (Fig. 10-4). His reaction to tuberculin skin test was strongly positive. Erythrocyte sedimentation rate was in the region of 100 mm/hr (Westergren). Rheumatoid factor was present in his serum, and many LE cell preparations were strongly positive. All other laboratory tests were unrevealing. Because the exudates in his fundus resembled tubercles, he was treated with isoniazid and PAS for possible miliary tuberculosis. It was considered that insufficient criteria were present to permit a diagnosis of SLE. The fever gradually fell by lysis and was normal after 3 weeks of antituberculosis therapy. During the next year a gradual and constant leukopenia developed in his peripheral blood, sometimes to as low as 1,500 leukocytes per cubic millimeter, with a very prominent lymphocytosis that accounted for 90 to 98 per cent of the total white blood cells. Two bone marrow examinations showed mild hypercellularity, with normal white cell precursors and a moderate increase in plasma cells to 10 per cent of the total. The serum γ-globulin levels were very high, accounting for up to 45 per cent of the total protein concentration. Immunoglobulin levels showed IgG 3,000 mg/100 ml, IgA 960 mg/100 ml, and IgM 180 mg/100 ml. These abnormalities in white blood cells and serum proteins persisted. Evidence of severe posterior column disturbance of the spinal cord first appeared a couple of years after his febrile episode, and during the following 5 years there developed a left-sided cerebellar disturbance and progressive dementia. The usual causes for such central nervous system disorders were excluded by appropriate testing. During his final illness, severe myopathy and hemolytic anemia appeared. At this time it was discovered that the positive serological reactions for syphilis were biologically false ones, and the entire clinical picture over the previous 8 years was seen to be that of SLE.

Mental illness in SLE. It has been obvious for a long time that psychiatric manifestations are very frequent in SLE [205, 348]. This observation has both clinical and theoretical significance. Its clinical importance has to do with the

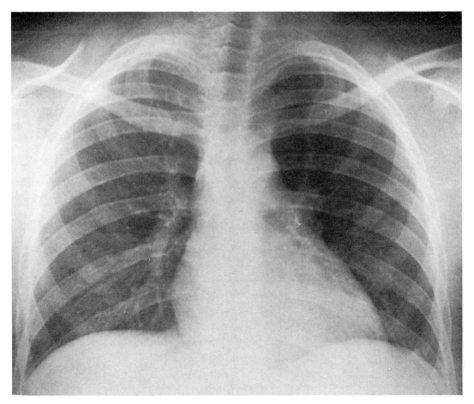

Fig. 10-3. Case 10-3, chest x-rays. A (above), 4/11/73: normal lung fields. B, 6/28/73: interstitial pneumonitis due to *Pneumocystis carinii*, with area resembling discoid atelectasis (arrow).

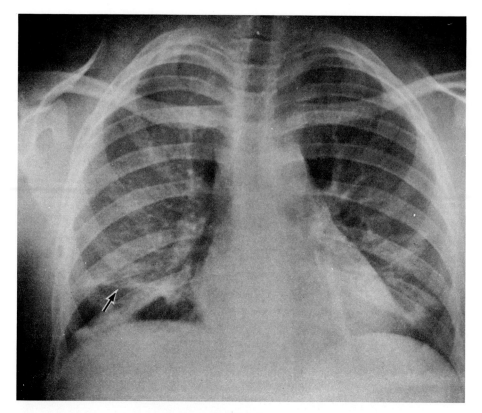

Fig. 10-3. B.

problem of determining whether psychiatric disturbances that occur during the course of SLE are due to the disease itself or to medication with corticosteroid. Psychotic manifestations due to either cause may be indistinguishable from those of the so-called "functional psychoses" or from those typical of organic brain syndromes. Abnormalities in the electroencephalogram or cerebrospinal fluid strongly favor SLE as the cause of the psychosis, but are present in only a minority of cases. The work of Petz et al [555] suggested that low levels of complement, especially the fourth component, in the cerebrospinal fluid are characteristic of the psychosis associated with SLE, and raised hopes of a ready mode of differentiating between the psychosis due to the disease and that induced by corticosteroids. More recent work, however, has indicated that many patients with SLE, even when there is no brain reaction, have lower than normal levels of cerebrospinal fluid complement, but that in the presence of psychosis due to the disease these levels are lowered even further [278]. Since it is not customary to establish baseline levels of cerebrospinal fluid complement in most patients with SLE, it is clearly not possible to interpret the meaning of low levels of cerebrospinal fluid complement during a psychotic episode. When an acute psychotic reaction occurs in a patient who is being treated with cortisone, it is my recommendation to increase the dose of cortisone unless it is already large, e.g., in excess of 100 mg daily of prednisone. This recommendation is based upon the fact, unexplained, that the psychiatric disturbance due to the disease itself usually

[handwritten note in top margin: ↑ STEROID-response 14 days if ⊖ rapidly tape]

responds within 14 days of instituting higher levels of cortisone; whereas the steroid-induced psychotic reaction may take many weeks or months to ameliorate in response to tapered doses of the drug. If, after 14 days of increased doses of cortisone, the psychotic reaction is no better, then the cortisone dose should be tapered rapidly and psychotropic drugs should be added.

The association between psychotic episodes and SLE is of theoretical interest in that careful post-mortem neuropathological examination of patients who had exhibited florid psychotic reactions during life have often shown no histopathological changes adequate to account for the psychotic disturbance [205]. That this observation may have relevance to the pathogenic mechanisms in functional psychoses is shown by the high prevalence of blood protein abnormalities in patients with schizophrenia [199] and the slightly increased prevalence of antinuclear factors in the blood of a mentally ill population [195]. The mechanism of the psychiatric disorder in patients with SLE untreated with corticosteroids is unclear. An interesting study by Atkins and coworkers [23] suggested that in SLE the choroid plexus filters out immune complexes in the same way as does the glomerular capillary network; their findings have been confirmed in experimental serum sickness [389]. Yet it is unclear how antigen-antibody complexes in the choroid plexus might account for functional psychotic behavior in SLE.

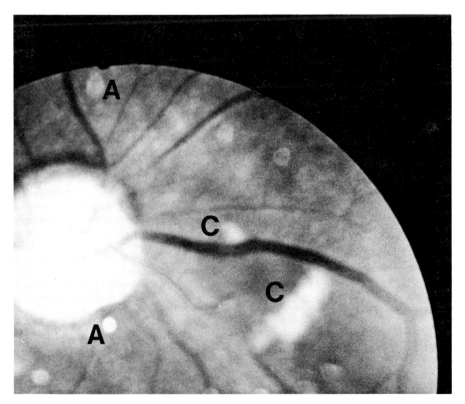

Fig. 10-4.   Case 10-4.   Cytoid bodies (c) simulating choroidal tubercles. Several camera-artifacts (A).

Many patients with SLE have major psychiatric disturbances antedating or immediately contemporaneous with the onset of the clinical manifestations of lupus. The following case is a good example.

Case 10-5. In a woman now 56 years old, although psychotic depression and a raised erythematous rash have been present recurrently since age 35, it was only after 20 years, at age 55, that the new appearance of polyarthritis, photosensitivity, and positive LE cell preparations permitted the diagnosis of SLE. The psychotic depression had appeared first, and seemed precipitated by the deaths of one of her sons and her two best friends when her house was consumed by a fire from which she herself managed to escape. A rash, which in retrospect was consistent with discoid LE, appeared shortly after the depression. Extensive psychiatric treatment, including electroconvulsive therapy, was required for control of the depression.

In their classic article, McClary and coworkers [454] pointed out that, in patients with SLE, masked depression is a common feature, and grief over the loss of or separation from a loved person is a frequent antecedent of clinical exacerbations. The reader is referred to Chapter 2 for a more detailed exposition of the role of the central nervous system in the pathogenesis of connective tissue diseases.

Myopathy. The frequency with which myopathy occurs during the course of SLE has been underestimated in the literature; 11 (17.2 per cent) of the 64 patients in this San Francisco population were so affected. In 10 (15.6 per cent), the myopathy was inflammatory in nature, i.e., polymyositis. Most often the polymyositis as part of SLE is mild, although on occasion it may cause profound weakness. The eleventh patient with associated myopathy had myasthenia gravis.

Parotid swelling as part of the SLE syndrome affected four (6.25 per cent) of the 64 patients. In all of the four, the glandular swelling was intermittent, lasting a few days or weeks at a time, and usually was only slightly painful. In one of the patients, who had generalized sicca syndrome, there was an acute inflammatory reaction in the gland with pain and tense swelling, and mild erythema of the overlying skin; the acute phase cleared spontaneously.

TESTS FOR ANTINUCLEAR ANTIBODIES AND LE CELLS IN THE DIAGNOSIS OF SLE

Although Fries and Siegel [226] matched the ARA criteria for diagnosis of SLE against a large population with various rheumatic diagnoses, and saw a considerable number of false-positive diagnoses of SLE, especially in patients diagnosed clinically as having scleroderma, Wegener's granulomatosis, or Felty's syndrome, Lie and Rothfield [423], Davis and coworkers [136], and Trimble and coworkers [686] observed a high concordance of the ARA criteria when these were tested in patients diagnosed clinically, like the ones whom we surveyed, as having SLE. It is clear that the ARA criteria may be misleading when applied to patients who have established diagnoses other than SLE; but where no definite alternative diagnosis is apparent, the proposed criteria are useful for confirming a provisional diagnosis of lupus. Pragmatically, the ARA criteria are valuable, as in the following case, by allowing the diagnosis of SLE when tests for antinuclear antibodies and LE cell preparations are consistently negative.

Case 10-6. A white woman was seen at the age of 31 years with severe thrombocytopenia, the platelet count being as low as 12,000/cu mm. Facial erythema had been present for many years; aside from this, there were no relevant physical findings. During the next 3 months, alopecia and polyarthritis appeared. Thus, she had a sufficient number of the preliminary criteria to permit the clinical diagnosis of SLE. Additional features included the appearance of papules over her cheeks, severe bloody diarrhea without evidence of abnormality on barium enema examination, and mild granularity in the bowel mucosa seen on sigmoidoscopic examination. Because it was impossible to control the platelet count with doses of prednisone as large as 120 mg daily, splenectomy was performed. Histopathological examination showed no onionskin fibrosis of splenic arterioles. During the next 6 years, seven separate tests for antinuclear antibodies and nine separate LE cell preparations were negative, as were results of tests for anti-DNA antibodies performed by radioimmunoassay in two separate laboratories.

The above case is of interest first, concerning the accuracy of the clinical diagnosis of SLE, and second, regarding the absence of serological findings that are usually considered necessary for the diagnosis of SLE. The clinical constellation—namely, thrombocytopenia of such severity as to require splenectomy, rash, polyarthralgia, and alopecia—is adequate for the diagnosis of SLE according to the ARA criteria; indeed, it is difficult to visualize any disease other than SLE that could account for this symptomatology. Although absence of antinuclear antibodies is exceptional in SLE, the LE cell preparation is frequently negative. Technical difficulties probably account for many instances of negative LE cell preparations; but no such excuse can be offered to explain failure to demonstrate antinuclear antibodies; on the contrary, the main problem with the ANA test system is the frequency of false-positive findings. An interesting case, reported by Salisbury and coworkers [598], was in a woman who had the combination of polyarthritis, Raynaud's phenomenon, and hemolytic anemia. Repeated LE cell preparations gave negative results. It was only when symptoms and signs of acute viral hepatitis developed, with hepatitis-associated antigen in her serum, that the LE cell preparation became positive and antibodies appeared for the first time, to native double-stranded DNA. Concurrently, antibodies developed which reacted with synthetic double-stranded RNA (poly I-poly C). As her hepatitis resolved, the LE cell preparation reverted to negative, and the titers of antibodies to RNA and DNA gradually declined to within normal ranges. Some time later, she had tuberculous meningitis and the LE cell preparation once more became positive.

We currently conceptualize the serological abnormalities as having major significance in the pathogenesis of the clinical features of SLE; under contemporary theory it is difficult to account for those cases in which the clinical picture is consistent with SLE but the serological abnormalities are persistently absent. On the other hand, we frequently see patients whose early clinical manifestations are consistent with SLE but in whom LE cell preparations and tests for ANA become positive only later in the course of the illness. In this connection, discoid LE is of interest because, although it is probably a limited form of the wider syndrome (see Table 10-3 and References 161, 256), the majority of patients with discoid LE have negative LE cell preparations, negative responses to tests for ANA, and negative titers of antibodies to DNA [443]. Three (4.7 per cent) of the 64 patients in this series who had criteria adequate for the diagnosis of definite SLE had test results negative for both ANA and LE cells. A report by Harbeck and coworkers [287] indicated that DNA binding by sera from some patients without lupus nephritis was higher than by sera from some patients with active lupus nephritis, and that certain patients with active lupus nephritis had normal C3 levels and no evidence of circulating DNA:anti-DNA complexes. The above considerations lead to the question, whether the presence of ANA and LE cells ought any longer to be held as *sine qua non* for the diagnosis of SLE.

PATTERNS OF SLE

The picture that develops from this study of idiopathic SLE as it exists in the community is of a common disease that has a relatively benign, long-term course. Besides the violent, quickly lethal mode from which the illness derives its evil reputation are patterns characterized by one or a few brief episodes, by an intermittently stuttering course, or by benign chronicity. The following experience illustrates a single, brief episode of SLE, without any further activity of the disease during lengthy follow-up:

Case 10-7. A 60-year-old white woman had been followed at this clinic for 4 years, during which the only significant abnormalities, noted by several observers, were hostility and bizarre behavior. She then had pleuritic chest pain and radiological evidence of a pleural effusion. Fifteen days later she complained of pain in both ankle joints, which were observed to be swollen. The only other significant sign was longstanding sunsensitivity. The erythrocyte sedimentation rate was 101 mm/hr (Westergren) and LE cell preparations were positive on two occasions. Treatment with prednisone was followed by complete remission of all manifestations. During the next 10 years there were no manifestations of SLE, but she took up to 5 mg of prednisone daily. Ten years after the acute episode, antinuclear antibodies were absent from the serum. Prednisone was then stopped, and during the following 4 years the patient remained perfectly well.

Of further interest in this case was the family history of cutaneous lupus in one sister and crippling arthritis in another, rheumatoid arthritis in one brother and Bright's disease in another.

The intermittently stuttering course that may be seen in SLE is exemplified by the following case:

Case 10-8. A white woman, born in 1914, received her medical care at our clinic and hospital from 1955 until her death from arteriosclerotic heart disease in 1972. In 1956, she was first observed to have the skin changes of lupus erythematosus over the hands and face. At about the same time, an erosion approximately 2 cm in diameter was seen in the buccal mucosa; she told of a similar erosion that had been present 4 years previously. Biopsy of the new erosion showed a heavy, band-like infiltrate of chronic inflammatory cells pressed against the surface of the lining epithelium. The rash extended and during the next 14 years she was seen on many occasions by four different dermatologists, each of whom concurred with the diagnosis of discoid lupus erythematosus. In 1959, she complained of pleuritic pain in the right side of the chest, which lasted for approximately 2½ weeks. Shortly after its cessation, she had pain briefly in the left shoulder. White blood cell counts were below 4,000/cu mm in 1955, and again in 1956 and 1957, on the later two occasions associated with negative LE cell preparations. The results of tests for ANA were negative in 1970, and positive in 1971 with an accompanying negative LE cell preparation. In 1964 a hematocrit reading was 30 per cent while the red blood cells were normochromic and normocytic; the serum iron level was 103 μg/100 ml. The patient died of myocardial infarction in April 1972.

One may classify the above case as systemic lupus erythematosus: the presence of cutaneous LE, leukopenia, recurrent stomatitis, pleuritic chest pain, joint pain, and an anemia that was possibly hemolytic, together provide sufficient criteria to place it in this category. Although from the clinical viewpoint it clearly represents almost pure discoid LE, the complete medical record, compiled over 17 years, demonstrates that on occasions widely separated in time there were several transitory manifestations of the systemic syndrome. Without the benefit of the complete medical record, this would undoubtedly have been labeled a case of pure discoid LE.

The benign, chronic form of the disease was seen in the following case:

Case 10-9. A black woman was first seen at age 35 years with a 17-year history of recurrent arthralgia that had affected most joints of the body, some of which had been swollen and warm. For the previous year she had had polymyalgia, and for a few months Raynaud's phonomenon with the stages of both pallor and cyanosis. Physical examination revealed striking weakness of the muscles of the shoulder and pelvic girdles. Muscle biopsy revealed marked variation of muscle fiber size together with an interstitial inflammatory infiltrate. The diagnosis of SLE was confirmed by the finding of a persistent leukopenia, the white blood cell count varying between 2,000 and 3,000/cu mm; and positive LE cell preparations.

During the next 7 years the polymyositis aspect persisted, as shown by varying degrees of muscle weakness and elevation of serum enzyme levels. In addition, there were frequent episodes of both pericarditis and pleuritis; the pleural friction rubs tended to be chronic and were heard for long periods. The roentgenographic appearances of diffuse interstitial fibrosis developed in the lung. A further interesting feature was recurrent, bilateral, acute parotitis. After 7 years of follow-up, the patient had hypocomplementemia, and mild chronic hemolytic anemia which required prednisone for control; but she was functioning reasonably well despite approximately 25 years of presumptively active SLE.

PREGNANCY AND SLE

A question frequently posed by both patient and doctor is whether pregnancy is contraindicated in the presence of SLE. Garsenstein, Pollak, and Kark [235] studied 21 patients in 33 pregnancies. Exacerbations of SLE were especially common during the first 8 postpartum weeks, being seven times as frequent then as in control periods in the same patients. Four of the 21 patients died, all of the four having severe renal involvement. However, the mortality rate during pregnancy was one death per 520 patient weeks of observation; whereas there was one death per 207 patient weeks of observation in nonpregnant women. This suggests that pregnancy does not cause an increase in the death rate from

SLE, despite an increased rate of exacerbation of the disease. Moreover, among women with lupus nephritis, the number of deaths during pregnancy was not greater than during the nonpregnant state. Estes and Larson [182] similarly concluded that pregnancy does not alter the course of SLE in the majority of cases. An interesting study by Siegel and coworkers [627] showed that the survival rates of women with SLE were lowest among the nonpregnant and highest among those who had had two or more pregnancies. This observation remains unexplained, but suggests that those who are able to conceive and maintain pregnancy may have less severe disease than those who are unable; alternatively, gestation may in some way contribute to survivorship.

OVERLAP BETWEEN LUPUS AND RHEUMATOID ARTHRITIS

Within the framework of our present understanding of the pathogenesis of lupus and rheumatoid arthritis, it is difficult to account for the occurrence of the two diseases in the same individual. Patients in whom the two conditions coexist are important because they suggest that SLE and rheumatoid arthritis are the poles of a similar underlying disease, in the same way that lepromatous and tuberculoid leprosy are polar forms of the same disease.

Case 10-10. At age 35, a white woman had skin lesions on fingers and toes that comprised a mixture of large bullae, erythema, scaling, and ulceration. The white blood cell count was 2,400/cu mm and she was mildly anemic, with hematocrit reading of 34 per cent. An LE cell preparation was negative on three occasions, and a test for rheumatoid factor was positive. A dermatologic consultant considered that the skin lesions were typical for lupus erythematosus; they cleared gradually during the next year. Three years later an inflammatory polyarthritis appeared, and at this time there were numerous hematoxylin bodies and rosettes in the LE cell preparation, but no classic LE cells were seen. Antinuclear antibodies were present. During the next 4 years her illness was dominantly one of arthritis. A nodule appeared over the right elbow; this was removed and histopathologic examination showed the appearances of a typical rheumatoid nodule. X-rays at this time showed severe erosive changes at the proximal interphalangeal joints with lesser changes at the metacarpal phalangeal joints (Fig. 10-5). Rheumatoid factor was still present in her serum; antinuclear antibodies were present, and antithyroid antibodies were present to a titer of 1:10.

OVERLAP BETWEEN SLE AND OTHER SYSTEMIC RHEUMATIC DISEASES

A subcategory of patients with SLE isolated by Sharp and coworkers [622] has been labeled by them as having "mixed connective tissue disease." The dominant clinical characteristics of this subcategory include arthritis or arthralgia, swelling of the hands reminiscent of scleroderma, Raynaud's phenomenon, myositis, lymphadenopathy, and hypergammaglobulinemia. Noteworthily, renal disease is absent. The characteristic laboratory finding is

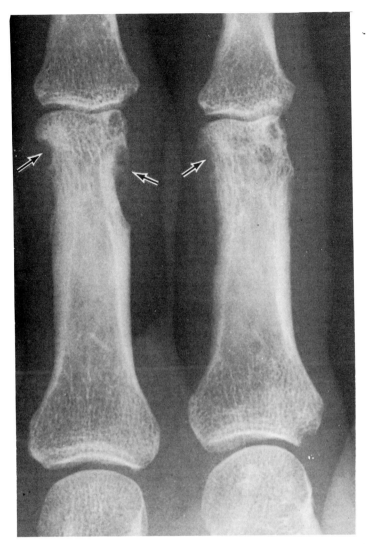

Fig. 10-5. Case 10-10. Systemic lupus erythematosus with erosions at second and third proximal interphalangeal joints, left hand.

serum antibodies directed against extractable nuclear antigen (ENA). This antibody is found in the serum of about 50 per cent of patients with active or inactive SLE; but Sharp and colleagues [622] found it in only two subjects among 407 controls, including 36 patients with rheumatoid arthritis, 25 with scleroderma, 12 with polymyositis, and 42 with other rheumatic diseases. In patients with mixed connective tissue disease, the serum antibody to ENA was eliminated by treatment with RNase; whereas it was unchanged by RNase in patients with SLE. Five of 25 patients with mixed connective tissue disease had positive LE cell preparations. The patients of this subcategory had an excellent response to corticosteroid therapy, and the prognosis appeared to be favorable.

A good example of mixed connective tissue disease was seen in the following woman.

Case 10-11. At age 40 years, a woman was first reported to show a weakly positive reaction to the VDRL test; the response persisted on sporadic testing over subsequent years. That the reaction was a biologically false positive one (BFP) was demonstrated on a later occasion by a negative response to the fluorescent treponema antibody test. Mild hypertension was first noted at age 45. Between the ages of 51 and 53, keratoconjunctivitis sicca developed, with excessive hair fall and generalized inflammatory polyarthritis. She was anemic, with a hematocrit reading in the region of 32 per cent. During the next 2 years her main difficulties were the widespread inflammatory polyarthritis, severe dryness of the eyes and mouth, chronic fatigue, severe vasospastic symptoms in the hands with digital ulcerations, and transitory myopathy as shown by myalgia and proximal muscle weakness. In addition, dyspnea developed, and evidence of interstitial pneumonitis. Pertinent laboratory findings included total serum proteins of 12.3 g/100 ml, of which 50.5 per cent was γ-globulin. Most of the increase in γ-globulin was accounted for by IgG: 5,370 mg/100 ml. Rheumatoid factor and antinuclear antibodies were present; anti-DNA antibodies were not. Anti-ENA titer exceeded 1:100,000. Chest x-ray showed mild pulmonary fibrosis. Pulmonary function tests revealed reduction of all volumes and of diffusing capacity, indicating severe restrictive lung disease and loss of alveolar capillary bed.

It remains to be seen, whether the presence of antibodies to extractable nuclear antigens defines a separate disease, as suggested by Sharp and coworkers [622]. One frequently encounters patients whose clinical features are those of several collagen diseases; antibodies to ENA are not always found in such people. I prefer to categorize these individuals as having "systemic rheumatic disease"; from the clinician's viewpoint the label is less important than knowledge of the component parts of the multisystem involvement. A case in point follows.

Case 10-12. A 53-year-old man had intermittent claudication, shown angiographically to be caused by atherosclerotic obstruction of the iliac arteries. He was allergic to penicillin, but had taken griseofulvin orally for onychomycosis continuously during the previous 10 years. Aorto-iliac endarterectomy and aortofemoral graft were performed. Postoperatively there developed fever and an infiltrate of the left lung. He was given three doses of cephalothin and then cephaloridine for 3 days. Four weeks after the operation he had pain in the knees; later, he had pain in the wrists and proximal interphalangeal joints. During the next couple of weeks, effusions appeared in the proximal interphalangeal joints, metacarpophalangeal joints, and one knee. At this time herpes zoster occurred over the right shoulder and right arm. Several small exudates were observed in his optic fundi. The erythrocyte sedimentation rate was 100 mm/hr (Westergren); peripheral leukocytes were 8 per cent eosinophils; serum protein was 25 per cent γ-globulin; IgG 1,800 mg/100 ml (normal, <1,500), IgA 270 mg/100 ml (normal, <250), IgM 270 mg/100 ml (normal, <150). Test results were positive for rheumatoid factor, negative for ANA, weakly positive for cold agglutinins (1:64). Serum complement (C3) level was normal. Muscle biopsy (Fig. 10-6) showed degenerative changes in the muscle fibers and intense foci of plasma cells, which were, for the most part, accumulated in a perivascular distribution.

During the next 8 months there developed cutaneous infarcts at his fingertips, skin ulcers in various sites, and proximal weakness in all four limbs; creatine phosphokinase was 1,100 U/100 ml, and response to the test for cryoglobulins became positive. Australia antigen was not found in the serum.

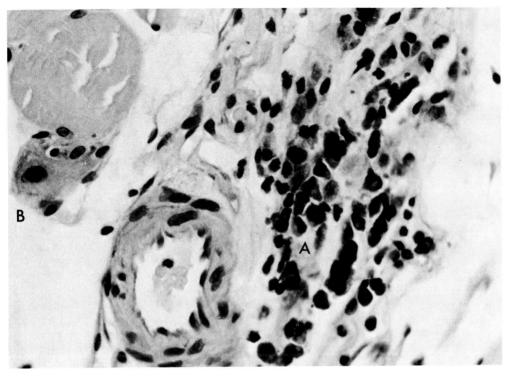

Fig. 10-6. Case 10-12. Mixed connective tissue disease. Muscle biopsy showing interstitial infiltrate of mainly plasma cells (A), and myopathic reaction (B) with proliferation and central migration of sarcolemmal nuclei.

Clinical improvement followed treatment with azathioprine and prednisone. Multiple premature ventricular contractions then occurred, and electrocardiogram showed evidence of bilateral partial bundle branch block. The cardiac arrhythmia was abolished by increasing the dose of prednisone. During the next 2 years the major systemic features of his illness gradually subsided and he was left with chronic joint pain and a nonspecific rash. When he was last seen, his main complaints were of polyarthralgia and Raynaud's phenomenon; he required 15 mg of prednisone daily to control his arthralgia. Response to test for ANA was positive for the first time; antibodies to ENA were, however, absent.

OVERLAP BETWEEN LUPUS AND LYMPHOMA

The picture of SLE as it appears in New Zealand black (NZB) mice is interesting because it bears close similarity to the disease in humans. Female mice are more frequently affected than males; there is a Coombs'-positive hemolytic anemia; various autoantibodies appear in the blood, and a glomerulonephritis develops that has all the characteristics of glomerulonephritis of human SLE [316]. The genetic predisposition is much more clearly defined in the murine than in the human disease; another difference is the very high rate of occurrence of malignant lymphoma, in approximately 20 per cent of the diseased mice [466]. Virus-like particles are found in various tissues in the mouse suffering from spontaneous SLE, just as in the human condition; similar particles are seen within the cells of the lymphoma tissue, and the lymphoma may be transmitted to other mice by means of cell-free filtrates. Although autoimmune phenomena, e.g., Coombs'-positive hemolytic anemia, are well-known accompaniments of malignant lymphoma in man, the appearance of malignant lymphoma in patients with collagen diseases is rather uncommon, and is certainly rare by contrast with its high frequency in NZB mice. One of our 64 patients with SLE is therefore of considerable interest because of the almost concurrent appearance in her of SLE and malignant lymphoma.

Case 10-13. A black girl born in 1955 was well until 1969, when two-phase Raynaud's phenomenon appeared. There were no further symptoms until 1972; polyarthralgia then developed and, at the end of that year, the first episode of what was to be recurrent pericarditis with central chest pain and consistent electrocardiographic changes. When hospitalized early in 1973, the patient was found to have Coombs'-positive hemolytic anemia, strongly positive response to test for antinuclear antibodies, negative LE cell preparations but hematoxylin bodies in the preparations, and a persistent pericardial friction rub. Chest x-ray showed an increase of the transverse cardiac diameter from 11 cm to 12.5 cm; this contrasted with the examination of 4 months previously, and was considered to represent pericardial effusion. In addition, there was a well-defined density adjacent to the right border of the heart, considered at the time to represent either a loculated pleural effusion or a pericardial cyst which communicated with the pericardial cavity. It was decided to observe the patient; but because the mass seen in the chest x-ray did not change, biopsy was performed approximately 6 months later and showed the cellular pattern of lymphocyte-depleted type of Hodgkin's disease, with malignant histiocytes, only a scattering of lymphocytes, and numerous classic Reed-Sternberg cells. At this time, the serum C4 level was only 12.0 mg/100 ml (normal, >25 mg/100 ml), and radioimmunoassay showed antibodies to DNA at 324 counts per minute (normal, <150 cpm).

The following patient is another who provides an example of the overlap between diseases of disturbed immunity or autoimmunity, and malignant lymphoproliferation.

Case 10-14. A man first seen at age 71 for complaints of fever, severe fatigue, polyarthralgia, polymyalgia, and a generalized papular rash with petechiae had enlargement of lymph nodes, liver, and spleen. Aside from a white blood count of only 3,500/cu mm, all laboratory studies, including bone marrow examination, were unrevealing. The episode cleared within 2 weeks and he remained well for the next 4 years. He then complained of dizziness, and impairment of vibration sensation and abnormal cerebellar signs were found in the legs. Extensive laboratory testing did not reveal the cause of these findings. One year later a cervical lymph node enlarged and was removed. Microscopic examination showed that it was so full of plasma cells as to suggest the possibility of myeloma. Serum protein electrophoresis, however, showed profound diminution of γ-globulin without monoclonal spike; and quantification of immunoglobulins showed a global decrease: IgG was only 280 mg/100 ml, IgA only 20 mg/100 ml. The bone marrow now showed a quantitative increase in eosinophils and reticulum cells without other abnormalities.

During the next year, thrombophlebitis, peripheral neuropathy, and generalized lymphadenopathy developed. There were progressive signs of a tumor at the cerebellopontine angle. In the cerebrospinal fluid, the total protein level was normal (17 mg/100 m), but the γ-globulin percentage was excessive, at 25 per cent. Severe leukopenia and anemia appeared, response to Coombs' test became positive, and there were signs of polymyositis. The patient died. Autopsy demonstrated diffuse enlargement of lymph nodes, found histopathologically to be from malignant lymphoma. The muscles showed myopathic changes. There was an acoustic neuroma which contained many foamy cells and no primary neuroma cells. There were demyelination of the posterior columns of the spinal cord, mild loss of Purkinje cells and gliosis of Bergman cells in the cerebellum, and marked demyelination of the peripheral nerves.

It is of considerable interest that this patient's eldest son showed abnormally low IgM, at 30 mg/100 ml; his IgG was borderline, at 790 mg/100 ml. This suggests the possibility that the basis of the patient's illness was an inherited disorder of the immune system.

OVERLAPS BETWEEN COLLAGEN DISEASES, LYMPHOMAS, AND DISORDERED IMMUNITY

The fact that an association, seemingly more than chance, exists between collagen diseases and lymphomas and between each of these nosologic categories and disordered immunity suggests the possibility of common pathogenesis. This possibility may be of heuristic value in unravelling ultimate causation of these illnesses: Fudenberg [229] postulated that somatic mutation of lymphoid cells, rendering them antigenically deficient, could induce in effect a graft within the host; and that the ensuing graft-versus-host reaction might be responsible for the polyarthritis, nephritis, and hemolytic anemia seen in autoimmune diseases. Whatever the final explanation of causation may be, a more immediate implication for the rheumatologist is that all of the collagen diseases share similar pathogenetic events; therefore, one should not insist too rigidly upon separation of these entities. Further, the questions should be posed, why one particular collagen disease develops rather than another—why rheumatoid arthritis rather than systemic lupus; why the patient with apparently established rheumatoid arthritis suddenly develops SLE; why the rarer reversal of SLE into localized rheumatoid arthritis; why the great rarity of the overlap between SLE and scleroderma? These issues seem more susceptible of solution by clinical than by laboratory observations; therefore, patients having these overlapping syndromes warrant most careful study.

THE DIATHESIS TO LE REACTIONS

In addition to patients with chronic discoid LE, groups of persons with several other conditions or symptoms might potentially swell the ranks of those with strong liability to SLE. High on the list would be those with idiopathic thrombocytopenia [346], with chronic biologically false positive serologic reactions for syphilis [292], or with hypertension. The question of hypertension as an antecedent of SLE was discussed by Alarcón-Segovia and coworkers [12], who studied 50 patients with hydralazine-induced SLE. Manifestations possibly indicative of a lupus diathesis were found in the past histories, or in previous clinical or laboratory data, of 37 (74 per cent) of the 50 patients but in only 13 of 100 hypertensive control patients. Indications of lupus diathesis included a past history of arthritis (22 per cent), arthralgia (10 per cent), myalgia (2 per cent), unexplained leukopenia (14 per cent), pleuritic pain (10 per cent), epilepsy (4 per cent), or false positive serologic reaction for syphilis (2 per cent). A family history of inflammatory rheumatic disease or possibly related conditions was found in 23 (46 per cent) of the 50 patients with hydralazine syndrome but in only eight of the 100 hypertensive controls. For 35 patients, follow-up data were available regarding the course of the syndrome after discontinuation of hydralazine therapy for an average of 4½ years. One or more clinical or laboratory manifestations of a state similar to LE persisted in 24 of the 35 patients. These manifestations included arthritis in seven, skin rash in six, pleuritis in three, fever in two; positive LE factor in nine, leukopenia in six, and anemia in two patients. Contrary to other reports, these workers saw renal manifestations in a significant proportion of patients with the hydralazine syndrome. They attributed the renal manifestations to the hydralazine reactions, not to the hypertension, because they subsided or disappeared on withdrawal of the drug. Alarcón-Segovia and his coworkers made the provocative suggestion that, since the hydralazine syndrome develops in between 8 per cent and 13 per cent of hypertensive patients treated with large doses of this drug, it is conceivable that the lupus diathesis is present in a similar percentage of all hypertensive patients [12].

Possibly relevant to the excess frequency of SLE in the black population is a study of mean white blood cell counts in 86,488 ambulatory patients who had multiphasic examinations as part of the Kaiser-Permanente Medical Care Program [222]. The lower limit of normal (2 standard deviations below the mean) for the leukocyte count in nonsmoking white women was 4,000/cu mm; in nonsmoking black women it was 3,200/cu mm. Even for the black women who smoked, the lower limit of normal was 3,400/cu mm. Although the antecedents for the leukopenia in the normal black female population are quite unknown, its existence corroborates the tendency to an excess of SLE in this segment of the population.

While it is natural to postulate genetic factors as contributing to the excessive frequency of SLE in black people, it is noteworthy that the occurrence of proved lupus in blood relatives of the patients in this series (aunts, mothers, daughters, or sisters) was only about 6.3 per cent. This figure is stated as approximate because two of the five relatives with lupus (mother and daughter) are each included in the 64 cases of definite SLE, so that the figure for familial prevalence could be given as five in 64 (7.8 per cent). Among these five relatives with lupus, four had SLE and one had chronic discoid LE. Only one of the five patients with SLE who had one or more relatives affected by lupus was black: this suggests no increased genetic influence in black people. The rarity of SLE in identical twins [55] further attests to the weakness of the genetic element in pathogenesis.

An obviously genetically determined factor that influences the emergence of lupus is the female sex. Table 10-2 shows that with increasing numbers of criteria for diagnosis of SLE, there is an increasing percentage of women. Although the figures did not reach statistical significance, the numbers were small, and the tendency suggests the possibility that being male protects against the fullblown systemic disorder even when the diathesis exists. The observation of histocompatibility antigens associated with SLE supports the possibility of a genetic contribution to the susceptibility for the disease. Grumet and coworkers [269] tested 40 patients and found the W15 antigen in 40 per cent, but in only 10 per cent of controls (p<0.005), and the HL-A8 antigen in 33 per cent of patients with SLE but in only 16 per cent of controls (p<0.025).

ROLE OF DRUGS, FOOD ADDITIVES, AND COSMETICS

Approximately 25 drugs have been reported as capable of causing positive LE cell preparations (Table 10-6). Only a few of these medicines, procainamide, hydralazine, diphenylhydantoin, and isoniazid, cause an LE syndrome with any frequency; the case reports of LE reactions associated with use of the other drugs in Table 10-6 are either very sparse or show only a tenuous relation between the

Table 10-6. Drugs Capable of Causing Positive LE Cell Preparations or SLE Syndrome (after Young et al [733]); the Number of Prescriptions for Each Drug Filled in an Outpatient Pharmacy and the Number of Patients Taking Each Drug, During a 6-Month Period*

	Prescriptions	Patients
Acetazolamide	279	122
Aminosalicylic acid	6	5
Chlorothiazide	1,504	971
Diphenylhydantoin	538	274
Ethosuximide	19	10
Griseofulvin	232	144
Hydantoins	0	0
Hydralazine	268	107
Isoniazid	286	157
Methyldopa	724	269
Oral contraceptives	4,313	2,507
Oxyphenisatin	6	2
Penicillin	2,577	2,109
Phenolphthalein	2	1
Phenylbutazone	691	557
Primidone	66	33
Procainamide	174	71
Propylthiouracil	100	41
Streptomycin	1	1
Sulfonamides	2,623	2,049
Tetracycline	231	179
Trimethadione	1	1
Totals	14,641	9,610

* Data based upon 145,263 separate prescriptions dispensed for 43,365 patients in a clinic that serves approximately 126,000 health plan members.

Table 10-7. Drug-use by a Population of 69,122 Adults. Percentages of Persons, by Decade of Life, Answering Yes

Age (years) Total number	Women						Men					
	20–29 6859	30–39 7028	40–49 9545	50–59 8349	60–69 4929	70+ 1341	20–29 4265	30–39 6813	40–49 8164	50–59 6800	60–69 3765	70+ 1264
	%	%	%	%	%	%	%	%	%	%	%	%
In the past *year* have you taken *any*:												
Asthma medicine, sprays or injections?	2.2	3.2	2.8	2.7	2.2	1.9	3.5	2.9	2.5	2.1	2.4	2.7
Codeine, morphine, Darvon, Percodan, or Demerol?	15.4	12.1	10.4	9.6	6.8	5.8	7.5	6.6	5.3	5.3	4.2	2.5
Cortisone type medicine?	3.3	3.9	6.2	7.5	6.9	7.2	2.6	4.0	4.9	6.5	5.6	4.0
Dicumarol, Coumadin or blood thinning pills?	0.1	0.1	0.2	0.4	0.7	0.8	<0.1	0.2	0.4	1.1	1.5	2.1
Digitalis or heart medicine?	0.1	0.3	0.6	0.1	4.6	8.6	<0.1	0.4	0.8	2.7	5.6	9.5
High blood pressure medicine?	0.5	1.2	3.4	8.4	14.3	21.0	0.4	0.9	3.4	7.1	10.6	12.0
Reducing medicine to try to lose weight?	16.4	15.8	15.7	12.2	7.9	3.6	3.4	3.9	3.2	2.3	1.6	1.1
Shots or pills to lose water from your body?	9.0	12.8	14.9	12.0	9.2	10.7	0.5	0.8	1.3	2.3	3.1	3.6
Hormones?	16.0	10.9	18.1	25.0	10.4	6.6	0.6	0.6	0.9	1.5	2.0	2.4
Insulin or diabetes pills?	0.4	0.2	0.7	1.1	18.7	1.8	0.3	0.4	0.9	2.4	3.0	3.4
Iron or anemia medicine?	17.0	14.8	13.8	9.1	7.0	9.5	2.8	2.7	3.1	3.5	4.0	3.7
Penicillin or other antibiotics?	29.5	22.8	17.2	15.4	12.8	7.8	21.9	19.0	14.0	11.9	10.5	6.7
Sulfa drugs?	9.5	7.7	6.7	5.9	5.7	3.9	3.3	0.4	4.0	4.3	3.7	3.7
Thyroid medicine?	7.4	9.9	10.6	11.6	10.5	8.8	1.1	1.7	2.2	2.7	2.9	2.1
Any of above?	66.2	62.2	61.4	61.8	55.1	56.9	35.8	34.5	32.3	36.7	39.5	39.1
In the past *year* have you *often* taken any:												
Antihistamines or allergy medicine?	8.0	10.8	10.8	8.4	7.4	4.2	6.9	8.7	8.1	6.4	5.4	2.4
Aspirin, Empirin, Anacin, Bufferin, etc.?	1.3	1.4	2.2	3.0	4.0	4.0	0.5	0.7	1.1	1.6	2.4	2.2
Benzedrine or dexedrine?	2.6	2.9	3.2	2.2	1.7	0.9	1.7	1.1	0.8	0.8	0.7	0.7
Phenobarbital or barbiturates?	2.4	3.8	6.4	9.4	11.9	15.2	1.4	1.9	3.3	5.0	6.1	5.9
Pain medicine?	10.1	11.7	13.7	15.3	15.9	17.4	6.3	7.5	8.3	10.3	11.4	12.0
Sleeping pills?	2.6	3.8	5.9	8.5	12.7	15.4	1.4	2.7	3.6	6.0	7.7	9.7

Stomach or digestion medicine?	8.2	10.0	12.8	15.2	17.4	16.8	9.8	13.3	15.3	15.5	13.4	14.6
Tranquilizers?	6.8	11.0	13.7	13.4	12.4	10.5	3.2	5.2	6.8	7.6	6.3	4.2
Any of above?	28.9	34.9	40.2	43.0	44.7	45.9	23.7	28.8	32.1	34.4	34.0	33.1
In the past *6 months*, have you *often* taken any:												
Cough medicine?	2.8	2.9	2.9	3.5	4.6	6.0	1.8	2.0	2.4	3.1	5.3	7.0
Laxatives or cathartics?	4.8	5.9	8.0	12.9	16.9	22.6	1.3	2.0	2.5	4.0	7.7	13.2

use of the drug and the emergence of LE. Nevertheless, the length of the list and the number of the incriminated medicines that are commonly prescribed draw attention to the strong possibility that drugs may be chief offenders among the environmental agents that cause LE reactions.

The magnitude of the problem is shown by the huge numbers of drugs prescribed in our society. During the 6-month period, July 1 to December 31, 1969, 145,263 separate prescriptions were filled in our outpatient pharmacy for 43,365 patients among our closed population of approximately 126,000 Health Plan members (Table 10-1). Our information suggests that about 20 per cent further prescriptions dispensed to Health Plan members were filled at other pharmacies. Table 10-6 shows the numbers of these dispensed medicines that have been incriminated as capable of causing a positive LE cell test response or actual lupus syndrome. It is astonishing that 14,641 (10.1 per cent) of all prescriptions dispensed were for medicines listed in Table 10-6, and that drugs of these categories were taken by 9,610 (22.2 per cent) of the total group of 43,365 patients. These figures do not include drugs dispensed to hospitalized patients! The drugs that are considered the most important as causing an SLE reaction, i.e., diphenylhydantoin, hydralazine, isoniazid, and procaine amide, accounted for 1,266 (0.9 per cent) of all prescriptions and were taken by 609 (1.4 per cent) of all patients receiving medicines. Sulfonamides, which are notorious causes of hypersensitivity, comprised 2,623 (1.8 per cent) of all prescriptions and were taken by 2,040 (4.7 per cent) of all patients receiving medicines. In their analysis of 1,193 cases of SLE, Lee and coworkers [405] concluded that drugs may have caused or activated the disease in as many as 12 per cent of the patients.

The figures in Table 10-7 should convince any reader who finds the data in Table 10-6 incredible, that ours is a society permeated by medicines. The data in Table 10-7 are derived from a self-administered questionnaire that was answered by 69,122 persons in the San Francisco Bay Area as part of a multiphasic health check taken between the years 1964 and 1968. The percentages listed indicate the proportions of positive answers to questions about use of those medicines listed in the left-hand column of the Table. In all decades of adult life, the high percentages of women and of men taking medicines is a source of both astonishment and consternation. As examples, among women aged 20-29 years, 9.5 per cent had taken sulfonamides during the previous year, 29.5 per cent had taken antibiotics, 16.4 per cent had taken reducing medicine to try to lose weight; 6.8 per cent had often taken tranquillizing drugs, and 2.4 per cent phenobarbital or barbiturates. Laxatives or cathartics were often taken during the previous six months by 4.8 per cent of women aged 20-29; and this percentage, like most of the others in the Table, increased with each decade of age.

Oxyphenisatin was shown to cause lupoid hepatitis in a convincing report by Reynolds, Peters, and Yamada [574]. Their observation is remarkably important because oxyphenisatin was a constituent of several widely used laxatives; moreover, the compound has been said to be the laxative ingredient of prunes, although Reynolds and coworkers [574] could find no definitive reports to prove this point. The urgent need for further studies along these lines to elicit antecedents of idiopathic SLE, e.g., proprietary medicines, cosmetics, food additives, etc., is stressed by the inference drawn by Reynolds and coworkers [574], that autoimmunity may not always be a factor in the perpetuation of lupoid hepatitis since their patients had marked improvement, without recrudescences, after stopping the oxyphenisatin. The potential importance of this observation for the management of patients with idiopathic SLE is obvious.

The enormous potential of food additives as causes of chronic hypersensitivity disorders has been discussed by Feingold [191], who calculated that more than 2,700 individual items are intentionally added to food; these include more than 1,600 synthetic flavorings, more than 30 different colors, plus preservatives, antioxidants, surface active agents, enzymes, etc. An unintentional food additive is penicillin, which is used both for prophylaxis and treatment of the udders of cattle; cows may be given huge quantities of penicillin by intramuscular injection every couple of weeks, and the drug is excreted into the milk. In studies of large groups of patients, it was found that 6.6 per cent of people gave a history of penicillin sensitivity, that an actual reaction to penicillin was observed in as many as 1.0 per cent of persons to whom this drug was administered, and that 0.87 per cent of patients who supposedly had never previously received penicillin experienced a penicillin reaction after having been given this medicine [594]. An important possibility exists that milk or its products contain residual penicillin and may thereby initiate or perpetuate a disease of chronic hypersensitivity.

The preponderance of women in groups of patients with SLE makes one wonder about the role of cosmetics in pathogenesis. By an industry count, 20 million women in the United States dye their hair [652]. Paraphenylene-diamine or one of its derivatives is the main dye used for the hair. Semipermanent dyes, which account for the greatest volume of sales in hair colorants, give colors that persist over six to ten shampoos before washing out. Such dyes are made with materials that have color in their own right; they are small molecules such as nitrophenylenediamines and nitroaminophenols, which penetrate the hair under mild conditions. Permanent hair colorants are based almost exclusively on oxidation dyes, the best known of which are p-phenylenediamine and p-toluylene-diamine. Geschickter and coworkers [242] applied n, n-dimethyl-p-phenylene-diamine in a 2 per cent oily solution, by repeated daily brushings to the shaved skin of rats. A variety of focal lesions resembling those seen in the collagen diseases was induced, including Aschoff-like bodies, rheumatoid nodules, capillary platelet thrombi, wire loops in the glomeruli, and focal fibrinoid degeneration. The dye commonly used in lipstick is eosin, which dyes tissues by binding to proteins. Burry [79] asked, "What happens to all that lipstick licked off all those lips?". Most of the eosin from the lipstick would be swallowed and, presumably, absorbed from the gastrointestinal tract.

In addition to using cosmetics, women differ from men by undertaking most of the household chores, including the domestic clothes' washing. Modern washing powders contain enzymes that are derived from bacteria. The enzymes are, of course, proteins and have been responsible for allergic manifestations [37]. It is very likely that traces of these enzymes remain in the washed clothes, from which they may be absorbed through the skin into the body of the wearer. Not only are traces of enzymes contiguous to the skin, but many modern clothing fabrics contain polymer fibers of one sort or another, and all of these so-called "polymers" contain traces of monomers, dimers, trimers, etc., which may potentially be absorbed via the skin. One wonders about the toxic potential of these monomers and dimers in view of the known hazards of the monomer vinyl chloride (See Chapter 12). The artificial fibers themselves contain light stabilizers, surfactants, enzymes, and additives used in the process of polymerization, plus, of course, dyes: if these molecules are absorbed via the skin, it is conceivable that they might initiate a hypersensitivity reaction or trigger the alternative pathway for activation of complement.

VIRUS-INDUCED LUPUS REACTIONS

Lupoid hepatitis provides a link between drug-induced and virus-induced LE reactions, and indicates the likelihood that the LE reactions to various stimuli differ only in detail. Mackay [435] stated that the criteria for diagnosis of lupoid hepatitis include jaundice that relapses or continues for at least 6 months, positive responses to tests for antinuclear and smooth-muscle antibodies, sustained increases of SGOT beyond 100 units/100 ml, and of γ-globulin beyond 2.0 g/100 ml, and piecemeal necrosis with lymphocytic and plasmacytic infiltration. The term, "piecemeal necrosis," describes the widespread necrosis at the border between the liver parenchyma and portal tracts, where groups of damaged liver cells become isolated to form rosettes. The concept of lupoid hepatitis has proved controversial: one opinion holds that lupoid hepatitis is merely idiopathic SLE complicated by viral hepatitis; the other view considers lupoid hepatitis to be an entity separate from idiopathic SLE. These two ideas are reconciled by the notion that lupoid hepatitis and idiopathic SLE are each LE reactions to different stimuli. The close similarity in the broad detail of these reactions is indicated by the facts that in lupoid hepatitis, 80 per cent of the patients are female, arthritis affects 50 to 60 per cent of the patients, and various rashes simulate those of idiopathic SLE [435]. Among the 20 patients with lupoid hepatitis analyzed by Maclachlan and coworkers [437], 16 had polyarthritis or polyarthralgia, four had pleurisy, three had pericarditis, four had a facial rash, one had alopecia, two had convulsions, three had renal lesions, 13 had either anemia, leukopenia, or thrombocytopenia, and 14 had positive LE cell preparations.

Searches for viruses in human idiopathic SLE have been inspired by several observations: the occurrence of an LE reaction in viral hepatitis; the finding of cytoplasmic myxovirus-like structures in the electron micrographs of various tissues of patients with idiopathic SLE (vide infra); the observation that the New Zealand mice with SLE reaction harbor murine leukemia virus, produce antibody to it, develop positive Coombs' test reactions at a time when viral antigen is produced, and have a cumulative mortality rate that rises in phase with antibody production [467]; and the general concept that viruses might be the initiating factors of autoimmune disease.

Myxovirus-like tubular structures in the glomeruli of a patient with lupus nephritis were first reported by Fresco [220]; the observation was confirmed by Györkey and coworkers [275]. These structures are considered to be morphologically similar to strands of nucleoprotein liberated from myxoviruses. Kawano and coworkers [371] saw such structures in 28 of 260 renal biopsies; 25 of the 28 specimens came from patients with SLE, and in two of the remaining three the histologic findings were consistent with SLE. Hurd and coworkers [330] observed the tubular structures in all of 42 renal biopsies from 35 patients with SLE, five of whom had normal kidney tissue according to light microscopy; the virus-like structures were also seen in biopsy specimens from 24 of 113 patients with renal disease not associated with SLE. Further evidence that the occurrence of these structures is not specific for SLE or other collagen disease was their presence, found by synovial biopsy, in a patient with pigmented villonodular synovitis [484].

There are elevated levels of antibodies to various viral antigens in SLE. Hollinger and coworkers [315], examining sera from 31 patients with SLE, saw significantly higher than normal mean titers of antibodies to measles, rubella, parainfluenza types 2 and 3, and reovirus type 2; their conclusions that patients with SLE have an overall hyperreactivity to viral antigens was confirmed in similar studies by Hurd and coworkers [329]. There was no increase of mean antibody titer to Epstein-Barr virus [556]; and neither hepatitis-associated antigen (HAA) nor its antibody (anti-HAA) was detectable [536] in sera of patients with SLE. Enthusiasm for the idea that specific infection may play a direct role in the causation of SLE is further dampened by the negative results of attempts to culture viruses or Mycoplasmas from synovial membranes and other tissues, including some that showed tubular structures [193, 553].

CHAPTER 11

Muscle Reactions

Most general internists and many rheumatologists are unclear in their minds about some of the important clinical aspects of muscle disorders. This chapter briefly covers the muscle diseases that are seen in the course of rheumatological practice, with especial emphasis upon their diagnosis and differential diagnosis, and with mention of some rarer entities of which the rheumatologist should be aware. The chapter is organized as follows: 1) the clinical recognition that a myopathy exists, 2) laboratory confirmation of the suspected myopathy, 3) classification according to cause, 4) the work-up for the cause of the myopathy, 5) the general nonspecificity of the findings from muscle biopsy, 6) the special problem of idiopathic polymyositis, 7) experimental contributions to current understanding of the pathogenesis of muscle reactions, 8) interference with the normal balance of the cycle of degeneration-regeneration of muscle cells as a unifying concept for the causation of muscle reactions, 9) the contribution of immune mechanisms to the pathogenesis of idiopathic polymyositis.

CLINICAL RECOGNITION THAT A MYOPATHY EXISTS

The term *myopathy* is used for a muscle disorder that originates directly from an influence upon muscle fibers rather than indirectly via the nervous system. In essence, the term is used to exclude a neurogenic causation of the muscle reaction, which may thus have its roots either in a primary affection of the muscle fibers or in a systemic, non-neurologic disorder.

The symptoms that alert the clinician to the presence of a muscle disorder are weakness and pain; rarely, there may be dark urine from myoglobinuria. Weakness is almost always present. For reasons that are not satisfactorily explained, it is the proximal muscles of the body that are worst affected; therefore, the patient complains of weakness in such activities as ascending or descending stairs, arising from a low chair or from a bathtub, or combing the hair. Muscular pain occurs more often early than late in the course of muscle disease. It is important, but sometimes difficult, to differentiate pain that arises primarily in the muscles, from pain that is referred to the muscles from neighboring joints. For example, in polymyositis, the patient may complain of pain in the mid-arm; whereas in primary affections of the shoulder joint, the complaint is typically of pain in the shoulder which radiates to the mid-arm; only an occasional patient with primary shoulder disease complains of pain localized to the mid-arm.

Many statements have been made in the literature concerning the relative frequency of weakness versus pain in patients with polymyositis; the precise frequencies of these symptoms are of little relevance to the clinician, who should be aware that either or both symptoms may be present in the individual patient.

Dark urine from myoglobinuria is an extremely rare manifestation of polymyositis; it was not present in any of 45 patients (Table 11-1) with polymyositis that I have seen during the last 9 years, although myoglobinuria in trace amounts has been detected immunochemically quite frequently in patients with polymyositis [353].

It is important for the rheumatologist to practice testing muscle strength in as many normal persons as possible; only thus will he be able to appreciate deviations from the norm. There are no easy substitutes for manual muscle testing, although we have found the following method useful: the patient lies supine and the following times in seconds are measured: 1) the duration of his ability to hold the head elevated from the couch, and 2) the duration of his ability to hold the extended leg at approximately 45° to the horizontal. Finally, the patient attempts to arise from the supine position unaided by the arms, which may be folded or held forwards. The results of these tests in 300 subjects without known myopathy and in 30 with known myopathy are shown in Figure 11-1. Although the normal persons and myopathic patients were separated partially by the results of the individual maneuvers, they were more clearly differentiated when the basis of comparison was a subnormal performance in two or more of the three tests. Only 7.4 per cent of the normal subjects, but 92 per cent of the myopathic men and 82 per cent of the myopathic women had two or more abnormal test results [206]. We have found these maneuvers especially useful in monitoring the progress of the muscle disorder.

In addition, each individual muscle group must be tested manually and rated, usually from $\frac{1}{5}$ to $\frac{5}{5}$, where $\frac{5}{5}$ represents normal strength. Generally, the muscles that show weakness earliest in acquired muscle reactions are the

Table 11-1. Classification of 200 Patients with Myopathy

		Number	Per Cent
Dystrophies		23	11.5
Idiopathic polymyositis		45	22.5
Endocrinopathies		31	15.5
Hypothyroidism	18		
Diabetic amyotrophy	6		
Other	7		
Connective tissue disease		31	15.5
Systemic lupus erythematosus	13		
Polyarteritis	8		
Rheumatoid arthritis	7		
Scleroderma	3		
Polymyalgia rheumatica		27	13.5
Miscellaneous causes		28	14.0
Cancer		10	5.0
Alcohol		5	2.5

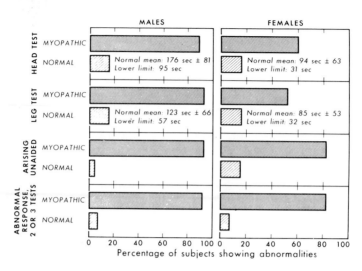

Fig. 11-1. Responses to muscle testing in 13 myopathic men, 17 myopathic women, and 300 controls (150 men, 150 women).

iliopsoas, hamstrings, deltoids, infraspinati, anterior neck, and anterior trunk muscles. In the dystrophies of the Duchenne limb girdle and facioscapulohumeral types, Walton [704] has noted that the earliest affected muscles are the pectorales, serrati, biceps, brachioradiales, quadriceps, hamstrings, and anterior triceps; he has observed that the deltoids remain comparatively unaffected in these dystrophies.

The question commonly arises, whether weakness in a given patient is psychogenic or has an organic basis. Useful differentiating points here are whether there is selectivity of muscle weakness, and whether the weak muscle groups are the ones mentioned above as being those most usually affected early. It is also important to mention that the adductor muscles of the thighs and the plantar flexors are among the last to be affected by most muscle disorders. Finally, it should be emphasized that there is no diagnostic specificity associated with the distribution of weakness in the various muscle groups aside from the special instance of familial dystrophies, which is mentioned in greater detail in a subsequent section.

CONFIRMATION OF A MUSCLE DISORDER BY LABORATORY TESTING, ELECTROMYOGRAPHY (EMG), AND BIOPSY APPEARANCES

Clinical Chemistry. Although creatinuria used to be emphasized as an important confirmatory feature of muscle wasting, this clinical tool has been virtually completely replaced by estimations of serum enzyme levels. The serum enzyme estimations that are readily available to the clinician are glutamic oxalacetic transaminase (SGOT), lactic dehydrogenase (LDH) with its isoenzymes, creatine phosphokinase (CPK), and aldolase. One or all of these may be elevated in the serum of the patient with a muscle disorder.

Some problems exist in the interpretation of the results of serum enzyme estimations. First, the levels may be entirely normal in rare instances of acute muscle inflammation; I have seen this in a patient with florid dermatomyositis even during acutely progressive weakness. Where the clinician suspects strongly that myositis or myopathy exists, he should make frequent estimations of the serum enzyme levels. Occasionally, only one of the several enzymes is elevated; a variation is elevation of several, but predominantly of one. In these instances, the pattern as it is first seen tends to remain characteristic of the disease for the particular patient; thus, occasionally the CPK may be predominantly elevated while the other enzyme levels are either only slightly high or normal. One should not be dogmatic about which of the serum enzymes is the most useful in diagnosing and following muscle disorders, because there is great variability from patient to patient. In general, however, the CPK is the most sensitive of the several enzymes in the various myopathies [504].

Other problems in the interpretation of serum enzyme levels are that these may be elevated in patients with neurogenic muscle wasting and weakness, especially when this is acute; in patients with central nervous system diseases of many sorts, especially after strokes or epileptic seizures [38, 159]; in patients with motor neurone disease [3, 714]; in patients with schizophrenic reactions [470]; in families of propositi who have malignant hyperpyrexia after anesthesia [333]; in persons with large muscle mass [233], and after mild exercise [359]. I have found that in some normal persons, minor elevation of CPK follows even manual muscle testing in the office. In borderline cases, therefore, it is preferable to ask the patient to have blood drawn for CPK analysis in the resting state on the day after the muscle testing procedure. It is superfluous to mention that intramuscular injections of any sort may elicit a rise in serum enzymes; this is well known to cardiologists, who insist that all injections be given intravenously to patients with suspected acute myocardial infarction, lest the serum enzyme levels be affected by intramuscular injections. It is important for the rheumatologist to recall that electromyography may elicit a transient rise in serum enzyme levels.

Electromyographic findings are useful in confirming that a muscle disorder is present. I rely upon the expert interpretation of the electromyographer, and will not discuss the patterns in any detail. Myopathic potentials have small amplitude, are of short duration, and may be polyphasic. As with most of the other test findings, the electromyographic results are not specific for any myopathy; although there may be some features suggestive of one rather than another. Two exceptions are the findings in myasthenia gravis, where there is gradual reduction in the height of the action potential seen on voluntary activity; and the reverse of this, in the Lambert-Eaton syndrome. The latter is most commonly observed in patients who have carcinoma of the bronchus and generalized muscle weakness. Myotonia has a very typical electromyographic appearance, which is seen most frequently, of course, in myotonia congenita or myotonia dystrophica, but is, rarely, also seen in polymyositis. Finally, a characteristic EMG pattern is seen in McArdle's syndrome.

The electromyogram, like the serum enzyme levels, cannot be relied upon absolutely to establish the diagnosis of myopathy. In our hands it has sometimes been normal in patients with muscle reactions proved by other means to be present. Nor should one be misled by the interpretation that the findings are more consistent with neuropathic than with myopathic abnormality, because such findings are not uncommon in patients with polymyositis. The reason is, presumably, that the inflammatory reaction in polymyositis may affect the nerve fibers coursing through the muscle bundle or the motor end plates themselves.

The appearances of the muscle tissue obtained at biopsy represent the final mode of confirmation that a muscle reaction is present. It is important that the clinician select for the surgeon the site to be sampled. The sampled muscle should be one that is weak and that has not been needled for electromyography. Where there is a great deal of muscle atrophy, it is preferable not to select the most atrophic muscle. The surgeon should be encouraged to remove a generous portion of muscle, approximately $3 \times 1 \times 3$ cm. The surgeon should tie the muscle specimen to a tongue blade so as to prevent distortion, and leave the specimen in isotonic saline for 10 minutes before placing it in fixative [572]. If facilities for performing enzyme histochemistry and electronmicroscopy on the muscle are available, it is important that the muscle tissues be appropriately handled, at the time of biopsy, for these studies.

The appearances upon light microscopy are entirely nonspecific [266]. Myopathic changes may characteristically include any of the following: marked variation in diameter of the muscle fibers; increased basophilia of the fibers, reflecting regenerative activity; floccular or hyaline changes, reflecting degeneration; increased numbers of sarcolemmal nuclei; central migration of sarcolemmal nuclei into the substance of the muscle fiber; interstitial accumulation of inflammatory cells, which may be seen invading the substance of the degenerating muscle fibers [266]. Interpretation of the muscle biopsy appearances is as fraught with difficulties as is interpretation of the EMG and serum enzyme levels. First, the biopsy appearances are not infrequently normal in the presence of clinically active muscle disease [146]. This is obviously due to a sampling difficulty; even repeated biopsy may find normal tissue in the presence of clinically active muscle disease [428]. Second, although the microscopic appearances of the tissue obtained at muscle biopsy were long held to be reliable in differentiating neuropathic from myopathic cases, it has been well established recently that myopathic changes may be seen in the muscle in both acute and chronic denervation [3, 157, 178]. These and other aspects of the nonspecificity of the appearances of muscle taken at biopsy are considered in greater detail in a subsequent section.

The early expectations that electronmicroscopy of muscle tissue would offer greater diagnostic specificity than does light microscopy have not been fulfilled. Although in rare congenital or familial disorders, the electronmicroscopic appearances have been useful and have defined new nosological categories such as megaconial and nemaline myopathies [177, 691] and central core disease [45], electron microscopy is not a useful tool in the investigation of the ordinary case of muscle disease. The ultrastructural changes are manifold and there is great overlap among the various muscle disorders.

Similarly, extensive studies of the enzyme histochemical staining reactions of muscle obtained at biopsy have yielded important information about fiber types, but the clinical value of the findings has been chiefly limited to the diagnosis of rare diseases [85, 118, 508]. We studied histochemical staining reactions for adenosine triphosphatase, phosphorylase, succinic dehydrogenase, nonspecific esterase, and acid phosphatase in muscle biopsy specimens from 58 patients with neuromuscular diseases, 26 patients with lung cancer who had no known myopathy, and 30 control subjects. The patients with neuromuscular disease included 14 with idiopathic polymyositis, five with one of the muscular dystrophies, one with familial amyotrophic lateral sclerosis, and 37 whose myopathy was associated with the following conditions: hypothyroidism (5), exogenous hypercortisonism (1), diabetic neuromyopathy (3), cancer (3), connective tissue diseases (9), or one of a group of miscellaneous disorders (16). Results were normal in virtually all patients and in all of the controls, with the exception that acid phosphatase staining was clearly reduced in 14 per cent of the myopathic patients, but was abundant in specimens from nonmyopathic controls, including those with lung cancer. Thus, while a nonspecific reduction in acid phosphatase staining intensity may be a helpful clue to the presence of myopathy, we cannot recommend routine enzyme histochemical staining of muscles on all patients with muscle disorder. Brooke and Kaplan [74] recently reported a nonspecific abnormality of fiber types in patients with polymyalgia rheumatica, but our findings have not been identical. Although there are histochemical differences between the appearances of muscles from patients with myopathies and those with neuropathies, we have not found this a clinically relevant observation and do not recommend the technique of enzyme histochemistry as necessary for this differentiation.

CLINICAL CLASSIFICATION ACCORDING TO THE CAUSE OF THE MUSCLE REACTION

It is important to emphasize that myopathy is a symptom-diagnosis that is confirmed by the laboratory, electromyographic, and biopsy findings discussed above, and that requires further study for its underlying cause. From the clinical viewpoint, the major grouping of patients is into those with a familial and those with a nonfamilial disorder (Table 11-2). The *familial disorders*, of course, are the so-called "dystrophies," not discussed here in detail, although the rheumatologist must be reminded that the current fashion is to divide the dystrophies into four major groups: the sex-linked, recessive, progressive muscular dystrophy of the Duchenne type which is seen in boys in their first few years of life but has a rare variant, the so-called "Becker type," of later onset and usually of a more benign prognosis; limb girdle dystrophy, which is usually autosomally recessive and has variable phenotypic expressivity with a pattern that tends to be characteristic for each family; facio-scapulo-humeral dystrophy, which is transmitted as an autosomal dominant characteristic; and dystrophia myotonica, of variable inheritance. About 10 per cent of dystrophies are of other types. As is mentioned in a later section, there are many resemblances between the dystrophies and idiopathic polymyositis, and a helpful tip for the clinician is to examine available family members for weakness and to take blood samples from them for serum enzyme levels. Quite frequently one obtains a negative family history for neuromuscular disease, yet the study of the family members shows that there are subclinical cases among the relatives. The diagnosis as to whether a patient's muscle reaction is familial or nonfamilial has obvious, important therapeutic connotations, as illustrated by Case 11-1.

Table 11-2. Clinical Classification of Causation of Myopathies

Familial
  Duchenne's disease
  Limb girdle dystrophy
  Facio-scapulo-humeral dystrophy
  Myotonic dystrophy
  Other dystrophies

Nonfamilial
  Sporadic dystrophy
  Metabolic disorders
  Toxins
  Neoplasm
  Infection
  Connective tissue disease
  Idiopathic polymyositis

Case 11-1. A 49-year-old man with a history of polyarthralgia of 7 years' duration stated that one elbow and the entire hands had been actually swollen, although lengthy observation at another clinic had not substantiated such swelling. Serious complaints were also made about pain and tenderness in the muscles of the arm, forearm, and thighs. There had been unsustained microhematuria about 5 years previously. Physical examination failed to show abnormal findings in any joints except the shoulders, which were painful on full abduction. All muscles tested showed normal strength. Rheumatoid factor was present, and CPK level elevated at 220 units. All other laboratory studies gave normal findings, including erythrocyte sedimentation rate, tests for C-reactive protein and for antinuclear antibodies, and thyroxine level. X-rays of affected peripheral joints and sacroiliac joints showed no abnormality. During the next several months, there was persistent moderate elevation of CPK levels. Electromyogram and muscle biopsy both showed normal findings.

Because of the symptom of polyarthralgia, the complaints of muscle pain, the high CPK levels, and the presence of rheumatoid factor, a tentative diagnosis of low-grade polymyositis was made. The patient was so incapacitated by his symptoms as to lose his job; in view of this indication of their severity, prednisone was given in doses of 20 mg daily. This did not affect the stiffness and soreness in his joints, nor did the CPK level fall. After a lengthy period of observation elsewhere, he was seen again, still complaining of marked myalgia. At that time he mentioned that his mother had had intermittent weakness of her muscles, and that his younger brother had muscle pains similar to his. The possibility of a familial disorder was therefore investigated, and confirmed when his younger brother, who was not available for physical examination, was found to have a CPK level of 325 units/liter. The patient was found to produce a normal rise in blood lactic acid after ischemic exercise. The nature of this familial muscle disorder remains uncertain.

Nonfamilial causes of muscle reactions include the following:

1. *Sporadic dystrophy.* Here, a characteristic picture of dystrophy is seen without a familial basis, and can be most confidently diagnosed where the pattern is that of Duchenne's dystrophy or dystrophia myotonica. The clinical pic-

ture of limb girdle dystrophy is so similar to that of polymyositis that clinical differentiation may be most difficult unless there are either the classic rash of dermatomyositis or accompanying rheumatic features such as arthritis, Raynaud's phenomenon, or abnormal serologic reactions.

2. *Metabolic abnormalities.* Endocrinopathy of almost any sort may be accompanied by myopathic features. Among the endocrine disorders, hypothyroidism is numerically the most important in my experience (Table 11-1 and Fessel [200]). The muscle complaints of patients with hypothyroidism may be those of pain or weakness; pain has been prominent in my patients [200]. The muscle biopsy may be frankly myopathic (Fig. 11-2), occasionally with interstitial inflammatory infiltrate. Of the 200 patients with muscle disease listed in Table 11-1, 18 (9 per cent) had hypothyroidism and the majority of these were not clinically hypothyroid when first seen. It is important that patients be repeatedly tested for hypothyroidism, because in some instances the laboratory tests showed frank hypothyroidism only after several months.

Case 11-2. A 53-year-old white woman complained that for approximately 9 months she had been experiencing attacks of fatigue, great chilliness, generalized myalgia, polyarthralgia, and depression, occurring about twice monthly and lasting for a couple of days each time. Physical examination showed no abnormalities in the muscles or joints.

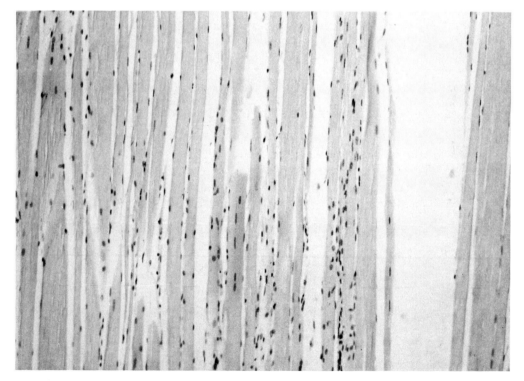

Fig. 11-2.   Hypothyroid myopathy. Separation of fibers by interstitial edema; variation in size of fibers; increase in number and central migration of sarcolemmal nuclei.

The skin was moderately dry and there was remarkable prolongation of the contraction phase of almost all of the deep tendon reflexes, reminiscent of myotonia. Percussion myotonia was elicited in neither the tongue nor the thenar muscles. The thyroid gland was of normal size, a trifle firmer than normal. The Achilles reflex half-relaxation time was 400 msec on two occasions (upper limit for euthyroidism, 380 msec).

During the next 15 months, eight estimations were made of serum thyroxine levels; on six occasions the level was below 4.0 μg/100 ml (two were 3.3 and 3.4 μg/100 ml); the two values above 4.0 were only 4.2 and 4.5 μg/100 ml. Fifteen months after the patient was first seen, the Achilles tendon half-relaxation time was 470 msec; and at about the same time the 24-hr uptake of radioactive iodine was 12 per cent, the lower limit of normal; the latter contrasted with a 24-hr radioactive iodine uptake of 27 per cent on the occasion of her first examination. Values for tri-iodothyronine uptake remained normal.

I have emphasized elsewhere [200] the importance of considering hypothyroidism in the differential diagnosis of acquired muscle reactions. This case illustrates the difficulties of reaching the diagnosis in some instances. It seems likely that this patient's glandular output of thyroid hormone fluctuated within a norrow range between normal and abnormal levels. It is also interesting that the tissue reaction noted symptomatically by the patient may be a more sensitive indicator of hypothyroidism than the tests of thyroid function currently available. This patient's symptoms were totally alleviated by eventual treatment with L-thyroxine.

Hyperthroidism is, contrariwise, also a well-known cause of weakness: Ramsay [569] found that 70 per cent of patients with hyperthyroidism had detectable weakness. Both hypercalcemia [24, 213, 560, 639, 696] and hypocalcemia [318, 543, 729] may be accompanied by myopathy. It is insufficiently recognized that hypophosphatemia—a frequent finding in hospitalized patients, which is readily reversible—may cause muscle weakness. It is commonly induced by intravenously administered glucose solutions, by vomiting [46], or by antiacids, which bind excessive amounts of dietary phosphate in the gut [429] (see also Chapter 4, page 000). Both hyperadrenalism [502, 550], including hyperaldosteronism [599], and hypoadrenalism [560] may induce a muscle reaction. A muscle disorder characteristic of diabetes mellitus is diabetic amyotrophy [427], considered in greater detail in a later section. Occasional cases of hyperinsulinism have been reported to have myopathic features [500]. Not surprisingly, pituitary disorders may have associated myopathy [418].

3. Such *toxins* as alcohol [381, 548, 549] and venoms [624]; such medicines as clofibrate [368], chloroquin [321, 336], colchicine [387], heroin and other addictive drugs [547], diazacholesterol [645], pargyline [735], and penicillamine [606] may cause muscle reactions.

4. *Neoplasms.* These are important causes of muscle disease. Although the mechanism is generally unknown, sometimes the tumor produces a hormonally active polypeptide, such as ACTH.

Case 11-3. Lung cancer had been diagnosed in a 78-year-old man one month before he was admitted to hospital because of weakness. The physical examination confirmed generalized muscle weakness, most severe in the proximal muscle groups; muscle biopsy showed severe myopathic changes. The serum potassium level of 2.1 mEq/liter and bicar-

though undoubtedly many patients labeled as having this disorder have been inadequately studied for the identification of a causative factor. The feature that permits one to be certain that the diagnosis is idiopathic polymyositis is the classic rash of dermatomyositis. This is seen more frequently in children than in adults. The violaceous rash of the eyelids and periorbital skin, together with the erythematous, scaly eruption over the extensor surfaces of joints, is quite characteristic, even pathognomonic. It is strange that this rash, especially the violaceous rash around the eyes, is not seen in any of the other connective tissue diseases.

Rheumatic symptoms, e.g., Raynaud's phenomenon or polyarthritis, are present in approximately 25 per cent of patients with idiopathic polymyositis [546]. Even these may be misleading, however, because a muscle reaction indistinguishable from that of idiopathic polymyositis may occur in any of the other connective tissue diseases. Whether a particular case is termed idiopathic polymyositis or one of the other connective tissue diseases will depend upon the relative prominence of the muscle disorder as contrasted with the other rheumatic manifestations. The problem arises mainly in rheumatoid arthritis, because the systemic manifestations and laboratory characteristics of systemic lupus erythematosus or polyarteritis allow these entities to be separated readily from polymyositis; and scleroderma with accompanying myopathy is equally readily identified.

It is worth noting that there are many overlapping features between idiopathic chronic polymyositis and the dystrophies. The differentiation between a sporadic (i.e., nonfamilial) dystrophy of the limb-girdle sort and idiopathic chronic polymyositis without rash or accompanying rheumatic symptoms may be very difficult. The changes in serum enzyme level and electromyogram are the same; the muscle biopsy in polymyositis may show either no changes or only degenerative ones without any cellular infiltration; and in muscular dystrophy one may see infiltrates of inflammatory cells (References 61, 505; and Cases 11-11, 11-12). It is important to study as many of the relatives as possible in such instances, to establish whether or not they have detectable muscle weakness or serum enzyme abnormalities. One should also take note of the muscle groups that are affected. In muscular dystrophy it is characteristic to see prominent wasting and weakness of certain muscle groups with complete normalcy of neighboring muscles. For example, it would not be uncommon to note profound wasting and weakness of, say, the biceps, with complete preservation of the triceps. This would be quite rare in chronic polymyositis, where the muscles contiguous with an actually atrophic muscle would almost always show some degree of wasting and weakness.

EXPERIMENTAL MODELS USED IN THE STUDY OF THE PATHOGENESIS OF MUSCLE REACTIONS

The multiplicity of causes of a pathological reaction in human muscles has been duplicated experimentally in animals. Iodides [84], chloroquin [9], plasmocid (an aminoquinoline) [559], x-irradiation [184], hyperoxygenation [96], and potassium depletion [382] have been shown experimentally to cause muscle reactions whose severity has varied from the earliest degenerative changes, seen only by means of the electron microscope, to extensive degenerative and regenerative changes together with inflammatory infiltration. The earliest alterations seen electron microscopically in these experimental models is selective destruction of the Z and I lines [559]. It is interesting that these represent the earliest changes seen both in human preclinical muscular dystrophy [540] and in dystrophic animals [95].

Nutritional deficiency of vitamin E has been extensively studied as an animal model resembling both human muscular dystrophy and human inflammatory muscle reactions of the sort seen in idiopathic polymyositis. It is interesting that the initial lesion here also is one of degeneration and necrosis, cellular infiltrate being present in the older lesions [357, 609]. The possible relevance of this is developed in a later section. Here it is only mentioned that vitamin E deficiency has never, with rare possible exceptions [33, 48], been demonstrated to be the cause of any human myopathy.

Hypersensitivity to muscle or to one of its components has been shown to be a cause of myositis in animals. In guinea pigs, injections of heterologous muscle with Freund's adjuvant was followed by a generalized myositis resembling that of human polymyositis [137]. Immunization of rabbits with isolated rat skeletal muscle membrane led to a myopathy characterized by muscle fiber degeneration and inflammatory cell infiltration [510]. Kakulas [356] was able to demonstrate that skeletal muscle cells in tissue culture were destroyed by lymph node cells obtained from rats immunized with heterologous muscle.

THE CONTRIBUTION OF IMMUNE MECHANISMS TO IDIOPATHIC POLYMYOSITIS

The occurrence of arthritis, Raynaud's phenomenon, and abnormal immunoglobulins in some patients with idiopathic polymyositis, the appearance of an inflammatory myopathy in patients with systemic lupus erythematosus and other connective tissue diseases, and the high prevalence of dermatomyositis in patients with congenital agammaglobulinemia are all intimations that immunity may play a role in the pathogenesis of idiopathic polymyositis.

Evidence for the presence of circulating antibodies directed against muscle tissue in idiopathic polymyositis is conflictive. Whitaker and Engel [716] found intramuscular vascular deposits of immunoglobulins and complement in patients with various muscular disorders; while Nishikai and Homma [515] saw positive results with immunodiffusion of purified myoglobin in seven of 11 patients with polymyositis but in no controls. We, however, were unable to differentiate between myopathic patients and controls when we sought for circulating antibodies to muscle by complement fixation, passive hemagglutination, and immunodiffusion; nor could we distinguish them by immunofluorescence studies, indirect or direct, looking for immunoglobulin and complement deposition in muscle tissue [203]. Circulating antibodies to myosin were found in the same percentages of patients and controls by Caspary, Gubbay, and Stern [91]. Relevant to this discussion was the report by Griggs and coworkers [267] of a patient who had classic dermatomyositis but a hereditary deficiency of C2.

Evidence for cellular hypersensitivity as a mechanism in idiopathic polymyositis is more convincing. Currie and coworkers [128] found that, when exposed to normal human muscle, lymphocytes from patients with active polymyositis showed a significantly greater response than did lymphocytes from patients with inactive polymyositis, other muscle wasting diseases, or no disease. When they exposed human fetal muscle cultures to lymphocytes from 18 patients with polymyositis, 83 per cent of the cultures were destroyed; whereas only 15 per cent of such cultures were destroyed upon exposure to lymphocytes from 15 patients with other muscle wasting diseases. Dawkins and Mastaglia [138] used a quantitative assay that depended upon the release of isotope from prelabeled cultures of chick-embryo muscle. Lymphocyte mediated myotoxicity was elevated in nine patients with active polymyositis but was normal in four patients with inactive disease. Indirect studies by Johnson, Fink, and Ziff [347] showed that when muscle pieces from patients with polymyositis were incubated with autologous lymphocytes, a lymphotoxin was produced which injured fetal muscle cells in tissue culture. Finally, Mastaglia and Currie [447] in electron microscopic studies of muscle from two patients with polymyositis, saw "activated" lymphocytes with bulky cytoplasm, some of which contained endoplastic reticulum, in contact with endothelium of small vessels.

One cannot, however, accept as conclusive the evidence that an immune mechanism plays an initiating role in idiopathic polymyositis. First, the results are conflictive concerning the presence of circulating antibodies. Second, the lymphocyte stimulation studies of Currie and coworkers [128] gave the same results in subjects with inactive polymyositis, muscular dystrophy, or no disease. In early muscular dystrophy, a prominent inflammatory response may be seen histologically [61, 84, 541]; cellular infiltration may also be seen in some myopathies of endocrine origin; it would be important to demonstrate that lymphocytes from such patients are not stimulated by exposure to muscle before concluding that the lymphocytic response in active polymyositis indicates a major or specific role for cellular immunity. The lymphocyte myotoxicity in active polymyositis was unrelated to the CPK levels in Dawkins and Mastaglia's studies [138]. It is puzzling, too, that the observations of Johnson, Fink, and Ziff [347] also showed no correlation between the lymphotoxin response and the activity of the polymyositis as reflected by the serum level of CPK. Moreover, Mastaglia and Currie [447] saw no "activated" lymphocytes in actual contact with muscle fibers, raising some doubt as to whether these were immunologically activated by muscle. Third, there are many examples, cited previously, of cellular infiltration into muscle as well as of fiber degeneration, in conditions other than idiopathic polymyositis. Among the most noteworthy is the experimental myopathy of vitamin E deficiency [609]. It is difficult to visualize a disorder of cellular hypersensitivity specific to idiopathic polymyositis when so many other muscle reactions in conditions without stigmata of disordered immunity are also characterized by infiltration with lymphocytes. Finally, one must account for those cases in which, despite great severity of the muscle reaction, there is no infiltration by inflammatory cells. A striking example was reported by Hill and Barrows [311]: although biopsy and necropsy studies each showed severe and widespread muscular degeneration, no inflammatory cells were seen in any of the microscopic sections. The argument fails, that steroid therapy may have destroyed the lymphocytes in the muscles, because the patient died despite therapy.

Whatever the final outcome of studies concerning an immunological component in the pathogenesis of muscle diseases, the question arises as to the point in pathogenesis at which an immunologic mechanism might become relevant. Any of the many stimuli mentioned as capable of causing a muscle reaction could so alter a component of the muscle fiber as to trigger an autoallergic reaction. One recalls, in this regard, the variety of virus-like particles that have been reported in the muscles of patients with polymyositis. These particles have had appearances of myxoviruses [103], picornaviruses [104], coxsackie viruses [449], and zoster viruses [519]. Viruses are currently considered likely as triggers of autoallergic reactions in connective tissue diseases. In any disease, the question is whether the immunological component is a mere epiphenomenon or a major element in pathogenesis.

Those cases of familial dystrophy that have a marked inflammatory element in the muscle as seen at biopsy are of considerable theoretical importance with regard to the question of primacy of an autoimmune mechanism in the pathogenesis of idiopathic chronic polymyositis. If we assume that 1) the dystrophies do not have a primary autoimmune component, and 2) there is no familial basis for a primary autoimmune reaction in muscles, then those instances of familially determined dystrophy which have an inflammatory element suggest that infiltration of muscle by lymphocytes and plasma cells such as appears in an autoimmune reaction can be a consequence of muscle degeneration rather than an initiating event. The following family is of considerable interest with regard to this question.

Case 11-11. A 30-year-old woman had first noted symptoms of muscle weakness at age 26 years, with gradual progression thereafter. Physical examination revealed a moderately severe degree of proximal muscle weakness affecting, especially, the pelvic girdle muscles. CPK level was 870 units (normal, <50). Muscle biopsy revealed marked myopathic changes with considerable variation of fiber size, increase in number of sarcolemmal nuclei, occasional central migration of the sarcolemmal nuclei, and degenerative changes in the muscle fibers. There was a prominent interstitial and perivascular infiltrate of lymphocytes and histiocytes which, in places, resulted in granuloma formation (Fig. 11-5).

The patient had a twin and an elder sister. I had opportunity to examine, briefly, the elder sister. She had been totally gray since age 12 years. Her eyes were blue, with brown pigmentation of the lateral half of the left iris. Physical examination revealed moderate weakness of the biceps brachii with normal strength in the other muscles of the shoulder girdle; moderate weakness of iliopsoas, adductor and abductor femoris, and quadriceps femoris, with normal strength of all other muscles. No laboratory tests were made.

The patient's twin sister was first observed to have muscle weakness at age 21 years, and when examined at another hospital at age 23 was found to have proximal muscle weakness and wasting, affecting especially the biceps brachii, brachioradialis, pectoralis, supinators and pronators of the hands, iliopsoas, quadriceps, hamstrings, adductors of the hips, and peroneal muscles. She had moderate pseudohypertrophy of both calves, and bilateral pes cavus was observed. The muscle biopsy of this twin was reported to show marked variation of muscle fiber size, cross-sectional diameters ranging from 9 to 90 microns; frequent internal migration of sarcolemmal nuclei; scattered fibers showed floccular changes with phagocytosis, and an infiltrate was seen, consisting of polymorphonuclear leukocytes, lymphocytes, and macrophages.

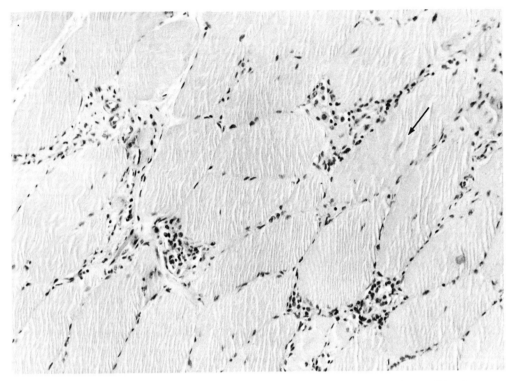

Fig. 11-5. Case 11-11, muscle. A (above), central nuclei; sarcolemmal nucleus proliferation; interstitial inflammatory infiltrate. Hematoxylin and eosin, ×130. B (page 202), degenerating fiber surrounded by histiocytes and lymphocytes. Hematoxylin and eosin ×400.

Three children of the paternal greataunt of these three patients were said to have muscular dystrophy. No further information was obtainable about the family members.

It is clear that this was a familial muscle disorder which would be classified as a limb-girdle dystrophy. Despite the marked inflammatory changes in the muscles, there were no other symptoms or findings to substantiate the possibility of familial chronic polymyositis: in neither of the two women examined by me was there any history or finding of joint disorder, of Raynaud's phenomenon, or of other symptoms suggestive of connective tissue disease. Nor did we find in the proposita any evidence of serological abnormality: there were normal levels of γ-globulin, and tests showed no evidence of rheumatoid factor or antinuclear antibodies.

A similar situation, without, however, the comforting evidence of a positive family history, was seen in the following case:

Case 11-12. A 47-year-old man had severe muscle wasting and weakness which had started at the age of 14 years. There was no known muscular disease in his parents, 14 siblings, his daughter, or his grandson. There was no history of dysphagia, significant joint disorder, or Raynaud's phenomenon. Physical examination showed generalized muscle weakness which was especially severe proximally and affected certain muscles more profoundly than others. The serratus anterior, latissimus dorsi, and pectoralis major and

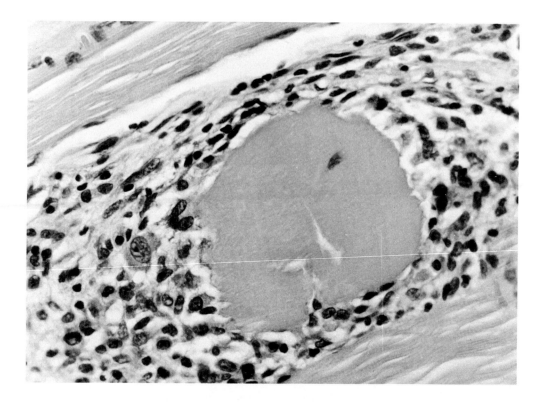

Fig. 11-5. B.

minor muscles were virtually absent, as were the opponens pollicis and abductor pollicis brevis bilaterally. Rhomboids and sternomastoids were very weak; deltoids, biceps, triceps, and iliopsoas muscles were moderately weak. Other muscles were of normal or almost normal strength. Tests showed no rheumatoid factor, antinuclear factor, or antibodies against thyroid or adrenal; CPK level was 191 units (normal, <50). Muscle biopsy showed mild variation in the size of muscle fibers, occasional fibers that were degenerating with the presence of local histiocytes and lymphocytes, some fibers with regenerative changes, occasional central migration of sarcolemmal cells, and accumulations of inflammatory cells that consisted mostly of lymphocytes together with a few histiocytes (Fig. 11-6). Treatment with prednisone, 30 mg daily for 4 months, caused no improvement in his strength.

It might be argued that this man had idiopathic chronic polymyositis; yet there were none of the occasional clinical concomitants of that condition, nor were any serological abnormalities observed. Moreover, the duration of illness, in excess of 30 years, would be exceptional for chronic polymyositis. I believe that the most likely diagnosis is a variant of facio-scapulo-humeral dystrophy, which has been found by Munsat and coworkers [505] to have an inflammatory element in some cases.

In summary, therefore, the evidence that leads one to question whether autoimmunity plays a prime role in the pathogenesis of idiopathic chronic polymyositis is as follows: first, the lack of inflammation in some patients with the disease; second, the laboratory studies that conflict with the reports of

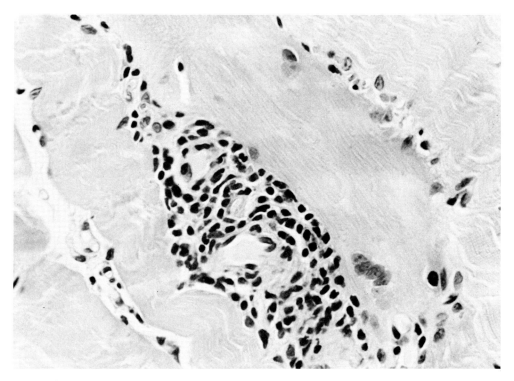

Fig. 11-6. Case 11-12, muscle. Sarcolemmal nucleus proliferation; perivascular lymphocytic infiltration. Hematoxylin and eosin, ×250.

humoral hypersensitivity reactions to muscle in this disease; next, the inflammatory reaction in cases of endocrinopathic myopathy; finally, the evidence from patients such as those described above, with a familial dystrophy and associated inflammatory cellular reaction seen on muscle biopsy.

INTERFERENCE WITH NORMAL BALANCE OF MUSCLE CELL DEGENERATION-REGENERATION CYCLE AS A GENERAL CAUSE OF MUSCLE REACTIONS: A UNIFYING CONCEPT OF CAUSATION

Although taught for many years, the concept that skeletal muscle is incapable of regeneration is now known to be incorrect [299]. There is, normally, a turnover of the muscle proteins [398], with slower turnover of the muscle nuclei: radioautography after injection of thymidine ^{3}H showed only one radioactive nucleus among about 50,000 [49]; but the nuclei labeled more rapidly after muscle injury. The acceleration in response to injury was reflected by the light microscopic observation that rows of aligned nuclei began to appear within 2 to 3 days after muscle transection; within 2 to 3 weeks, the muscle appeared histologically normal [399].

The demonstration of a process of muscle turnover in healthy animals, i.e., that a cycle of degeneration-regeneration occurs in health, implies that derangement of that cycle may occur, resulting in disease. This suggests a rational hypothesis for the manifold causes of muscle reactions in man and animals: *A muscle reaction occurs when the normal balance between muscle degeneration and regeneration is upset.* Muscle tissue is peculiarly liable to such imbalance because of its poor capacity for regeneration. Thus, an increase in degeneration—as after exposure to drugs or toxins, or after any anatomical-physiological disturbance of the muscle fiber—in this tissue, whose regenerative response is limited, would be manifest clinically and histopathologically as a myopathy.

It is necessary to emphasize the great structural complexity of the muscle fiber, with its actomyosin filaments, sarcotubular system, lysosomes, mitochondria, sarcoplasm, myoglobin, and sarcolemmal nuclei, as well as the enormous number of both aerobic and anaerobic metabolic processes performed by the muscle cell. Some of these anatomical and physiological processes are more vulnerable to injury than others; and it is obvious that injury to certain of them, for example, lysosomes, may be more potentially dangerous to the integrity of the muscle fiber as a whole than is damage to others. Nevertheless, one may conceptualize the muscle fiber as vulnerable to a myriad of toxic processes and as having only very limited histopathologically represented responses to all.

Denny-Brown [145] proposed that total failure to regenerate after injury is an inherent defect of the dystrophic muscle fiber. Walker [701], using a radioautographic method to estimate turnover time for replacement of muscle nuclei in dystrophic mice, showed that fiber degeneration is much more rapid than regeneration, and questioned whether an imbalance between these two processes could be at the root of hereditary muscular dystrophy. Simon and coworkers [633], studying muscle protein turnover in dystrophic mice, found that muscle protein loss resulted not from defective protein synthesis, but from accelerated protein turnover and, by inference, from degeneration. Gilbert and Hazard [245] obtained histopathological evidence that in both muscular dystrophy and polymyositis there is continuing necrosis; and that an ineffective process of regeneration in muscular dystrophy constitutes one of the main differences between the two conditions. Hudgson, Pearce, and Walton [320] concluded from studies of persons with preclinical muscular dystrophy, that the histopathological evidence showed a defect in the regenerative process. Mastaglia, Papadimitriou, and Kakulas [448] suggested that the muscle fiber has only a limited potential to regenerate, and that its regenerative capacity may become quickly exhausted. Shafiq and colleagues [615] saw electron microscopic evidence of a more widespread regenerative process in polymyositis than in dystrophy. Studies of denervated skeletal muscle by Pearlstein and Kohn [544] suggested that loss of muscle substance in that condition resulted primarily from acceleration of degradation, rather than from a defect in synthesis. Thus, there is some evidence to support the concept of an imbalance between the two processes of degeneration and regeneration as a basis for muscle disease.

To the rheumatologist, the importance of the above considerations is that, although idiopathic chronic polymyositis may be a homogeneous entity, there can be little doubt that the group of patients we currently designate as having this condition is heterogeneous. The numerous causes of degeneration of muscle fibers have already been cited. We should devote as much effort as possible to elucidating the causative factors that may be responsible for the muscle disorder in each patient, before concluding that his process is idiopathic.

CHAPTER 12

Sclerodermatous Reactions

INCIDENCE AND PROGNOSIS

Scleroderma is one of the rarest of the connective tissue diseases. During the 17-year period encompassed by Kurland and coworkers' [394] survey of the 50, 000 residents of Rochester, Minnesota, only eight cases occurred, giving an incidence rate of 1.2 per 100,000; the prevalence rate was 10.5 per 100,000.

The disease has a high mortality rate. A study by Medsger and coworkers [463] of 223 patients diagnosed in Pittsburg, Pennsylvania, and of 86 patients diagnosed in Memphis, Tennessee, showed the surprisingly low cumulative survivorship of only 35 per cent at 7 years. The death rate in older patients, even after allowance is made for the natural rise in mortality with age, was high, as it was in males and in black persons with the disease. Involvement of lungs, heart, and kidneys was in each instance independently correlated with decreased survival. A similarly poor prognosis was found by Farmer and coworkers [188]: follow-up information on 236 patients with scleroderma revealed that 115 (48.7 per cent) had died, the average interval between diagnosis and death being only 41.2 months. A fast erythrocyte sedimentation rate at the time of diagnosis was an ominous sign: 40 died among the 57 patients whose erythrocyte sedimentation rate exceeded 50 mm/hr (Westergren). It is well known that sclerodermatous involvement of the kidneys is a particularly malignant condition. Almost no patient with so-called "scleroderma kidney" survives beyond 9 months. Five patients died from scleroderma in our hospital during a 5-year period: two from scleroderma kidney, one from severe malabsorption syndrome due to diffuse bowel involvement by the disease; the two others had extremely severe associated myopathy, one dying from cardiomyopathy, the other from disseminated intravascular coagulation. Both patients with skeletal myopathy died within 18 months of onset of the disease, suggesting that the association of skeletal myopathy with scleroderma is an ominous prognostic sign.

Case 12-1. Raynaud's phenomenon first appeared in a black girl at age 14 years. Within a few weeks, gangrenous changes occurred at the tips of several fingers and her hair started falling. When first seen shortly thereafter, she had increased skin pigmentation over several parts of the body, and patchy decrease of pigmentation in other parts. Results of tests for cryoglobulins, cold agglutinins, rheumatoid factor, antinuclear antibodies, and immunoglobulins G, A, and M were all either negative or within normal limits. Within a few weeks, definite sclerodermatous changes became evident in the hands and distal portion of the forearms. An interesting physical sign that is occasionally found in scleroderma was observed; namely, palpable crepitus over the flexor tendon sheaths at the wrists. (Such crepitus may also occur in the anterior compartment of the legs, where it is probably caused by fasciitis rather than by tendinitis; it may be heard on auscultation with the stethoscope, but this must be interpreted cautiously because a minor degree of friction may be heard in normal subjects.) About 6 months after the Raynaud's phenomenon commenced, a severe degree of proximal muscle weakness appeared, accompanied by high serum enzyme levels (CPK, 535 units/100 ml) and evidence of myopathy on biopsy. Two months thereafter, treatment was started with prednisone, 40 mg daily. The dose was soon increased to 80 mg daily because of the rapidly progressive muscle weakness and associated loss of 20 pounds. Almost exactly one year after her illness had commenced, a brain syndrome suddenly developed, characterized initially by what appeared to be a catatonic state, followed rapidly by signs suggesting a lesion in the pons. The major laboratory abnormalities found at this time were a decreasing platelet count and some degree of fragmentation of the red cells in the peripheral blood. Heparin was given intravenously as treatment for the presumed disseminated intravascular coagulopathy, but the patient died within 2 days. Autopsy confirmed the presence of platelet thrombi in the pons and elsewhere.

CLINICAL AND PATHOLOGICAL ASPECTS

The typical clinical picture of scleroderma is too well known to warrant detailed description, but some less widely recognized facts about the disease are worth mentioning: The diagnosis should not rest upon the presence of thick, bound-down skin over the fingers, a phenomenon termed *sclerodactyly,* because this may be seen in chronic Raynaud's phenomenon of any cause. In scleroderma, the cutaneous thickening appears proximal to the metacarpophalangeal joints, favored sites being the dorsa of the hands and forearms. It is also seen on the sides of the neck, the front of the upper part of the chest, and the shins; perhaps most typical is the appearance produced when the skin of the central portion of the face is affected, causing taut lips and a pinched nose. *Telangiectases* are common and should be sought on the palms and fingers and inside the mouth; they do not necessarily affect only skin that is clearly sclerodermatous.

A *generalized hyperpigmentation* may be so severe as to suggest the possibility of Addison's disease. I was once asked to confirm a diagnosis of Addison's disease in a patient who, when examined, was seen to have obvious advanced scleroderma without any evidence of adrenal insufficiency. Often the hyperpigmentation is localized to the dorsa of the hands and forearms, the sides of the neck and the cheeks—those same sites of predilection for the skin thickening. In black patients one sometimes sees areas of increased pigmentation side-by-side with vitiligo.

Raynaud's phenomenon tends to be more severe and chronic in patients with scleroderma than in those with any other condition. This was the initial manifestation of scleroderma in 32.5 per cent of the 271 patients with scleroderma studied by Farmer and coworkers [188] and was present at some time in 81.2 per cent of them. Scleroderma was the underlying diagnosis in 36 (26.2 per cent) of the 137 patients with Raynaud's phenomenon studied by Velayos and coworkers [694]. It should be noted that all of these 137 patients were hospitalized; whereas *idiopathic* Raynaud's phenomenon was the diagnosis in only 28 (20 per cent) of the 137 hospital patients, this would be the most prevalent diagnosis in outpatients with Raynaud's phenomenon. It is of interest that trauma, as from cold or an occupational injury, and occlusive arterial disease between them accounted for the Raynaud's phenomenon in 15.3 per cent of the cases reported by Velayos and coworkers [694]. The arteriographic findings do not differentiate the various causes of Raynaud's phenomenon, unless a localized block, as from atheroma, is shown. In most instances, the ulnar artery is narrowed or occluded; the radial artery and common digital arteries tend to be spared, but the proper digital arteries are stenosed or totally occluded (Fig. 12-1, and Reference 132).

Aperistalsis of the esophagus (Fig. 12-2) is related in an uncertain fashion to the presence of Raynaud's phenomenon and not specifically to scleroderma.

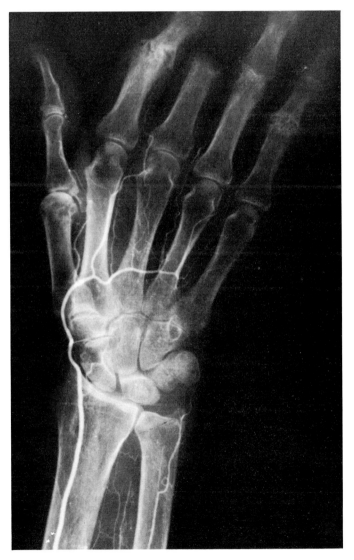

Fig. 12-1.   Arteriogram of patient with scleroderma and Raynaud's phenomenon. Note occlusion of ulnar artery at level of distal ulna, great narrowing of most common digital arteries, and virtual obliteration of all proper digital arteries.

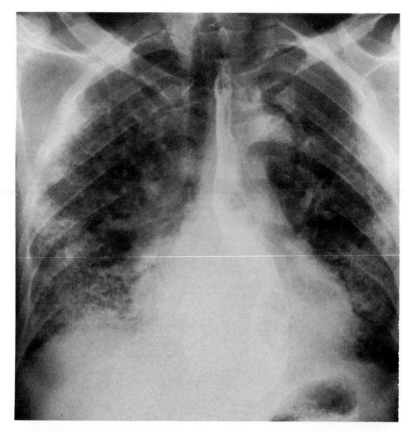

Fig. 12-2.   Scleroderma. Dilated esophagus; diffuse interstitial pulmonary fibrosis.

Among 30 patients with Raynaud's phenomenon and aperistalsis of the esophagus studied by Stevens and coworkers [660], 20 had scleroderma, five had other connective tissue disease, and five had no evidence of a multisystem disorder. D'Angelo and coworkers [133], on the contrary, saw muscle atrophy and/or fibrosis in the esophagus of 74 per cent of patients with scleroderma but in none of the controls; these histopathological changes were less prevalent in the small intestine (48 per cent) and large bowel (39 per cent).

Calcinosis cutis, seen in about 10 per cent of patients, affects usually the fingers and hands, less often the skin over other bony prominences such as the free border of the ulna, the olecranon process, and the acromion process. The calcium deposits may erode through the skin, producing a chalky discharge. In recent years, the term *CRST syndrome,* acronymous for calcinosis, Raynaud's phenomenon, sclerodactyly, telangiectasia, has become popular. This is sometimes held to be a newly observed combination but was, in fact, described some forty years ago by Thibierge and Weissenbach [674] and the eponymous term was used in the older literature.

Lung involvement, especially with diffuse interstitial fibrosis (Fig. 12-2), is particularly characteristic and common; parenchymal fibrosis and/or pulmonary arterial thickening was seen in 81 per cent of the cases studied at autopsy by d'Angelo and coworkers [133]. The *skeletal muscles* may be involved, as in Case spondylitis, a second son had Reiter's disease, and the third son had Reiter's disease followed by rheumatoid arthritis.

It is difficult to avoid the conclusion that the conditions commonly labeled "collagen diseases" may not be true diseases, i.e., entities having distinct cause and unvarying, identifiable clinical pattern. They may, rather, be tissue reactions to a variety of pathogenic agents. These tissue reactions are very closely related to one another, and more than one may occur in the same patient. Klemperer himself stated [380] that "all we wanted to express originally was that in certain diseases, anatomical investigations reveal conspicuous alterations of the intermediary substances of the connective tissue in a systematic manner." The preferred nomenclature would be rheumatoid *reaction,* due to, e.g., psoriasis, or idiopathic; lupus *reaction,* due to, e.g., procainamide, or idiopathic; angiitic *reaction,* due to, e.g., penicillin hypersensitivity, or idiopathic; myopathic *reaction,* due to, e.g., hypothyroidism, or idiopathic; sclerodermatous *reaction,* due to, e.g., carcinoid, or idiopathic.

CHAPTER 14

Uncommon Syndromes and Diseases

A number of exceptional conditions warrant discussion both on account of their intrinsic interest and because their diagnosis depends upon awareness of their general features. At some time in the future, when computers assume the more difficult tasks with which we now burden our memories, rare diagnoses will become easy to make. At present, however, the mind must remain prepared for them, in which condition, according to an aphorism attributed to Pasteur, it will be favored by chance.

RELAPSING POLYCHONDRITIS

It is interesting, how frequently a trained observer with a carefully prepared mind may gloss over as unimportant, some small detail of the history or physical examination which, in retrospect and subsequently, proves to be the key to the diagnosis. In the first of the following cases of relapsing polychondritis, the diagnosis could have been made a couple of months earlier had the relevance been recognized of the cellulitis of the bridge of the nose. It was not until inflammation in an ear occurred for the second time that the correct diagnosis was realized. Awareness of the presence of an unusual degree of monocytosis and hyper-α_2-globulinemia in the first case allowed the correct diagnosis to be made in the second case without delay.

Case 14-1. A 58-year-old man was investigated for a prolonged fever of unknown cause, which had been accompanied by some night sweats and pleuritic-type chest pain. Aside from the fever and tachycardia, the physical findings were remarkable only for the observation of cellulitis at the tip of the nose, which apparently had commenced earlier over the bridge of the nose and had been attributed by the patient to the use of spectacles. The erythrocyte sedimentation rate was 123 mm/hr. The serum α_1-globulin of 7.0 per cent was high; and the α_2-globulin of 22 per cent was considerably elevated. Bone marrow examination showed such increased numbers of monocytes that the hematologist entertained the possibility of monocytic leukemia. Coombs' test was positive. Results of extensive further testing were entirely normal including urinalysis, blood chemical analyses, liver function tests, antinuclear antibodies, tests for rheumatoid factor, cryoglobulins, x-rays of the chest and bones, and numerous sputum tests for tuberculosis and fungi. Complement fixation tests were negative for histoplasmosis and coccidioidomycosis.

In the absence of any other discernible cause, the possibility of temporal arteritis was considered because of the very fast erythrocyte sedimentation rate and the unusually high level of α_2-globulin. Biopsy of the artery did not confirm this diagnosis.

The patient was discharged from the hospital, still febrile, and was seen approximately one month later. While he had been in the hospital, the ear adjacent to the each limb. Her temperature was 41° C (105.8° F); pulse rate, 100/min. The liver was palpable 5 cm below the costal margin. Electrocardiograms showed a high-grade atrioventricular block with periods of atrioventricular dissociation and captured beats. There were periods of sinus conducted beats with a long PR interval.

Bilateral esotropia was noted on the next day; evidence of weakness of the external rectus and superior rectus muscles appeared in both eyes. These defective ocular movements disappeared completely by the third hospital day. In the meantime the temperature had become normal, presumably through the influence of prednisone, 60 mg/day. The patient was discharged from the hospital taking prednisone, 30 mg/day, but required readmission 8 days later because her temperature was 40° C (104° F) and she had bizarre ocular movements. This time, there was no stable sort of disordered movement, but a chaotically disconjugate motion of the eyes, particularly when the patient attempted to look at an object that was not perfectly in front of her. Intravenously administered edrophonium had no effect on the eyes, and electromyography likewise gave no evidence of myasthenia. As previously, she awoke with entirely normal eye motion on the third morning after the abnormal ocular movements had started.

Because these two episodes of disordered eye movements had occurred at times of fever, the effect of artificially raising the body temperature was tested: the patient was wrapped in an electrically warmed blanket. Disordered eye movements began within 30 minutes. During the first such test, they were present for approximately 8 hours and disappeared completely within 1½ hours after removal of the blanket. A second test again induced disturbed ocular motion; an electroencephalogram during the period of disturbance remained normal.

During this second stay in hospital she showed evidence of an organic brain syndrome: difficulty in initiating sentences, inability to complete an entire sequence of a series of numbers, inability to subtract correctly 7 from 100, impairment in recent memory, visual and auditory hallucinations, impaired intellectual functioning, concreteness with literal interpretation of proverbs, and occasional confabulation.

Many studies were made during these two hospital stays. The white blood cell count was 4,900/cu mm, 16 per cent stab forms and 76 per cent polymorphonuclear cells. The hematocrit was initially 36 per cent but fell transiently to 28 per cent, when the reticulocyte count became 3.5 per cent, and serum haptoglobin was undetectable; responses to Coombs' test were negative. Serum glutamic oxalacetic transaminase was elevated, between 53 and 130 units (normal, <40 units); LDH was as high as 500 units (normal, 120 units), with a normal distribution of isoenzymes.

The latex test showed rheumatoid factor. Antinuclear antibodies were absent from the serum; serum protein electrophoresis and quantitative studies of immunoglobulin showed normal values.

Responses to the following tests were either negative or within normal limits: urinalysis; serum sodium, potassium, chloride; glucose tolerance curve, blood urea nitrogen and creatinine, analysis of the cerebrospinal fluid (1 lymphocyte/cu mm; protein, 26 mg/100 ml), serum creatine phosphokinase, sulfobromophthalein retention test (5 per cent). X-rays of the chest and skull as well as two brain scans showed no abnormality.

Qualitative lipoprotein electrophoresis during the acute panniculitis showed a very intense β band, but the pattern became normal after the panniculitis had subsided. Serum triglycerides were 220 mg/100 ml; cholesterol, 182 mg/100 ml.

A biopsy specimen was taken from an area of panniculitis and the underlying muscle. The muscle fibers were entirely normal, and no evidence of vasculitis was seen. Histochemical staining gave normal results for adenosine triphosphatase, phosphorylase, succinic dehydrogenase, nonspecific esterase, and acid phosphatase. There was a normal distribution of muscle fiber types. The fat lesion typified Weber-Christian disease, showing intense infiltration of the fat lobules and the fat septa by polymorphonuclear leukocytes, histiocytes, lymphocytes and, rarely, plasma cells. Immunofluorescent microscopy did not demonstrate increased deposition of IgG in the panniculitis lesion.

After a relatively uneventful year, jaundice appeared; the temperature was 40° C (104° F). The white blood cell count was 2,000/cu mm (polymorphonuclears 80 per cent, lymphocytes 12 per cent, monocytes 8 per cent); the hematocrit reading fell to 34 per cent; serum total bilirubin rose to 8.0 mg/100 ml (direct reacting bilirubin 6.1 mg/100 ml); serum alkaline phosphatase, to 140 King-Armstrong units; SGOT, to 1,900 units. Within 3 weeks all of these abnormalities had almost completely resolved, but after another 2 weeks the patient was admitted to the hospital because her temperature was 41.1° C (106° F), she was again deeply jaundiced and the liver was enlarged and extremely tender. Depression of the skin overlying the left buccinator fat pad was observed for the first time; this resembled lipodystrophy but might have been liposclerosis in healed panniculitis. The serum total bilirubin was 9.0 mg/100 ml (direct reacting bilirubin, 6.9 mg/100 ml); serum alkaline phosphatase, 130 King-Armstrong units; SGOT, 3,100 units; prothrombin time was 26 per cent of normal. There was evidence of hemolysis: the hematocrit reading fell to 29 per cent, reaction to Coombs' test was positive, haptoglobin was undetectable and, later, a reticulocyte count was 3.5 per cent. Other pertinent laboratory findings were normal levels of glucose-6-phosphate dehydrogenase, plasma cholesterol of 354 mg/100 ml, total protein of 7.1 g/100 ml (40 per cent γ-globulin by electrophoresis), and a negative response to test for antinuclear antibodies.

The dose of prednisone was increased to 60 mg daily and the temperature rapidly became normal. The liver shrank and the laboratory test results improved. When the patient had been in the hospital for 2 weeks she was almost anicteric (total bilirubin 1.9 mg/100 ml) and the SGOT had fallen to 102 units; only then was the prothrombin time sufficiently normal to permit needle biopsy of the liver. This showed marked bile stasis in the biliary canaliculi, normal hepatocytes, and no inflammatory changes. The patient recovered and has remained well, without prednisone, for the past 6 years.

In 1965, Milner and Mitchinson [479] could find only 11 reported cases of systemic Weber-Christian disease confirmed by necropsy; they added a twelfth. All authors have emphasized that the typical lesions, i.e., inflammation and necrosis of fat followed by fibrosis, may occur in virtually any visceral site where there is adipose tissue. Favored sites are the retroperitoneal, mediastinal, pericardial, and pretracheal locations.

The liver is commonly involved by systemic Weber-Christian disease. Among the 12 patients whose courses were summarized by Milner and Mitchinson, 10 had fatty change or patchy necrosis of the liver. The patient reported by Arnold and Bainborough [19] had lipogranulomatosis along the course of the large vessels within the liver, and similar lesions infiltrated Glisson's capsule in the patient observed by Nakagawa and Takayanagi [509]. Mostofi and Engleman's [496] patient, like mine, had a moderate proliferation of bile ducts; theirs also had hepatic necrosis.

Some of the systemic aspects of the disease may be interpreted as merely mechanical, secondary to involvement of visceral fat. In this category are probably the obstructive jaundice in my patient; the bone involvement simulating multiple myeloma in Doel's [153] patient; liposclerosis in the retroperitoneal space producing the picture of retroperitoneal fibrosis [618]; and symptoms of a cerebral tumor in the patient with fat necrosis of a dural lipoma [19].

Other manifestations, however, are clearly not mechanically based, but related to the underlying pathophysiology. These include the anemia and leukopenia, both of which are quite common in patients with Weber-Christian disease without other systemic manifestations. My patient had three separate episodes of hemolytic anemia, one at the time of a positive response to Coombs' test; this has not been reported in Weber-Christian disease. Her leukopenia was less severe than that of Steinberg's second patient, whose white blood cell count was as low as 1,200/cu mm [658].

It is difficult to understand the basis of the intermittent complete heart block in my patient, another hitherto unreported occurrence. Although involvement of myocardial fat may happen, as in Hutt and Pinniger's [332] patient, it seems unlikely that this would cause an intermittent and variable type of heart block unless the lesion were of sufficient degree to produce evidence, which was lacking, of damage to contiguous myocardial muscle. Although one of her early attacks might have induced a tiny lesion in the cardiac conducting system, the possibility exists of an intermittently occurring metabolic disorder affecting conduction.

Likewise, the brain disturbance evidenced by the organic mental syndrome and the chaotic ocular movements can hardly be attributed to involvement of adipose tissue. The most likely explanation for the eye disorder is an area of acute demyelination within the brain stem, related to the hemolysis and heart block. Both its transience and its reproduction by artificial elevation of body temperature favor acute demyelination, even though electrophoresis of the cerebrospinal fluid showed normal γ-globulin levels. Another possibility is of fat embolism from fat necrosis outside the nervous system. The patient reported by Milner and Mitchinson [479] had fat embolism to the lungs.

The pathogenesis of this disease is unknown. Observers have incriminated several factors as precipitating either the onset or the recurrence of the disease: use of iodides, bromides, penicillin, or insulin; avitaminosis, and various infections. An animal model was studied by Duran-Reynals [168] in rabbits which he had injected with the Brown-Pearce tumor, the Shope fibroma, vaccinia, several species of bacteria, and some noninfectious materials. Lesions indistinguishable from those of human Weber-Christian disease appeared; there were also hemorrhagic and necrotic lesions within muscles in which fibrotic nodules later developed. The fat lesions were mainly in the abdomen along the psoas muscles from the groin to the kidneys; occasional lesions were in the peritoneal cavity attached to the intestine, liver, or bladder. The disease was epidemic in the rabbits and a viral etiology was suspected because the disorder was transmitted more rapidly and with greater incidence by extracts of the masses than by extracts of control materials.

The nosology of Weber-Christian disease is unclear. It is usually classified as a rheumatic disease because some patients have joint pain or effusions. Panniculitis may be seen in systemic lupus erythematosus and in any cutaneous vasculitis affecting the hypodermis. Yet it is noteworthy that necrotizing vasculitis is not a feature of Weber-Christian disease even though minor endarteritic or perivasculitic changes may be seen in or close to the panniculitis. Lupus factor and rheumatoid factor, often present in systemic rheumatic diseases, were absent in my patient, who did, however, have an epidose of acute hemolytic anemia associated with a positive response to Coombs' test.

ERYTHROMELALGIA

Erythromelalgia is a rare disease in which redness and warmth of the hands or feet, more usually the latter, may be associated with burning pain. The pain may be induced by dependency or other forms of venous congestion, by warmth, or even by light pressure. During an attack the feet are bright red, and tender to the slightest touch. Elevation usually relieves the pain, but hardly affects the redness. It is not clear whether this should be regarded as a disease in its own right or a syndrome with little specificity, as was believed by Lewis [419]. The following patient was referred by a generally knowledgeable internist as possibly having gout or a collagen disease.

Case 14-6.   A 49-year-old man had been experiencing recurrent attacks of pain and redness in fingers and feet. The episodes occurred every few days and were rapidly and lastingly relieved by only 325 to 650 mg of aspirin. He was observed during an attack. The foot and ankle were dusky red and warm; there was distinct swelling of the pulps of the toes and definite, slight swelling of the subcutaneous tissue of the entire foot and ankle. Normal or negative results were obtained on testing for erythrocyte sedimentation rate, C-reactive protein, rheumatoid factor, antinuclear antibodies, serum protein electrophoresis, blood uric acid, and x-rays of the hands and feet. Urine serotonin level was normal.

Another case accorded with the classic description of erythromelalgia as given by Telford and Simmons [673].

Case 14-7.   A 42-year-old man complained of intermittent swelling and color change of both feet and their toes, lasting several months at a time. This had been occurring only for one year. The skin of the affected feet was variously dusky red or cyanotic. The pain was of a burning character, much aggravated by dependency, and there was exquisite tenderness to the lightest tough so that during the height of an attack the patient could not tolerate the pressure of the bedclothes on his skin. There was some alleviation by elevation of the legs.

Babb, Alarcón-Segovia, and Fairbairn [25] reported 51 cases of erythromelalgia seen at The Mayo Clinic during the years 1951 to 1960. Associated conditions, considered possibly causative of the syndrome, were seen in 21 patients; these included polycythemia in nine, systemic lupus erythematosus in one, and rheumatoid arthritis in one. As in Case 14-6, a single dose of 650 mg of aspirin relieved the symptoms in some of their patients for as long as 4 days. Eleven of their 17 patients with primary erythromelalgia and 14 of the 18 patients with secondary erythromelalgia, or 70 per cent of the total who used aspirin, responded well to this small dose.

Two facts suggest the possibility that prostaglandins might mediate erythromelalgia. Prostaglandins E_1, E_2, and $F_{1\alpha}$ and $F_{2\alpha}$ induced wheal and flare responses in human skin [647]. Secondly, prostaglandin production was abolished in platelets from three subjects by the end of the first hour after they had swallowed 650 mg of aspirin, and this effect lasted for as long as 3 days [384, 638].

NONTRAUMATICALLY INDUCED SYSTEMIC FAT EMBOLISM

Patients with multisystem diseases of obscure cause are frequently referred to the rheumatologist, with the question whether they have a collagen disease. In the differential diagnosis of multisystem disease one must include the following: chronic infection, especially mycobacterial or fungal; sarcoidosis or other idiopathic chronic granulomatosis; disseminated cancer, especially lymphoma; amyloidosis; endocrine disorders, particularly hypothyroidism; avitaminoses; paraproteinemias; chronic disseminated intravascular coagulation; and microembolism. Microemboli are often thrombi from leg or pelvic veins, aggregates from infected heart valves, or platelet aggregates from prosthetic heart valves; sometimes they are tiny fragments of atheroma (see Fig. 11-3). It is not widely recognized that fat embolism may be systemic and not confined to the pulmonary circulation, and that fat embolism may occur without apparent trauma.

Case 14-8. A 41-year-old white man was first seen for the complaint of loss of hearing on the right for 2 weeks and blurred vision on the left for 3 days. He drank alcohol only occasionally and in moderation, and had had no known contact with liver toxins.

He was obese, measuring 1.58 m (5'6") and weighing 130.9 kg (288 pounds). Blood pressure was 170/90. On different occasions during the next 3 months, the retinal arteries of both eyes were found to have marked but variable perivascular sheathing, and to contain brilliantly refractile, silvery particles within their lumina, which shifted in their positions and were interpreted as microemboli. The vessels distal to these microemboli were often apparently bloodless. Figure 14-1 illustrates some of these changes.

Hearing loss in the right ear was interpreted as caused by a sensorineural lesion because a vibrating tuning fork held at the vertex (Weber's test) was heard on the left but not on the right side. The initial chest x-ray showed a small infiltrate in the left lung, which had disappeared 5 days later.

Each of the following further evidences of microembolism appeared transiently during his 2-month stay in the hospital: paresthesiae affecting the right arm and right side of the face; pain in the left calf; a period of confusion, inappropriate affect and impaired memory, lasting 2 days and associated with diffuse abnormalities in the electroencephalogram which were absent from a later electroencepahlogram; and signs of pyramidal tract dysfunction on the right side.

Before the microemboli were seen in the retinal vessels, a tentative diagnosis of polyarteritis had been made; but a muscle biopsy did not confirm this diagnosis. After the retinal emboli were observed, it was believed that atheromatosis was the cause of his complaints. However, angiography of the aortic arch, the major arteries in the neck and the intracranial arterial system showed no arteriosclerosis.

Plasma cholesterol was 238 mg/100 ml; triglycerides were 220 and 540 mg/100 ml on different occasions, and lipoprotein electrophoresis showed an increase in the pre-β fraction. Analytical ultracentrifugation of the serum lipoproteins showed Sf 0-12 of 426 and Sf 12-400 of 305 mg/100 ml, which are normal values. Fasting blood sugar was 91 mg/100 ml; the 1-hour value was 203, the 2-hour 234 mg/100 ml.

During an episode of left calf pain that lasted for a day, the creatine phosphokinase was 93 units (normal, <50); it became normal, at 19 units, a few days later.

Platelet counts varied from normal to as high as 785,000/mm, but platelet electrophoretic mobility and adhesiveness were normal, as were results of the following

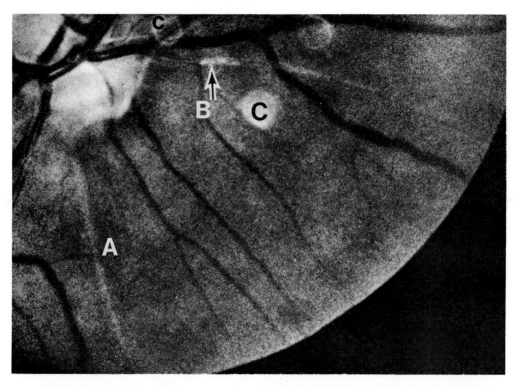

Fig. 14-1.   Case 14-8.   Retinal fat embolism. An empty, "ghost" vessel is seen at A; distal to discrete embolic particles at B, segments of the vessel are empty. The large circular white areas, C, are artifacts from the camera.

studies: hematocrit, white blood cell count, urinalysis, creatinine, serum glutamic and pyruvic oxalacetic transaminases, alkaline phosphatase, sulfobromophthalein retention test, isotopic scan of the liver, blood viscosity, fibrinogen, cryoglobulins, antinuclear antibodies, and VDRL test for syphilis.

In view of the patient's obesity, fat embolism was then considered as a cause of the microemboli in his retina, and presumably in other areas. Fat globules were found in five sputum specimens but none were seen in four urine samples. Attempted percutaneous needle biopsy of the liver was unsuccessful because the abdominal subcutaneous fat was so thick.

The patient's diet was then restricted to 800 calories daily; dicoumarol was given for anticoagulation, and the administration of dipyridamole was begun because of the high platelet count, even though platelet adhesiveness and mobility had been found normal. His complaints ceased and the retinal lesions cleared during his 2 months' stay in the hospital. He took the above therapy for about 6 months. He was observed periodically, and remained well until 6 years later, when anemia and weight loss prompted further studies, which disclosed lymphosarcoma of the spleen; at laparotomy, the pancreas was seen to be infiltrated by the neoplasm and there was fat necrosis in this area.

Zenker's original observation [741], in 1862, of traumatically induced systemic fat embolism in a patient with multiple rib fractures and a lacerated fatty liver, has been repeated many times in patients with bone fractures. Fat embolism may also occur after extensive trauma to subcutaneous fat, and after severe burns or frostbite. The reader is referred to the encyclopedic review by Groskloss [268] of the literature between about 1880 and 1930, the period when most of the important observations relevant to this subject were made, and ideas of pathogenesis conceived. What is sometimes called "atraumatic fat embolism"—although it seems possible that some degree of trauma might precede embolism—is seen in patients with fatty liver [291] and in patients with bone marrow infarction from sickle cell crisis [378].

Hartroft and Ridout [291], and Owens and Sokal [534] induced fatty livers in rats by means of choline-deficient diets, and gave histopathologic evidence that fat globules in the liver parenchyma can rupture into the central sinusoidal veins and reach the systemic arterial tree after passage through the lungs. Lynch et al [433] correlated the amount of fat in the liver and the presence of fat emboli within the lungs or brain in a series of chronic alcoholic patients studied at autopsy. They also found that among 51 patients with alcoholic psychosis 48 had fat globules in their sputum. They considered that embolism to the brain from a fatty liver might sometimes cause delirium tremens and epilepsy in alcoholic patients. Fat embolism in the absence of obvious trauma has also been seen in both endogenous and exogenous hypercortisonism [312, 351]. In such cases, fatty liver, known to result from chronic administration of corticosteroid drugs [490], is presumably the source of the embolized fat.

The source of the fat emboli in our patient is not determined. It is possible that the lymphosarcoma which indirectly caused retroperitoneal fat necrosis was already present; but such dormancy would be unusually long for this neoplasm. We could not obtain a liver specimen, but responses to all of the chemical tests of liver function were normal, and he drank little alcohol. Despite this, he might have had a fatty liver because he was enormously obese. Yet one wonders why the subcutaneous fat itself might not serve as a source of fat embolism. One can readily visualize fat globules being squeezed and ruptured into adjacent veins by local pressure upon the buttocks when a very fat person sits down. One may speculate, whether fat globules are normally squeezed into the blood stream from various sites such as ribs, abdominal organs, and subcutaneous fat; if this indeed happens physiologically, the mechanism that ensures their prompt emulsification must be defective in Case 14-8 and in those subjects—as many as 50 per cent in some series [268]—found to have fat embolism at postmortem examination. An extension of this concept is the possibility that blood lipids may become demulsified. Lehman and McNattin [407] found that trauma had played no role in half of all subjects found to have fat embolism at postmortem examination; and Lehman and Moore [408] calculated that the amount of fat in the marrow of a femur is insufficient to induce the symptoms of fat embolism. They studied the plasma as a source of embolic fat (although the word "embolic" here may be etymologically incorrect, its meaning is clear). They showed that ether, histamine, and extracts of necrotic muscle could destroy emulsions *in vitro,* and that ether could promptly induce fat embolism *in vivo.* They therefore proposed that demulsification of the blood fats could contribute in whole or in part to fat embolism either in the presence or in the absence of trauma. The earliest example of this in diabetic lipemia was probably contributed by Saunders and Hamilton [602] in 1879.

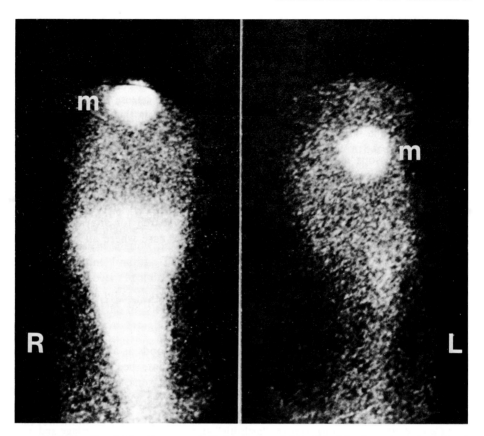

Fig. 14-2.   Case 14-9.   Bone scan. Ewing's sarcoma of right tibia. M = isotopic markers placed over tibial tubercles.

several years, for which she used an occasional aspirin tablet. About 2 weeks before the petechial rash had appeared, she had increased the quantity of aspirin from 1 tablet every 2 or 3 days, to 2 tablets daily.

Physical examination in April 1971 demonstrated swelling and pain in the fifth right metacarpophalangeal joint and in the second left terminal interphalangeal joint, with some pain to pressure in a few of the metatarsophalangeal joints. Aside from the presence of fading petechiae, the remainder of the physical findings were within normal limits.

Pertinent laboratory findings included 5 per cent eosinophils in the peripheral blood, γ-globulin level of 22.3 per cent, and a positive test for rheumatoid factor. Responses were negative to tests for Coombs' reaction, antinuclear antibodies, cold agglutinins, and cryoglobulins. X-rays of the hands and feet showed no abnormalities. Biopsy of the skin at the site of the petechial eruption demonstrated acute vasculitis.

She was placed on a salicylate-free diet and within one week felt much better. She noted, then, that previously she had drunk liberal quantities of wine, and had used skin creams, both of which contain large amounts of salicylates.

Follow-up during the next 4 years showed absolutely no recurrence of her polyarthritis. There were occasions when a few petechiae recurred, but she was always able to relate these to the inadvertent ingestion of foods that contained salicylate, e.g., vinegar or citrus fruits. She was so impressed by the remission of her polyarthritis, and by the clear relation between the recurrence of petechiae and salicylate-containing foods, that she adhered rigidly to her diet during the 3 years of follow-up. Repeat blood tests for rheumatoid factor in 1972 and 1973 were both negative.

The nature of intolerance to aspirin is of interest. Samter and Beers [600] pointed out that aspirin-sensitive patients are able to take *sodium* salicylate with impunity; and that the existence of antibodies to acetylsalicylic acid has not been demonstrated unequivocally. The usual manifestations of intolerance to aspirin comprise angio-edema, rhinitis, and bronchial asthma. Samter and Beers proposed that these effects were from a direct action of aspirin upon peripheral chemoreceptors, and not from an antigen-antibody reaction. They were unable to explain certain features of the syndrome of intolerance to aspirin, namely the frequent presence of nasal polyps and urticaria. Swineford and Bray [664] reviewed 111 reports of adverse effects of aspirin listed in the *Index Medicus* during a 4-year period. In only eight of these reports were the manifestations considered to be of the sort ordinarily seen from an immunological reaction; and six of these eight referred to urticaria, angio-edema, and asthma. Thus, it appears that true allergy to aspirin or salicylates is uncommon. There is, unfortunately, no laboratory test system to prove allergy to aspirin; nevertheless, it seems likely that salicylate allergy was responsible for the inflammatory polyarthritis and cutaneous vasculitis in Case 14-11.

CHAPTER 15

The Community Hospital Laboratory in Diagnosis of Rheumatic Diseases

Although the spectacular advances in rheumatology have been made through the facilities of research laboratories, the facilities of the community hospital laboratory are generally ample for diagnosing and following rheumatic patients. All of the needed studies are usually available, and those that are as yet unavailable to the community laboratory have not been tested in adequate numbers of patients or in sufficiently various conditions to make the findings easily interpretable.

HEMATOLOGIC STUDIES

Hematocrit. In rheumatoid arthritis, the hematocrit reading is usually in the region of 30 to 35 per cent; it is occasionally as low as 25 per cent without evidence of gross gastrointestinal blood loss. The anemia is usually normocytic and mildly hypochromic. Serum iron levels are diminished in proportion to the activity of the disease; total iron binding capacity is low, in contrast to the situation in iron deficiency anemia. Bone marrow iron stores are normal. Many investigators have found slightly decreased rates of red blood cell survival, but these findings have no clinical relevance.

When anemia is present in systemic lupus erythematosus, one should seek evidence of hemolysis. The reaction is often positive to Coombs' test with antigammaglobulin serum; but in some cases of frank hemolysis, the reaction to Coombs' test with this reagent is negative. This is because in certain instances sublytic fixation of complement to red cells occurs together with antibodies to red cells, and such erythrocytes are not hemolysed outright. The detection of binding of complement components to the red blood cell may require use of specific antisera to one or more of the human complement proteins. It is necessary to ascertain that the laboratory uses a Coombs' reagent that contains antisera both to γ-globulin and to complement. If, however, the anticomplement component of the reagent is insufficiently powerful, many instances of hemolytic anemia in systemic lupus erythematosus will be labeled as Coombs' negative.

White blood cell count. In adult rheumatoid arthritis, leukopenia is rare, and when present should alert one to the possibility of systemic lupus erythematosus rather than rheumatoid arthritis. In juvenile rheumatoid arthritis, leukocytosis is quite common and may be so considerable as to suggest the possibility of leukemia. White blood cell counts of 30,000 or even 50,000/cu mm are not exceptional.

Leukopenia affects about 40 per cent of patients with systemic lupus erythematosus at some during the course of the illness. The ARA criteria require leukopenia of <4,000/cu mm on two or more occasions, as a qualification toward the diagnosis of systemic lupus erythematosus [115]. There are important differences in mean leukocyte counts according to sex, race, and smoking habits [222]: higher mean counts are found in women than in men, in whites than in blacks, and in smokers than in nonsmokers. Four thousand white blood cells per cubic millimeter is the lower limit of normal for white nonsmokers of both sexes; but the lower limit of normal for nonsmoking black men is 3,300 and for nonsmoking black women 3,200/cu mm.

Monocytosis. Maldonado and Hanlon [442] studied patients whose relative monocyte count exceeded 15 per cent and whose absolute count exceeded 500/cu mm. Among 160 patients with monocytosis according to these criteria were 16 (10 per cent) with collagen diseases, mostly rheumatoid arthritis.

Eosinophilia. Mild eosinophilia may be seen in any of the connective tissue diseases but is especially characteristic of polyarteritis nodosa. The highest eosinophil counts, sometimes reaching 70 to 80 per cent, are seen in allergic granulomatosis.

Platelets. Thrombocytopenia, defined as a platelet count of <100,000/cu mm, affected 11.4 per cent of the patients with systemic lupus erythematosus studied by the Diagnostic and Therapeutic Criteria Committee of the ARA [115]. Low levels of platelets should also alert one to the possibility of the rare thrombotic thrombocytopenic purpura. Contrariwise, thrombocytosis, defined as counts >400,000/cu mm, was found to be due to collagen disease, principally rheumatoid arthritis, in 18 of the 82 patients with such high platelet counts studied by Levin and Conley [413]. Selroos [612] saw platelet counts exceeding 400,000/cu mm in 35 (29 per cent) of 120 patients with rheumatoid arthritis, in seven (32 per cent) of 22 with ankylosing spondylitis, and in nine (15 per cent) of 62 patients with other connective tissue diseases. A specific example, Wegener's granulomatosis, was given by Fauci and Wolff [189]: seven of 18 patients had thrombocytosis with a mean platelet count of 1,007,500/cu mm, in a range of 540,000 to 1,630,000/cu mm.

ACUTE PHASE REACTANTS

The erythrocyte sedimentation rate (ESR) is the acute phase reactant that is usually measured. Experience has shown that the Westergren method is superior to others. Early studies revealed some patients with normal ESR by the Wintrobe method but very fast ESR by the Westergren technique [248]. Everyone recognizes the value of the finding of a fast ESR. However, a common error is to assume that a normal ESR excludes the possibility of serious disease. We have often seen patients with active systemic lupus erythematosus, including one in severe lupus crisis, and patients with active rheumatoid polyarthritis, whose ESR was normal by the Westergren method. The fastest ESR's are seen in multiple myeloma, Waldenström's macroglobulinemia, polymyalgia rheumatica, and giant cell arteritis. In these conditions, the ESR often exceeds 120 mm/hr (Westergren method). A remarkably slow ESR, even zero, should alert one to the possibility of cryoglobulinemia.

One of the main problems in interpretation of ESR is the patient's age. Studies show that by the time a patient reaches age 60, the Westergren ESR may normally be as high as 30 mm/hr. It is not clear how high the ESR may normally reach after the age of 60; it is likely that a further 10 mm/hr per decade of age may be added to the normal value at age 60.

It is no longer fashionable to measure other acute phase reactants, such as fibrinogen, C-reactive protein, haptoglobin, α_2-macroglobulin, and hexose-bound proteins, e.g., sialoprotein. On occasion, however, when the ESR is normal and one is looking for another measure of disease activity, these acute phase reactants may be useful factors to follow in measuring the efficacy of therapy.

SERUM CHEMISTRY

Serum uric acid. It is crucial to understand that there are important differences in findings according to whether the laboratory uses a manual colorimetric, automated colorimetric, or ultraviolet spectrophotometric (uricase) method of analysis. The colorimetric methods give mean values between 0.5 and 1.0 mg/100 ml higher than the uricase method. There is great variation between laboratories, even when using the same technique; the widest variation occurs with the manual colorimetric method. We have found statistically significant differences between the mean values obtained by similar instrumentation and method in laboratories at our San Francisco and Oakland clinics (see Table 5-1). Moreover, there is a marked variation across time. For all these reasons, it is not acceptable for the laboratory to quote a normal range from the literature; each laboratory must establish its own normal ranges, and must repeat such studies from time to time.

Serum calcium and phosphorus levels. These should be estimated in all but the most obvious or trivial cases because of the arthropathy, myopathy, or neuropathy that may accompany derangements in these levels.

Serum thyroxine. Important rheumatic manifestations accompany both hyperfunction and hypofunction of the thyroid gland. Hypothyroidism is more often the cause of rheumatic complaints and is more difficult to diagnose than is hyperthyroidism. More recent studies suggest that thyroid stimulating hormone, now readily measurable by radioimmunoassay, provides the most useful measure of hypothyroidism.

SERUM ENZYMES

Lactic dehydrogenase. This is an important enzyme in suspected muscle disease. It has five isoenzymes, labeled 1 to 5 according to the rapidity of their electrophoretic migration, the fastest (i.e., most anodal) being number 1; the slowest (i.e., most cathodal), number 5. Each isomer is a tetramer having different combinations of two major subunits, A and B. LDH 4 and 5 are the principal isoenzymes in skeletal muscle and liver; LDH 1 and 2 are the principal isoenzymes in the heart, red blood cells, and kidney. The percentage of LDH 4 and 5 tends not to rise until the absolute level of LDH exceeds approximately four times normal.

Creatine phosphokinase. The serum creatine phosphokinase (CPK) level is widely recognized as among the most useful of the various blood enzymes for the diagnosis of myopathy. This topic is covered in greater detail in Chapter 11. Here, it will only be mentioned that interpretation of high levels must be made with knowledge of the several conditions other than skeletal myopathy or cardiomyopathy that may cause a rise in serum CPK activity, including various disorders of the central nervous system, among them acute stroke and epilepsy; acute psychotic states; muscular exercise and electromyography; acute pulmonary embolism, and hypothyroidism. An advantage of studying CPK rather than serum glutamic oxalacetic transaminase or LDH levels in the diagnosis of myopathy is that CPK is not influenced by minor degrees of liver disease or anemia as are the latter. On the other hand, in idiopathic polymyositis, the CPK may occasionally be normal when other enzyme levels are increased; in muscular dystrophies the CPK is the most sensitive test [504].

SEROLOGIC STUDIES

Serum protein electrophoresis. Serum protein electrophoresis is widely performed but has very little, if any, value because virtually every abnormal pattern is nonspecific. The only specific pattern of rheumatologic interest is that of agammaglobulinemia; even this must be further studied in terms of specific immunoglobulin deficiencies. The presence of a monoclonal spike in the region of the β- or γ-globulin fractions must be investigated as possibly due to multiple myeloma, benign monoclonal gammopathy, primary macroglobulinemia of Waldenström, or one of the many causes of secondary macroglobulinemia.

Immunoelectrophoresis. This study is almost never indicated for routine clinical investigation except in an attempt to demonstrate that a peak in the electrophoretic pattern is monoclonal rather than polyclonal.

Quantitative immunoglobulin levels. Knowledge of quantitative levels of immunoglobulins is of far greater utility than the immunoelectrophoretic pattern because 1) levels of specific immunoglobulins are absent or low in so-called "agammaglobulinemia,"which is more usually hypogammaglobulinemia, or 2) the level of an immunoglobulin of a single species is greatly increased in a monoclonal gammopathy. The study has virtually no other clinical value.

Cryoglobulins. These are mostly IgG, occasionally IgM. While cryoglobulins usually reflect a generalized dysproteinemia, they may occasionally represent specific paraproteins as in myeloma or macroglobulinemia. When present in large quantities, cryoglobulins may cause clinical difficulties by mechanically impairing the peripheral circulation. While it is usually necessary to cool the serum to approximately $+4°$ C in order to demonstrate cryoglobulins, they sometimes precipitate at much higher temperatures, even as close to body temperature as 35° C; the clinical syndromes that result may then be especially severe. Rarely, the cryoglobulin consists of a mixture of IgG and IgM; here, the IgM has rheumatoid factor properties. These so-called "mixed cryoglobulins" are, in effect, circulating immune complexes and may cause any of the manifestations of immune complex deposition disease, including nephritis and cutaneous purpura.

Complement components. At the time of this writing, the C3 and C4 components of complement are readily estimated by means of immunodiffusion; whereas tests for levels of other complement components are not readily available in the community hospital laboratory. The major value of serum complement component levels is in following the activity of systemic lupus erythematosus. Lupus nephritis, an example of immune complex disease, is frequently accompanied by low serum complement levels because of the consumption of complement by the circulating immune complexes. In the presence of known lupus nephritis, the finding of low serum complement levels is particularly ominous because it demonstrates either current activity or the potential for early future activity of the nephritis. There is no substantial evidence to show that a low serum complement activity is necessarily ominous in systemic lupus erythematosus in the absence of known nephritis; but in all of such patients with this problem that I have followed, serious activity of their lupus has developed within 6 months. Therefore, serum complement levels should be carefully monitored at regular intervals in all patients with systemic lupus erythematosus. They represent the best yardstick of activity of the disease that is currently available. Serum complement levels may be low, too, in other immune complex deposition diseases, such as chronic serum sickness or the arthritis associated with the early phases of serum hepatitis.

Chronic false positive serologic tests for syphilis. Approximately 10 per cent of patients with systemic lupus erythematosus have chronic false positive reactions to serologic tests for syphilis (STS). Contrariwise, mass screening studies have shown that a high percentage of patients exhibiting a biologic false positive reaction to STS, as shown by systems utilizing nontreponemal antigens, eventually have a connective tissue disease, most often systemic lupus erythematosus. Positive reactions in the fluorescent treponemal antibody system may also be nonsyphilitic in origin in patients with systemic lupus erythematosus; in such cases, the fluorescent pattern is bumpy instead of linear.

Serum viscosity. Hyperviscosity is rarely of clinical importance in collagen diseases, but may be of major concern in multiple myeloma or Waldenström's macroglobulinemia. A clinical clue to its presence is seen in widely dilated, sausage-like retinal veins.

Histocompatibility antigens. Testing for histocompatibility antigens is beyond the scope of the community hospital laboratory, but it is possible to arrange for such studies to be performed by a number of specialized laboratories. It is appropriate to mention them here because a number of reports have shown such a strong association between a specific histocompatibility antigen (HL-A antigen W27) and both ankylosing spondylitis and Reiter's syndrome, that the possibility has been suggested of using the presence of the W27 antigen as a diagnostic test for these diseases.

The chromosome region that governs histocompatibility includes a series of separate loci, termed HL-A, that control different structures in the cell membrane. It is possible by serologic means to detect some of these antigenic structures in the cell membrane. The histocompatibility genes act as dominant autosomal traits. There is a close genetic linkage between the histocompatibility genes and the immune response genes. An association has been observed between certain HL-A antigenic phenotypes and the occurrence of some diseases. The significance of these associations is uncertain, but two ways in which heightened susceptibility to disease might result from possession of certain histocompatibility genes are: 1) shared antigens between the cell membrane antigens determined by histocompatibility genes and a foreign protein, e.g., virus, causing immunological tolerance to the virus, 2) control by the genetically linked immune response gene, of the host's reaction to the antigenic determinants of a virus [457]. Another possible mechanism to account for the association between particular HL-A antigens and certain diseases is that HL-A antigen, which is on the cell surface, has a molecular configuration that enhances selective binding by a virus or other pathogenic agent [457].

Brewerton and coworkers [70] identified HL-A antigen W27 in 72 (96 per cent) of 75 patients with ankylosing spondylitis and in only three (4 per cent) of 75 controls. Among 60 first-degree relatives of the patients, 31 (51 per cent) had HL-A antigen W27; 15 of the 30 female relatives were positive for the antigen. Similar results were obtained by Schlosstein and coworkers [603], who observed the W27 antigen in 35 (88 per cent) of 40 patients with ankylosing spondylitis and in 8 per cent of controls.

Morris and coworkers [492] found HL-A antigen W27 in 24 (96 per cent) of 25 patients with Reiter's syndrome, in only 8 per cent of 1,863 controls, and in none of 12 patients with gonococcal arthritis. Brewerton and coworkers [72] observed the W27 antigen in 25 (75 per cent) of 33 patients, Amor et al [16] in 37 (80 per cent) of 46 patients, and Woodrow [732] in 13 (65 per cent) of 20 patients with Reiter's syndrome.

A hint that the specificity might not prove to be quite so clear as the above results indicate came from a brief report by Aho and coworkers [10], who found HL-A 27 antigen in all of five patients with gonococcal arthritis: since they also identified the antigen in 20 of 22 patients with Yersinia arthritis, and Friis and Svejgaard [227] observed this antigen in three of five cases of Salmonella arthritis, it was postulated that the possession of this genetic determinant might predispose to infectious arthritis in general. This possibility raises many questions about the role of infection in the pathogenesis of those conditions that have a strong association with histocompatibility antigens.

ANTINUCLEAR FACTORS

Antinuclear antibodies. The use of fluorescein-labeled antigammaglobulin antisera, causing fluorescence of nuclei to which antinuclear antibodies are attached, is a technique available in most community hospital laboratories. The method is rapidly performed and quite sensitive, but lacks the specificity of the LE cell preparation. A variety of patterns of nuclear fluorescence may be observed: diffuse or homogeneous; speckled; outlined, peripheral or shaggy; and nucleolar. Despite some controversy on this point in the literature, there seems to be little specificity attached to any pattern except, possibly, to the outlined and nucleolar. The outlined pattern seems best correlated with the presence of antibodies to DNA in the serum and, thus, with active systemic lupus erythematosus. However, one should not infer activity of this disease merely on the basis of the presence of an outlined pattern of nuclear fluorescence. The nucleolar pattern of fluorescence is seen especially often in scleroderma, but may be noted in other conditions, particularly systemic lupus erythematosus. The specificity of the antinuclear antibody test system is increased by using a dilution of serum. The problem, a general one in laboratory medicine, is that increasing specificity of the test system causes concomitant decrease in sensitivity. Since the antinuclear antibody test is so readily performed, it is useful as a screening reaction, and it is highly desirable that a screening test system be as sensitive as possible, even at the expense of specificity. In our own studies, among 218 undiluted sera from individual patients with positive responses to tests for antinuclear antibodies, 24 were positive at serum dilutions of 1:10 with fluorescence >2+. Eight of these 24 sera, and only three of the remaining 194 sera, were able to induce positive LE cell preparations. In our laboratory, therefore, the serum dilution 1:10 seems the most useful in terms of correlation with positive LE preparation; each laboratory must determine the optimum dilution for the system in local use.

Positive results for antinuclear antibodies are seen in the following percentages: systemic lupus erythematosus, 95 per cent; rheumatoid arthritis, 30 per cent; other connective tissue diseases, 30 per cent; chronic bronchitis, 20 per cent; various thyroid diseases, 10 per cent; patients hospitalized for various medical conditions, 20 per cent. It is important to note that antinuclear factors are found in more than 75 per cent of normal sera if the top fraction of the frozen, then thawed, unmixed serum is used for the test [396].

Although the measurement of antibodies to DNA by radioimmunoassay is not yet a standard procedure in the community hospital laboratory, it seems probable that it will become routine within a few years. This is an important assay because it quantifies the antibody titer more accurately than is possible by other methods; a purified antigen is used, and the technique is relatively straight-forward. It has become clear that the sera of patients with diseases other than systemic lupus erythematosus have binding specificity for native DNA. This is not surprising, considering the nonspecificity of the antinuclear antibody assay by the fluorescent antibody technique. Among 182 sera from patients with diseases other than systemic lupus erythematosus, Hasselbacher and LeRoy [295] saw significant DNA binding by radioimmunoassay in sera from patients with viral hepatitis, chronic glomerulonephritis, acute glomerulonephritis, nephrotic syndrome, polymyositis, rheumatoid arthritis, and diffuse vasculitis. Aside from the questions that this finding raises about the role of DNA antibodies in the pathogenesis of systemic lupus erythematosus, it serves as a timely warning against diagnosing that disease on serological grounds alone.

LE cell preparations. The preparation and examination of slides for LE cells is both tedious and time-consuming, so that in many community hospital laboratories the results, especially when negative, are unreliable; for this reason, the LE cell test has been largely replaced by tests for antinuclear antibodies.

The recognition of LE cells in the bone marrow represented another landmark in rheumatology; indeed, in medicine itself. The history of the discovery of the LE cell by Hargraves [288] has been described by him in a paper to which the interested reader is directed. The key observation was in the bone marrow of a patient with systemic lupus erythematosus, reported by Dr. Hargraves as follows: "The outstanding thing in this bone marrow is the phagocytic reticulo-endothelial cells which contain a blue-staining hyaline-like material which we have not previously observed . . . . This material stains from a light blue to a very dark, almost indigo blue." In retrospect, Dr. Hargraves recalled reporting a bone marrow 3 years previously as follows: "Peculiar, rather structureless globular bodies taking purple stain. This is not diagnostic." The presence of positive LE cell preparations is almost specific for systemic lypus erythematosus, but it must be recalled that LE cells may be seen in 5 per cent or more of patients with rheumatoid arthritis depending upon the assiduity of the search for them, and that they are occasionally seen in other connective tissue reactions. They may also be observed in patients with chronic active hepatitis, and occasionally in patients with cirrhosis; in patients with drug reactions, e.g., to penicillin, sulfonamides, isoniazid, and diphenylhydantoin; and, of course, in drug-induced lupus, especially from procainamide and hydralazine (see Table 10-6).

Sometimes puzzling to the clinician is an LE cell preparation that is reported as showing hematoxylin bodies and rosettes, but no LE cells. In order to understand the significance of this finding, one should recall the mechanism of formation of the LE cell. The lupus factors enter the cells, especially the mononuclears, causing the nuclei to swell and be extruded from the body of the cell. These altered nuclei are termed *hematoxylin* (sometimes *hematoxophil*) *bodies* because they stain dark blue with hematoxylin dye; they are chemotactic and they attract microphages, the polymorphonuclear leukocytes, which become arrayed around each hematoxylin body in the shape of a rosette. The LE cell results when one of the microphages finally engulfs and phagocytizes the hematoxylin body. When one suspects systemic lupus erythematosus, the presence of abundant hematoxylin bodies should encourage one to make many more LE cell preparations in the expectation of obtaining a positive result.

Rheumatoid factors. Rheumatoid factors are autoantibodies, usually IgM but occasionally IgG, having anti-IgG specificity. The discovery of rheumatoid factors and the demonstration that they are autoantibodies represent landmarks in rheumatology, and some historical background may be of interest. In 1930, Cecil, Nicholls, and Stainsby [97] reported that sera of patients with rheumatoid arthritis caused agglutination of certain strains of streptococci. In subsequent years it was shown that various other bacteria, including pneumococci, enterococci, and staphylococci were also agglutinated by sera of patients with rheumatoid arthritis. It seemed, therefore, that the agglutinating activity of rheumatoid sera was the result of a nonspecific agglutinating factor rather than of specific bacterial agglutinins. Then, in 1940, Waaler [700] reported that sera from patients with rheumatoid arthritis were able to agglutinate sheep red blood cells that had been sensitized with small amounts of rabbit anti-sheep cell serum. Further studies of this phenomenon were published in 1948 by Rose and coworkers [589]. As a result, the so-called "sensitized sheep cell test" came to be called the Rose-Waaler reaction. Subsequently, several variations of this reaction system were devised, all depending upon some carrier particle, whether sheep red blood cells, human group O rhesus-negative red blood cells, bentonite particles, or latex particles. One of the most convenient systems, still in wide use, is the latex fixation test devised by Singer and Plotz [636], in which latex particles form a nidus around which the agglutination between γ-globulin (fraction II of human serum according to the Cohn method of fractionation) and rheumatoid factor agglutinate in such a fashion as to be macroscopically visible. If the reaction is performed in test tubes, serial doubling-dilutions may be made and a titer obtained; in a widely used modification, the reaction is performed on a slide and allows merely a statement that rheumatoid factor is present or absent.

Rheumatoid factors as measured by latex agglutination reactions are present in approximately 70 per cent of adult patients with peripheral rheumatoid arthritis, in approximately 30 per cent of patients with the combination of rheumatoid arthritis and psoriasis, and in about 30 per cent of patients with juvenile rheumatoid arthritis. Patients with rheumatoid nodules almost always have rheumatoid factor in the serum; so do patients whose joints show radiological evidence of erosions, unless they have juvenile rheumatoid arthritis, associated psoriasis, or ankylosing spondylitis. It cannot be sufficiently emphasized that the presence of rheumatoid factor in the serum does not establish the diagnosis of rheumatoid arthritis, because the factor is present in about 30 per cent of patients with other collagen diseases, in a high percentage of the family members of patients with rheumatoid arthritis, in 20 or 30 per cent of patients with various liver diseases, in as many as 50 per cent of patients with various lung diseases including chronic bronchitis, tuberculosis, or sarcoidosis; and, in general, rheumatoid factor may be found in any condition with associated hypergammaglobulinemia. Tests for rheumatoid factor may become transiently positive during active subacute bacterial endocarditis; and with increasing age there is a stepwise increase in positivity of tests for rheumatoid factor so that approximately 80 per cent of patients over the age of 80 have positive reactions even though they do not have rheumatoid arthritis. In the general population, positive latex agglutination on slide tests for rheumatoid factor were found in 2,870 (2.6 per cent) of 110,886 persons studied in our multiphasic program; there were similar numbers of positive reactions in females (2.7 per cent) and in males (2.6 per cent).

A positive reaction to test for rheumatoid factor in a member of the general population is a true positive, i.e., implies rheumatoid arthritis, in only 26 per cent of instances. This statement derives from the following reasoning: Assume that 1 per cent of the general population has rheumatoid arthritis, that 2 per cent of the general population has falsely positive reactions to test for rheumatoid factor, and that the test gives positive results in 70 per cent of patients with rheumatoid arthritis. Then, among 1,000 members of the general population there will be 10 (1 per cent) with rheumatoid arthritis, of whom 7 (70 per cent) react positively to tests for rheumatoid factor; and there will be 990 (99 per cent) without rheumatoid arthritis, of whom 20 (2 per cent) show positive reactions to test for rheumatoid factor; thus, among the 27 persons who react positively to test for rheumatoid factor in this general population of 1,000 persons, only 7 (26 per cent) have rheumatoid arthritis; the other 20 have falsely positive reactions.

For all of the preceding reasons, it is strongly recommended that the diagnosis of rheumatoid arthritis be made on clinical and radiological grounds rather than on the basis of the presence or absence of rheumatoid factor in the serum.

NITROBLUE TETRAZOLIUM (NBT) TEST IN SYSTEMIC LUPUS ERYTHEMATOSUS WITH FEVER

The differential diagnosis of a fever in patients with systemic lupus erythematosus is often difficult. Although fever may be part of active systemic lupus, the patient is often being treated with corticosteroids and so is liable to acute infection. The NBT test is not routinely performed in most community hospital laboratories, but it shows such promise of discriminating infectious from noninfectious causes of fever, that it may become more widely available. The test depends upon the reduction of pale yellow NBT to blue-black formazan crystals by peripheral blood neutrophils in the presence of bacterial infection. The studies of Matula and Paterson [451] showed an excellent separation of patients with infection from those without, by this test. Dr. Matula (personal communication) observed that the NBT test was uniformly negative in 10 patients with systemic lupus erythematosus who had no infection, and in one patient with systemic lupus and active tuberculosis; it was positive in six patients with systemic lupus and acute bacterial infection. An additional patient with systemic lupus and hyperpyrexia from lupus crisis had two negative and two positive test results. These are sparse findings but suggest that in febrile patients with systemic lupus, a negative response to the NBT test gives strong support to the probability that the lupus itself is the cause of the fever.

SYNOVIAL FLUID ANALYSIS

Although academic rheumatologists have given analysis of synovial fluid a crucial place in the investigation of arthritis, its practical value is somewhat limited. In chronic arthritis, analysis of synovial fluid permits the differentiation of inflammatory from noninflammatory conditions; sometimes such differentiation may be achieved without this examination. It is in acute arthritis that examination of synovial fluid is most valuable because it differentiates infectious synovitis and crystal-induced synovitis from other conditions.

In chronic noninflammatory arthritis, as from degenerative joint disease, the synovial fluid has a clear color, is viscous, does not clot spontaneously, has a white blood cell count of <3,000/cu mm with fewer than 15 or 20 per cent polymorphonuclear leukocytes, and has a total protein content that is usually <3.5 g/100 ml. A normal degree of viscosity may be inferred by ejecting some of the fluid from the syringe and noting that the expelled fluid remains in a solid column for about 2 inches before breaking up into droplets; a fluid of low viscosity breaks up into droplets almost immediately upon leaving the tip of the syringe. The presence of a normal-looking mucin clot, after addition of an equal volume of 2 per cent acetic acid, is another sign that the synovial fluid is noninflammatory, but this test may be omitted if the others are performed.

An inflammatory synovial fluid, e.g., from a patient with rheumatoid arthritis or Reiter's syndrome, is turbid, may clot spontaneously, has poor viscosity, contains >3,000 white blood cells per cubic millimeter with a much higher proportion of polymyorphonuclear leukocytes than in the noninflammatory fluid, has a total protein content >3.5 g/100 ml, and forms a poor mucin clot. Phase microscopy has shown that the polymorphonuclear leukocytes in synovial effusions may contain inclusion bodies; although these were at one time considered to be indicative of rheumatoid arthritis, they have been demonstrated in a wide variety of arthritides [22, 648, 693, 724].

In acute arthritis, the two crucial tests of the synovial fluid that must be made immediately are 1) the sugar content, which is very low in infectious arthritis, less than one-half the blood level, and 2) the examination under polarized light for crystals. The cell count may be quite misleading, because enormous numbers of white blood cells, 300,000 or even 500,000/cu mm, with a predominance of polymorphonuclear leukocytes, may be seen in noninfectious inflammatory conditions such as rheumatoid arthritis, gout, and Reiter's syndrome. The fluid is best examined for crystals by a polarizing microscope, with which most community hospital laboratories are unequipped; it may be done in a less satisfactory fashion by inserting polarizing material into the eyepiece and above the condensor of an ordinary laboratory microscope, and changing the axis of the polarized light by rotating the eyepiece. The urate crystals in gout are bright yellow in one axis of the polarized light and bright blue in the other; i.e., urate crystals are intensely birefringent. In contrast to these, the calcium pyrophosphate crystals of pseudogout are only weakly birefringent, i.e., the blue and yellow colors are not particularly intense. If the polarizing microscope is used, urate crystals may be seen to be negatively birefringent; i.e., they are

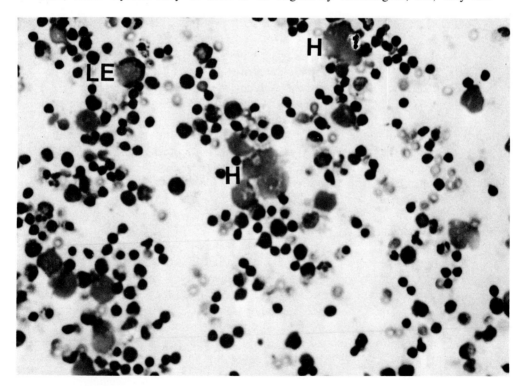

Fig. 15-1. Pleural effusion from patient with systemic lupus erythematosus. H = hematoxylin bodies; LE = lupus erythematosus cell. Hematoxylin and eosin ×325.

yellow when the long axis of the crystal is parallel to the axis of slow vibration of light; whereas the pyrophosphate crystals are positively birefringent, i.e., yellow when the long axis of the crystal is perpendicular to the axis of slow vibration of light.

Study of the total complement level of synovial fluid provides interesting and possibly important information; but the community hospital laboratory can usually provide only C3 and C4 levels, which are of little help in differential diagnosis (see Table 9-1).

PLEURAL FLUID ANALYSIS

In rheumatoid arthritis, the pleural fluid glucose level is exceptionally low, even lower than in cases of infection; in systemic lupus erythematosus, the pleural fluid glucose level is normal [88]. Pleural fluid complement levels may be very low in patients with rheumatoid arthritis or systemic lupus erythematosus. The pleural fluid is one of the few sites in which LE cells may form *in vivo* (Fig. 15-1), and an occasional case of systemic lupus erythematosus has been diagnosed on this basis by an alert cytologist. The cytology of the pleural fluid in rheumatoid arthritis is discussed in Chapter 9.

CHAPTER 16

Drug Treatment of Rheumatic Diseases

Any discussion of the drug therapy of the rheumatic diseases is complicated by the number of factors for which treatment is to be given, which are common to several or all of these disorders. It is further complicated by the applicability of the available forms of therapy to a variety of diseases of this category. The present discussion has for the most part been arranged according to disease. Preceding those divisions are five sections relating to treatments that are so widely applicable as to make totally arbitrary any attempt to place them under the heading of a selected disorder. An outline is furnished to facilitate the finding of specific subjects:

WIDELY APPLICABLE THERAPIES

  I. Nondrug therapy of rheumatic diseases
 II. Some comments on certain analgesic, antipyretic, and anti-inflammatory drugs
    A. Aspirin
    B. Codeine
    C. Indomethacin
    D. Phenylbutazone and oxyphenbutazone
    E. Chloroquine
III. Intra-articular steroid injections
    A. Injection of the knee
    B. Injection of the subacromial bursa
    C. Injection of the ankle joint
    D. Injection of the humeral epicondyles
    E. Injection of the carpal tunnel
    F. Injection of the wrist joint
    G. Injection of trigger finger
 IV. Systemic corticosteroid therapy
    A. General principles
    B. Precautions
    C. Adverse side effects
  V. General comments on the use of cytotoxic agents in rheumatic disease

TREATMENT OF SPECIFIC DISORDERS

 VI. Drug therapy of rheumatoid arthritis
    A. Gold
    B. Orally administered corticosteroids

NONDRUG THERAPY OF RHEUMATIC DISEASES

It is beyond the scope of this book to discuss the nondrug therapies of rheumatic diseases, but a brief statement is pertinent about the two chief forms of nondrug treatment—physical therapy and orthopedic surgery. Therapeutic exercises and appropriate splinting are the main contributions of physical medicine to this field; machines that deliver rays, vibrations, or electric currents have no place in the treatment of arthritis. The role of orthopedic surgery in rheumatic therapy is still being defined; before recommending a surgical procedure for joint disease, the internist should convince himself that the patient's functional impairment is such as to justify not only the general risks that attend operation, but also the possibility of failure. It is seldom proper to permit surgical correction of deformities for cosmetic reasons only; many patients have amazingly good function despite severe deformities and are often disappointed by the only slight improvement induced by surgical intervention. Synovectomies do not cure rheumatoid arthritis but may afford relief of pain for a year or so; the development of prosthetic joints is in its infancy and this form of treatment should be reserved for the very worst cases.

SOME COMMENTS ON CERTAIN ANALGESIC, ANTIPYRETIC, AND ANTI-INFLAMMATORY DRUGS

Aspirin, although in use for about a century, remains the drug of first choice in almost all cases of musculoskeletal pain: one makes no apology for reminding the reader of this because the author himself often forgets it. Yet, perusal of the remainder of this chapter demonstrates the sometimes gruesome adverse effects of drugs more powerful than aspirin. The more undesirable side effects of aspirin—gastric erosions with gastrointestinal bleeding, interference with platelet function, and hepatocellular injury [611, 730, 742]—occur rarely in contrast with the huge amounts of aspirin used by the population. According to the Boston Collaborative Drug Study [416], the annual incidence of hospital admissions for major upper gastrointestinal bleeding attributable to heavy regular use of aspirin is only 15 per 100,000 users; and gastric ulcers attributable to heavy regular use of aspirin affect only 10 per 100,000 users per year. Patients usually can tolerate the mild labyrinthine symptoms of subtoxic doses of aspirin.

Codeine is an excellent analgesic and addiction to it is rare. This drug has been more abused by its underuse than by its overuse.

Indomethacin is a valuable drug for any form of acute or chronic arthritis. It is both anti-inflammatory and analgesic. The usual daily dose for an adult is 150 mg; 75 mg is ineffective in most patients. In those who experience nausea or dizziness from the drug, a single bedtime dose of 100 mg taken with an antacid is often well tolerated and gives antiarthritic effects that are prolonged into the next day. The main side effects are gastric intolerance, dizziness, headaches, and psychological disorders; but the frequency of these adverse reactions has been exaggerated.

Phenylbutazone and its derivative, *oxyphenbutazone,* are considered by most rheumatologists to be extremely dangerous drugs, owing to the risk of aplastic anemia. Statistics on adverse reactions to phenylbutazone and oxyphenbutazone are available from the British National Health Service [121] for the year 1964, in which one death was attributed to phenylbutazone per 140,000 prescriptions of the drug, and one death attributed to oxyphenbutazone per 100,000 prescriptions of the drug. It is convenient to combine these rates as one death attributed to one or other of the two drugs per 120,000 prescriptions. Assuming that the drugs were used chronically with an average daily dose of 3 tablets, and that each prescription was for 100 tablets, then the 120,000 prescriptions would have been given to 10,000 patients during the year and the death rate attributable to the two drugs was one per 10,000 patients per year. This figure is probably an underestimate because adverse reactions to drugs are generally neither recognized nor reported as frequently as they occur. On the other hand, a comparable figure was obtained by Böttiger and Westerholm [63], who studied the population of a small town in Sweden where all drug purchases were entered into a computer. Phenylbutazone and oxyphenbutazone caused nine cases of thrombocytopenia with one death, 14 cases of aplastic anemia with seven deaths (this may be compared with only five cases of aplastic anemia with four deaths from chloramphenicol), and eight cases of agranulocytosis with three deaths. Clearly, phenylbutazone should be avoided in the long-term treatment of arthritis; and it is generally no better than indomethacin for short-term treatment.

Chloroquine. The anti-inflammatory effects of chloroquine were established in a controlled trial [439], but numerous reports of blindness from a pigmentary retinopathy led to disuse of the drug. More recent reports have suggested that the risk of blindness is dose related and may be minimized by using only 200 mg daily; further, it is held that strict ophthalmological supervision, measuring visual fields with a 1-mm red object or by electroretinography, can warn of impending visual loss and permit cessation of chloroquine treatment before irremediable damage has occurred. Nevertheless, few patients will accede to use of the drug when the risks to vision are frankly explained to them. Nor is chloroquine so effective that its loss from the arsenal of medicines is a serious matter.

It seems reasonable to consider using either chloroquine or phenylbutazone in rheumatoid arthritis after the disease has failed to respond to corticosteroids and the question of using cytotoxic agents is being debated. In view of the potentially devastating adverse reactions from chloroquine and phenylbutazone, an informed consent should be obtained before commencing long-term therapy with these drugs.

INTRA-ARTICULAR STEROID INJECTIONS

Joint injection should be performed with meticulous asepsis. The skin overlying the joint should be scrubbed for 5 minutes with an organic iodine preparation, and a strict no-touch technique used. The rate of occurrence of joint infection following injection is extremely low; one of my colleagues estimates that during the past 20 years he has injected approximately 7,000 joints and recalls only one case of sepsis. Perhaps one patient in every 100 experiences a so-called "post-injection flare," an acute inflammatory disorder that lasts from 1 to 3 days and presumably is a reaction either to the corticosteroid crystals or to the vehicle. There is evidence that frequent injections into the same joint—as often as, say, once monthly—hastens degenerative changes [99]. Therefore, indications for intra-articular injections of corticosteroids should be conservative, and one ought to avoid injecting the joint more often than three or four times yearly unless the inflammatory process is particularly resistant and severe.

The sites I have found most useful for injection therapy are the knee, the subacromial bursa, the ankle, the humeral epicondyles, the carpal tunnel, the wrist, and the flexor tendon sheaths of the fingers. Brief instructions follow for injections in these places.

Injection of the knee is best accomplished via the medial approach (Fig. 16-1). The patient lies supine with the leg extended. The skin is first scrubbed for 5 minutes with an organic iodide solution. The needle is inserted posterior to the patella at its superomedial aspect. Two milliliters of local anesthetic, lidocaine 2 per cent, is used to infiltrate the skin and subcutaneous tissues down to the capsule of the knee joint. If one injects slowly whilst inserting the needle, it is easy to recognize the capsule by its slight resistance both to advancement of the

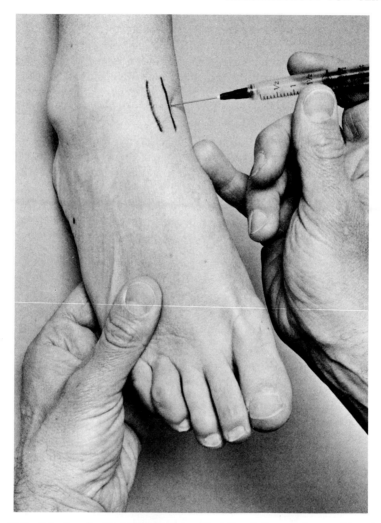

Fig. 16-3.   Injection of ankle (tibiotalar) joint. Black lines indicate surface marking of tendon of tibialis anterior.

terior to the epicondyle lest any crystalline material track posteriorly into the vicinity of the ulnar groove and induce a chemical neuritis.

Injection of the carpal tunnel is an easy procedure if the surface markings of the carpal tunnel are kept in mind. Beginning at the distal wrist crease, the tunnel extends approximately 1 inch into the palm of the hand. The median nerve enters the carpal tunnel deep to the tendon of palmaris longus; this tendon is easily identified, being the medial one of the two tendons that stand out on the volar surface of the wrist when it is flexed against slight resistance. To inject the tunnel, a 25-gauge needle is placed with its tip approximately ¾-inch distal to the distal wrist-crease in a line continuous with that formed by the palmaris longus tendon; the needle is angulated approximately 45° to the palm, and it is inserted to a depth of about 1 cm in a posterosuperior direction (Fig. 16-4). It is important to use a soluble rather than a crystalline steroid, in order to avoid the risk of inducing a chemical neuritis from a foreign-body reaction. A mixture of 4 mg decadron phosphate and 1 mg lidocaine in 1 ml of saline solution is convenient. The median nerve itself has a strong perineurium, so that it is extremely unlikely that the needle might transfix the nerve during the course of the injection.

The wrist joint is injected, after the usual 5-minute scrubbing with organic iodide, via a dorsal approach. The radiocarpal joint may be entered by inserting a 25-gauge needle a couple of millimeters below the dorsal tubercle, which lies in line with the radial border of the middle finger (Fig. 16-5). The tendon of extensor pollicis longus winds around the medial (ulnar) side of this dorsal tubercle and the needle should be placed slightly medial to this tendon, where there is a space between it and the common sheath of extensor digitorum and extensor indicis. Holding the hand in flexion, pronation, and ulnar deviation opens the joint space and facilitates the insertion of the needle. For this smaller joint space, it is best to use a more concentrated suspension of corticosteroid, e.g., 40 mg/ml, diluting 0.5 ml with 0.5 ml of 2 per cent lidocaine.

The tendon nodule and tenosynovitis that cause *trigger finger* overlie the metacarpophalangeal joints in the palm: at about this point, the flexor tendon sheaths for the second, third, and fourth digits become discontinuous from the common sheath. Therefore, the best place to insert the needle into the sheath for injection of the trigger finger is at the proximal phalanx. A 25-gauge needle is placed midway between the volar flexion creases of the metacarpophalangeal and proximal interphalangeal joints in the center of the phalanx. It is directed proximally, and posteriorly at an angle of 45° to the phalanx. About 0.5 cm of the needle's length is inserted and the same solution as that used in the wrist joint

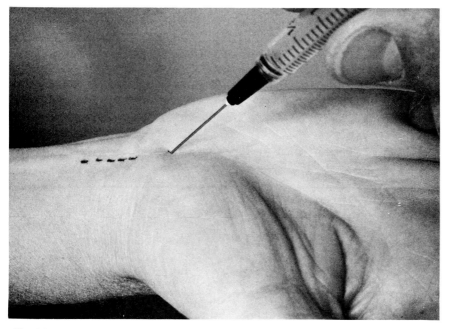

Fig. 16-4.   Injection of carpal tunnel. Black lines indicate surface marking of tendon of palmaris longus.

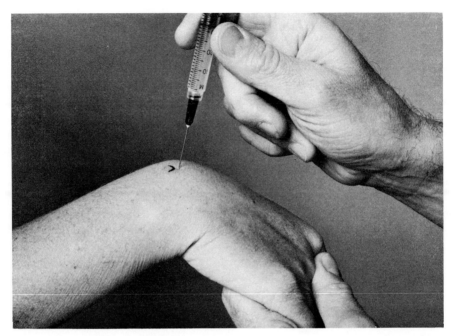

Fig. 16-5. Injection of wrist (radiocarpal) joint. Black V-mark indicates surface marking of dorsal tubercle of radius.

is injected. During the injection, the proximal end of the tendon sheath opposite the metacarpophalangeal joint is palpated and felt to expand.

SYSTEMIC CORTICOSTEROID THERAPY

General principles. There are three interdependent indications for commencing systemic therapy with corticosteroids. First, a trial of conservative therapy, for a period appropriate to the severity of the condition, should have failed. Next, systemic corticosteroid therapy should be considered only when there is inflammation both of considerable degree, and in too many joints to make intra-articular steroid injections practicable. Finally, whatever the degree of inflammation, resulting functional incapacity should be sufficient to cause hardship; this hardship may be economic, as in the case of a wage-earner, or domestic, as in the case of a housewife.

Precautions. Three main precautions must be observed in all patients receiving corticosteroids. A skin test for tuberculosis must always be performed before initiation of therapy. If the response is positive, isoniazid prophylaxis must be given for at least as long as corticosteroids are used. If there is a past history of peptic ulcer, a rigid antacid regimen must be insisted upon and strict dietary precautions instituted. A major contraindication to the use of oral corticosteroid therapy is a currently active peptic ulcer. An occasional patient with an ulcer must receive steroids; hourly antacids as well as the strict diet should then be given. One should be especially cautious in giving corticosteroids to patients with osteoporosis; although there are no statistics to prove this point, it is reasonable to suppose that these are the patients most liable to collapse fractures of vertebrae, so that tapering and withdrawal of the drug as soon as possible is most urgent.

Adverse side effects. The adverse reactions from oral corticosteroids are too well known to warrant tabulation. The following have been the most frequent and bothersome problems in our own practice. Potassium depletion may be severe, especially when diuretics are given concomitantly. Activation of tuberculosis has been seen in several instances when corticosteroid medicines have been given injudiciously, without isoniazid coverage, to patients known to have positive reactions to tuberculin skin test. It is my practice to continue isoniazid prophylaxis for a full year in patients with such positive reactions, even where corticosteroid therapy is stopped before the end of the year.

Posterior subcapsular cataracts are occasionally sufficiently bothersome to necessitate their extraction. It is worth noting that there seems to be no sound evidence for the existence of two complications of corticosteroid therapy that used to be postulated; namely, steroid pseudorheumatism, and steroid-induced vasculitis.

If the appropriate precautions are observed and the principles of therapy outlined above are closely followed, there is little to fear from corticosteroids. Indeed, in my opinion, unwarranted prejudice against these drugs causes them to be withheld too often, with consequent economic and social hardship. Justification for this statement is shown in Table 16-1, produced with the aid of a computer, which groups 924 patients with rheumatoid arthritis into 170 (18.4 per cent) who were given prednisone and the remainder who were not given prednisone, during a 6-year period of study. The major, and most frequently cited, complications of systemic corticosteroid therapy—peptic ulcer, hypertension, psychiatric disorders, and fractures—are tabulated for each group of patients. Only peptic ulcers and fractures were slightly more common in the group treated with prednisone, and in neither instance was the difference statistically significant. It is noteworthy how frequent were all of these associated conditions, even in the group that was not given prednisone: hypertension affected 15.0 per cent; psychiatric disorders (with depressive reactions predominating), 8.2 per cent.

GENERAL COMMENTS ON THE USE OF CYTOTOXIC AGENTS IN RHEUMATIC DISEASE

The three major classes of cytotoxic compounds are 1) the alkylating agents; for example, cyclophosphamide and chlorambucil, 2) the purine analogs; for example, 6-mercaptopurine and its derivative, azathioprine, 3) the folic acid antagonists, such as methotrexate. Drugs from each of these major categories have been found to suppress the primary and secondary humoral immune responses, delayed hypersensitivity, and experimental autoimmune diseases such as experimental allergic encephalomyelitis and spontaneous systemic lupus erythematosus in NZB mice. These agents could interfere with several of the phases of the immune response mechanism; namely, the handling of antigen, the differentiation of the immunocyte, the proliferation of B lymphocytes, and the efficacy of the T

Table 16-1. Potential Adverse Effects of Prednisone in Rheumatoid Arthritis. The Data are from 924 Patients with Rheumatoid Arthritis, Studied for 6 Months.*

	No Prednisone N = 754		Prednisone N = 170	
	No.	%	No.	%
Peptic ulcer	22	2.9	9	5.3
Hypertension	113	15.0	20	11.8
Psychiatric disorders	62	8.2	12	7.1
Fractures	44	5.8	12	7.1

* In no instance was the difference in percentage between the two treatment groups statistically significant.

lymphocyte activities. Current information suggests that all three classes of drug suppress the primary immune response; that azathioprine influences T cells more than B cells, and has a weak anti-inflammatory effect; and that cyclophosphamide has a stronger antiproliferative effect on B cells [328, 436, 657]. Investigators are considering the use of combined cyclophosphamide and azathioprine in selected patients with rheumatic disease, in view of the foregoing considerations as well as the finding of a synergistic effect in the treatment of the lupus-like nephritis seen in NZB/W mice [237, 279]. Before proceeding with a description of the results of these drugs in the treatment of human rheumatic diseases, it is proper to emphasize Steinberg's [657] warning: information about the effects of long-term use of these drugs in controlled series of patients with non-neoplastic disease does not exist. Short-term benefits may ultimately be outweighed by long-term risks. *It seems proper to give the drugs only in situations in which meaningful information as to their efficacy can be obtained.*

Practical goals for the use of cytotoxic agents in rheumatic diseases are 1) to suppress the disease, 2) to reduce steroid dose, and 3) to use them as additions to other drugs. One should consider their use only when there is life-threatening or seriously crippling disease; where the lesions appear clinically to be potentially reversible; where there have been intolerable side effects or failure to respond to conventional therapy; where there is no active infection; where the hematologic status is satisfactory; where meticulous follow-up is feasible, and where objective evaluation of results is possible. Finally, because of the most serious potential adverse reactions from these medicines, an honestly informed consent must be obtained from the patient.

Toxic side effects that are common to most of these agents include the following: bone marrow failure that may be irreversible; oral ulcers; gastrointestinal intolerance; hair-fall, especially severe with cyclophosphamide; cystitis that may be hemorrhagic with bladder necrosis, and is severe with cyclophosphamide; infection, especially pulmonary infection with cytomegalovirus, *Pneumocystis carinii,* candida, aspergillus, nocardia, and pseudomonas; induction of new tumors, expecially malignant lymphoma; reactivation of old neoplasms; liver damage, especially frequent with methotrexate; anovulation from ovarian fibrosis, especially with cyclophosphamide; and azoospermia, also especially common with cyclophosphamide. The possibility of very long-term adverse reactions that are unknown at present has been emphasized by Decker [140], who pointed out that it took about 20 years to recognize a relation between x-ray therapy and leukemia in ankylosing spondylitis, about 10 years to recognize that cataracts might be steroid-induced, and about 5 years to suspect that chloroquine could induce retinopathy.

DRUG THERAPY OF RHEUMATOID ARTHRITIS

Gold. The role of gold in the treatment of rheumatoid arthritis remains debatable. The controversy that still surrounds the use of gold salts in this disease is illustrated by the surprise that was expressed by many physicians who participated in a controlled trial [123], at the failure of their study to demonstrate a greater beneficial effect of the gold therapy. Explaining the small number of patients ultimately enrolled in their trial, the Cooperating Clinics Committee of the American Rheumatism Association (CCC,ARA) pointed out that some clinics may have been reluctant to enroll their patients because they were not convinced that gold is an effective mode of therapy; whereas others may not have participated because of their feeling that gold is efficacious and they did not want to withhold it. Many experienced clinicians maintain that gold therapy is undoubtedly efficacious, especially in patients with early rheumatoid arthritis accompanied by much joint inflammation; others consider that the small advantage that has been demonstrated to accrue to patients treated with gold over those treated with placebo in controlled trials is inadequate to justify the known toxic side effects, which include drug-induced hepatitis, nephrotic syndrome, stomatitis, dermatitis, and death from agranulocytosis. Some enthusiasts have even stated that the occurrence of toxicity is a favorable omen that a drug-induced remission of the arthritis will occur; this point, however, was not confirmed in a controlled trial [573]. There have been two good, controlled trials of gold salt therapy given for 6 months to patients with rheumatoid arthritis, one by the Empire Rheumatism Council (ERC) of Great Britain [252]; the other by CCC, ARA [123]. The study of the ERC was the larger of the two, comparing 90 patients treated with gold, with 95 controls; the CCC, ARA study compared only 36 patients treated with gold, with 32 controls. In each of these trials, each patient received a total of 1 g of gold over a period of 6 months. When assessed at the end of that course of therapy, the patients treated with gold in the British study were significantly better than the controls, according to both their own and their physicians' estimates: they had significantly fewer newly-active joints and reactivating joints, and significant improvements also occurred in the grip strength, blood hemoglobin level, and erythrocyte sedimentation rate. At the 6-months' assessment in the American study, the only significant improvement in the gold-treated patients was in erythrocyte sedimentation rate, although the trend in the various other measurements was towards improvement. The British observations were the more extended ones: 18 months after starting gold salt therapy, the various advantages were retained by the treated group, but after 30 months the differences between the treated and untreated patients were no longer present. In the American study, six patients received gold therapy at monthly intervals for a further 18 months; there was no significant improvement in this group over those not given such prolonged therapy. In the British study, 16 patients received second courses of gold injections starting at the eighteenth month; they did no better subsequently, either functionally or in radiologic progression, than did those 20 patients who received second courses of placebo injections. A third controlled study was recently reported by Sigler and coworkers [631]: they gave gold on a chronic basis for an average of 28 months and observed significant benefits upon synovitis as well as upon rate of progression of radiologic changes at the 2-year point of follow-up.

In summary, gold is a toxic drug. The short-term results of a 6-month course of treatment are variable: the British study showed benefit, the CCC, ARA study showed no benefit. The results of continued therapy seem equally variable: the British and CCC, ARA studies showed no benefit from continued therapy; the study by Sigler showed both clinical and radiological benefit after longer treatment.

Orally administered corticosteroids are used in the therapy of rheumatoid arthritis in accordance with the general principles outlined above. There are three major objectives in adjusting dosage. First, one should initiate and maintain the smallest dose of prednisone possible, preferably 7.5 mg or less daily, seldom 10 mg, and rarely as much as 15 mg per day. Second, one's aim is to reduce the pain to a tolerable level rather than to abolish it completely, if elimination of pain requires doses larger than those mentioned. Finally, at every encounter with the patient one must insist that he attempt to taper, and, if possible, to withdraw the medicine as soon as the desired effects have been attained.

Penicillamine has been used experimentally for the treatment of rheumatoid arthritis for about 10 years in the United States. A double-blind, multicenter controlled trial in England [503] showed considerable benefit from the drug in patients with acute, severe rheumatoid arthritis. No patients were removed from the treatment group because of progression of the disease; whereas 17 per cent of the control group were removed because of deterioration in the patients' condition. All measurements except radiographic changes in the small joints showed greater improvement in the patients treated with penicillamine, and the degree of improvement was usually statistically significant. According to the results of this trial, penicillamine is an effective form of treatment for active rheumatoid arthritis. The further progress of the original group of 85 patients treated with penicillamine, some of whom completed 5 years of treatment, was reported later [139]. Most benefit appeared during the first year of treatment, after the end of which there were significant improvements in morning stiffness, hemoglobin, erythrocyte sedimentation rate, and titer of rheumatoid factor. The authors stressed the low incidence of side effects when doses of the drug were kept low, 300 to 600 mg/day. It is considered that the patients chosen for use of penicillamine (which is still an experimental drug in the United States) should be those with early rather than advanced rheumatoid arthritis, in whom the disease has remained active and progressive despite simpler measures. Adverse side effects are rare; they include aplastic anemia and nephrotic syndrome that is probably on the basis of immune complex deposition.

Cytotoxic drugs. The use of alkylating agents for the treatment of rheumatoid arthritis was reported in sporadic cases and uncontrolled series since the early 1950's. The first controlled trial was reported in 1970 by CCC,ARA [122]. They chose patients with "definite" or "classic" rheumatoid arthritis whose disease was of at least 2 years' duration. A required condition for the trial was failure to improve in response to salicylates and another antirheumatic agent, such as gold salts or corticosteroid drugs, during the 6 months before the trial commenced. Twenty patients received a large dose of cyclophosphamide, up to 150 mg daily; 28 received a small dose of the drug, up to 15 mg daily. The trial was continued for 32 weeks. Six measures of disease activity were made: morning stiffness, grip strength, numbers of painful joints, numbers of swollen joints, time taken for a 50-foot walk, and erythrocyte sedimentation rate. The patients who received the larger dose of cyclophosphamide showed a greater reduction than those on the smaller dose, in each of these six measures except for the erythrocyte sedimentation rate, which was virtually the same in the two groups. The clearest distinction was in the number of painful joints; by the end of the study, two patients receiving large doses of cyclophosphamide had no painful joints, and five had no swollen joints; no such freedom from articular findings was seen in the patients receiving small doses of cyclophosphamide.

In a further study by the CCC, ARA [124], it was shown that doses of cyclophosphamide of 75 mg or less per day were ineffective, in contrast with doses between 75 and 150 mg/day. In the studies by the CCC, ARA, the major side effect of cyclophosphamide was bladder irritation with hemorrhagic cystitis, seen in two patients; a major degree of hair loss was noted in one-third of the group receiving a large dose; herpes zoster developed in two patients; *two patients on the small-dose schedule in their second study died of infection.*

A smaller controlled study of cyclophosphamide with average daily dose of 117.5 mg was reported by Townes, Sowa, and Shulman [683]. All of 11 patients receiving the drug showed improvement; increasing activity, of the disease was observed in most patients after cross-over to placebo. However, of the 11 patients on the drug, six had hematuria, four severe alopecia, three amenorrhea and menopausal symptoms, and two had either thrombocytopenia or herpes zoster. Lidsky, Sharp, and Billings [422] observed no benefit from cyclophosphamide in smaller doses, up to 1 mg/kg/day for 1 year. Aside from mild leukopenia (the lowest white blood cell count was 3,100/cu mm), these authors saw no significant adverse reactions at this low dose level.

The purine analog, azathioprine, has been tested in a double-blind cross-over study of 17 patients with "classic" rheumatoid arthritis resistant to conventional therapy [690]. After 6 weeks, patients receiving azathioprine showed significant improvement in articular index, count of total active joints, count of synovial effusions, and grip strength. Rash, nausea, and hair-thinning occurred in four of the 17 treated patients.

SYSTEMIC LUPUS ERYTHEMATOSUS (SLE)

Corticosteroids. The major causes of death from SLE are involvement of kidneys, brain, and lungs. It is the general belief of experienced clinicians that corticosteroids have been most beneficial in the urgent control of the acute lupus crisis—severe exacerbation of the disease in multiple systems, often accompanied by hyperpyrexia and profound general toxicity; before the introduction of corticosteroids this was a common cause of death in SLE, but is now a rare one. Likewise, it is the general impression that lupus brain and lung disease respond favorably to corticosteroids; but there are no controlled studies to prove this point. The basic principles for the use of corticosteroids in SLE differ in no way from those already outlined: when they are required, they should be prescribed in the smallest effective doses and withdrawn as soon as the indication for their use has been controlled. The need to taper the dose slowly must be stressed. For reasons that are unclear, a severe flare of SLE may occur if the corticosteroid is withdrawn too rapidly. At high dose levels, e.g., prednisone 60 mg or more daily, one may taper the dose by 10 mg each week; upon reaching a daily dose of 40 mg, the tapering process should slow so that only 5 mg/day is withdrawn every 2 weeks. One should consider this requirement in judging the starting dose of the drug.

Treatment of lupus nephritis. Confusion surrounds this topic for several reasons. The groups of patients reported in the major studies of treatment of lupus nephritis have been highly selected so as to include, generally speaking, those having SLE with the most severe features (see Chapter 10). There are ethical and practical difficulties in maintaining patients with SLE without any sort of therapy, and there are no reports of studies in which very long-term treatment was contrasted with the effects of no treatment in a simultaneously studied control group. Because of the inherent variability of SLE, there are serious problems in matching treated with untreated patients.

Corticosteroids and immunosuppressants. One of the few attempts at a prospective study of defined steroid therapy in lupus nephritis was that of Kagen and Christian [354]. They randomly assigned 36 patients to one of two steroid treatment groups: in the first group, 16 patients were to receive at least 50 mg of prednisone daily for 6 months; six of these patients could not continue this schedule. In the second group, 20 patients were treated according to their physicians' decisions; 18 of them received some steroid, two received none. After 1 to 4 years of follow-up, three deaths had occurred in each group.

The problem of the concomitant control group is paramount because, as our own findings (see Chapter 10) and those of others suggest, either the prognosis of renal lupus is not so serious as has been believed, or the selection of patients influences the outcome. Nanra and Kincaid-Smith [511], for example, studied 72 patients with lupus nephritis, 63 (87.5 per cent) of whom had diffuse proliferative nephritis, including 38 with histologically severe forms. During follow-up periods with a mean of 4.4 years (range, 1 month to 17 years), only 13 (18.1 per cent) of the patients died, only two of these from renal failure. Closely similar figures were reported by Striker and coworkers [663], who concluded that glucocorticoids and immunosuppressive drugs have little effect on the eventual outcome in most patients with diffuse or membranous lupus nephritis. A nearly identical mortality rate to that observed by Nanra and Kincaid-Smith [511], 19.9 per cent deaths among 31 patients with diffuse proliferative nephritis treated aggressively during follow-up periods averaging 4.7 years, was considered a favorable result by Epstein and Grausz [179]. Clearly, the interpretation of the results of therapy in lupus nephritis depends upon data from local control patients.

Cytotoxic drugs. In studying the treatment of SLE, an experimental model that has been most useful is the NZB/W mouse, which develops a disease that resembles human SLE in being characterized by antibodies to nucleic acids and immune-complex glomerulonephritis. Various studies have shown that cyclophosphamide, azathioprine, and prednisone modify this experimental disease [236, 279]. Dubois [160], in one of the earliest studies in humans, found that seven of 11 patients with lupus nephritis improved when treated with nitrogen mustards. In a randomized but not blind trial, Sztejnbok and coworkers [668] showed that in 21 patients with SLE to whose therapy azathioprine was added, 2.5 mg/kg/day, the morbidity and mortality rates were markedly less than in 19 of 21 controls. The measures of advantage included decreased steroid dose; decreased numbers of hospitalizations; no deaths in the treatment group, whereas there were six deaths (three from renal insufficiency) among the controls; and improved renal function.

Steinberg and coworkers [656] made a controlled trial of cyclophosphamide over a 10-week period in 13 women with lupus nephritis. They studied six measurements: antibodies to DNA, C3, urine sediment, 24-hour urine protein, creatinine clearance, and extrarenal minifestations. In nine treatment trials on the drug, improvement occurred in 34 of the 54 total measurements; whereas in six placebo trials, improvement was seen in only five of the 36 measurements. Donadio and coworkers [155], on the contrary, showed no such benefit after a controlled study lasting 6 months. All of their patients had diffuse proliferative glomerulonephritis, and renal biopsy was performed in each patient before treatment and after 6 months of therapy. All of the 16 patients received large doses of prednisone: 60 mg daily for the first 2 months, tapering to 20 mg daily by 6 months, and averaging 40 mg daily for the 6-month period. Seven of the 16 patients received in addition azathioprine, 2 mg/kg/day. There was significant improvement in the biopsy appearances of the renal tissue from both groups; glomerular fluorescence was unchanged before and after treatment in five patients from each group. Likewise, creatinine clearance, abnormalities of urine sediment, proteinuria, hypocomplementemia, and high titers of antinuclear antibodies showed improvement in most patients, but none of these correlated completely with the improvement seen on renal biopsy. Donadio and coworkers [155] concluded that the addition of azathioprine does not improve the short term results of treatment of lupus nephritis. Further complicating the use of azathioprine in lupus nephritis is a report that discontinuation of the medicine is frequently followed by exacerbation of the SLE [621].

In summary, studies during the past 10 years have shed little light upon the question of how best to manage lupus nephritis. The benefits of corticosteroid therapy have not been certainly shown, but such treatment is probably indicated where tests demonstrate deterioration of renal function in patients with diffuse proliferative glomerulonephritis. The indications for use of cytotoxic drugs are even less certain, and it is dubious whether these should be used except in the most desperate situations. The dictum, *primum non nocere,* must be constantly repeated.

SYSTEMIC ANGIITIC REACTIONS

Corticosteroids. Information concerning the efficacy of corticosteroid treatment for idiopathic angiitis, including periarteritis nodosa, is scanty and reported studies have been poorly controlled; but on the whole, the observations support the use of these drugs in this condition. The British Medical Research Council [462] collected 21 cases of periarteritis nodosa in which treatment had been with prednisone, and compared them with 19 untreated cases. After 3 years, 13 treated but only seven untreated patients were still alive; this apparent advantage to the treated group disappeared when patients with hypertension were excluded. Among the 41 patients with periarteritis nodosa studied at autopsy by Moskowitz and coworkers [494], three of the 10 who had had significant steroid therapy, and only one of the 31 who had not received significant steroid therapy showed healed or healing lesions. Intensive corticosteroid therapy had been given to 110 of the patients with periarteritis nodosa studied by Frohnert and Sheps [228]. Using the life-table method to calculate expected survivorship, they found a 5-year survival of 48 per cent for the treated patients and 13 per cent for the untreated ones; in the treated group, the survivorship curve declined only gradually so that at 10 years the expected survival was 42.4 per cent. Hypertension and renal disease were the main determinants of prognosis: the presence of one of these cut survivorship by about a fifth in comparison with the entire treated group. The presence of asthma, pneumonia, chronic bronchitis, or eosinophilia with associated respiratory symptoms made no difference to outcome.

WEGENER'S GRANULOMATOSIS

The results of cytotoxic drug therapy for Wegener's granulomatosis have been most encouraging. When generalized, this disease is almost always rapidly fatal. An early report showed the benefit of the combination of azathioprine and duazomycin A [362]. Raitt [567] treated six patients with generalized Wegener's granulomatosis, with corticosteroids and a cytotoxic drug, either an alkylating agent or a purine antagonist. Five of the patients were alive after a minimum of 15 months and a maximum of 96 months of observation. Similar encouraging results have been obtained by Fauci and coworkers [190], and by Novack and Pearson [522].

IDIOPATHIC POLYMYOSITIS

A number of patients with idiopathic polymyositis undoubtedly recover without treatment. This may account for the differences between the impressions of prognosis held by physicians at large university or other referral centers, and those expressed by physicians who practice in the community. It is not only patients with the mildest affection who recover spontaneously. One of my patients who had moderately severe weakness, and in whom biopsy showed severe necrosis of large areas of muscle, refused all drug therapy except salicylates. After 3 years he had totally recovered strength, and the following 4 years brought no recurrence of his polymyositis.

Corticosteroids. When they analyzed their experience with 279 patients with polymyositis, Winkelmann and coworkers [727] found that the remission rate had not been affected by the use of corticosteroid drugs; but that distribution of patients into the categories of better, worse, or dead had been favorably influenced by the use of cortisone. They found no benefit from cortisone in doses smaller than 50 mg/day. Rose and Walton [586] compared the survival rates of their patients treated with cortisone, with the rates for untreated patients reported in the literature. They considered that steroids gave a definite overall advantage, and advocated a minimum period of treatment of 2 years. Vignos, Bowling, and Watkins [697] drew similar conclusions from their experience with 38 cases.

I have given corticosteroids to those patients in whom the rapidity and severity of the course seemed ominous, especially if pharyngeal and respiratory muscles were involved. Recommendations vary as to the starting dose and duration of therapy. The starting dose depends upon the severity of the disease at the time; although I have found 40 to 60 mg of prednisone daily to be appropriate for most patients, occasionally it has been necessary to double or quadruple this dose in order to control the disease. The duration of therapy depends entirely upon response; I have been able to withdraw corticosteroids after as few as 3 months, but one patient still requires treatment after 8 years because of continued disease activity. One should carefully taper the dose of corticosteroids, and monitor the clinical and serum enzyme response to the new lower dose before continuing the process of withdrawing the medicine.

Cytotoxic agents have appeared to be therapeutically effective in individuals or small series of patients with polymyositis. Malaviya, Many, and Schwartz [441] gave methotrexate to four patients, including three who had been resistant to corticosteroid therapy; all had a good outcome. Good results from methotrexate in five of seven patients with polymyositis resistant to corticosteroids were reported by Sokoloff, Goldberg, and Pearson [643]. Arnett and coworkers [18] agreed that methotrexate was a useful adjunct to corticosteroids in resistant cases but found toxicity a serious limiting factor; methotrexate pneumonitis appeared in two of their five patients and contributed to the death of one.

Azathioprine has been used with favorable consequences [41, 459]; however, variable results from methotrexate, azathioprine, or cyclophosphamide were obtained by Currie and Walton [129] and by Haas [276]; and Fries and coworkers [225] saw no effect from cyclophosphamide in eight patients with polymyositis.

In summary, the general experience is that cytotoxic drugs may sometimes be useful in selected cases of polymyositis. These agents should be reserved for patients in whom the disease progresses despite adequate corticosteroid therapy, or in whom corticosteroids have caused serious adverse effects.

PROGRESSIVE SYSTEMIC SCLEROSIS (PSS)

The dermal and tissue fibrosis of PSS is not ameliorated by corticosteroids. However, a prolonged phase of dermal inflammation, which is rare, may be helped by corticosteroids; these drugs should also be tried if there is a prominent element of either polymyositis or angiitis accompanying the PSS.

RAYNAUD'S PHENOMENON

An attempt should be made to alleviate Raynaud's phenomenon when it is distressingly frequent and painful, or when ischemic ulceration or necrosis of the digit tips has occurred. General recommendations, such as avoidance of cold or of vibrating instruments, use of mittens or gloves, and termination of tobacco smoking, are obvious. Tranquilizing drugs are occasionally helpful where emotional stress is an important precipitant of the vasospasm. Surgical sympathectomy had a vogue two or three decades ago, but the long-term results have been disappointing [244]; despite this, the current fashion is for medical sympatholysis with reserpine or methyl dopa.

Reserpine. Abboud and coworkers [1] reported amelioration of Raynaud's phenomenon after the intra-arterial administration of reserpine. Romeo and colleagues [584] confirmed these findings. Willerson et al [723] showed short-term improvement in superficial blood flow to the digits after intra-arterial reserpine in patients with Raynaud's disease or Raynaud's phenomenon, and similar results after reserpine given orally were obtained by Coffman and Cohen [114]. In most observers' experience, including my own, few patients can tolerate oral reserpine in doses sufficiently large to be efficacious: the most distressing side effects of doses exceeding 0.25 mg two or three times daily are nasal stuffiness, depression, and impotence.

It is difficult to assess the long-term results of therapy in Raynaud's phenomenon, which is affected by the amount of current emotional stress and by ambient temperature, and which sometimes seems to vary capriciously for no identifiable reason. Thus, it is not surprising that the claims for a beneficial effect of intra-arterial reserpine have been disputed. Siegel and Fries [630] and McFadyen and coworkers [458] each made double-blind cross-over studies of intra-arterial reserpine and saline solution in patients with Raynaud's phenomenon. Neither saw any significant differences between the treatment and the control groups at the 1-month follow-up point. However, de la Lande and coworkers [142] showed that after intra-arterial reserpine administration, the blood flow to the hand is maximally increased at about 1½ hours and returns to baseline at 24 hours; i.e., the effect lasts hours or a day, rather than several days or weeks.

In light of the studies that show improvement in superficial blood flow to the digits after intra-arterial reserpine in patients with Raynaud's phenomenon, it seems reasonable to offer this treatment where digital necrosis is threatened. I have used it in a half-dozen such patients, and consider that it has averted gangrene in them; but one must be very cautious in drawing conclusions from limited personal experience. The patient should be hospitalized; 1 mg reserpine, diluted in 5 ml saline solution, is injected slowly into the brachial artery of the affected limb. The patient is kept in hospital for 24 hours to ensure stability of the blood pressure. In desperate cases, the injection may be repeated every 24 to 48 hours until the threatened digit seems to be out of danger.

Methyl dopa. The best drug for the oral treatment of Raynaud's phenomenon is methyl dopa because, unlike reserpine, this may be given in doses that are large enough to be apparently effective without causing intolerable side effects. Varadi and Lawrence [692] found that methyl dopa could prevent episodes of Raynaud's phenomenon during both experimental exposure to cold and normal wintertime exposure to cold. They saw improvement in 31 of 42 patients, two-thirds of whom had scleroderma. The drug is started in a dose of 0.25 g three times daily, and gradually increased to a maximum of 1.0 g three times daily, depending upon clinical response and side effects.

GOUT AND ASYMPTOMATIC HYPERURICEMIA

Acute gout. The efficacy of *colchicine* in the treatment of acute gout is well known. *Indomethacin* is often preferred by patients because its side effects are less violent and the drug is as effective as colchicine: most patients experience 50 per cent alleviation within 24 hours of starting indomethacin. A schedule that generally works is 50 mg every 6 hours for eight doses, then 50 mg every 8 hours for 5 days. For those few patients who experience no relief from indomethacin, one may in rare instances use *phenylbutazone,* starting with 600 mg daily and tapering to total withdrawal by the sixth day. Most patients prefer indomethacin to phenylbutazone, and the serious risk of aplastic anemia is far less from indomethacin.

Long-term treatment of gout with a drug that lowers serum uric acid should be started only when the acute attacks are inconveniently frequent; or when tophi, renal function impairment, or renal stones are present (see, also, Chapter 4). *Probenecid* has been used for about 20 years and seems to have no serious long-term hazards; therefore this is usually the drug to start with. *Allopurinol* has unknown long-term hazards and should not be used as the initial agent except in those patients with impaired renal function or renal stones. The addition of two or three colchicine tablets daily will further reduce the frequency of acute attacks.

Asymptomatic hyperuricemia. I want to emphasize that I advise against treating asymptomatic hyperuricemia at any level of serum uric acid.

GONOCOCCAL ARTHRITIS

Penicillin. The gonococcus is always sensitive to penicillin, so that this is the standard drug for therapy. Penicillin enters the septic joint freely and the levels of the drug in joint fluid and serum are comparable [512]; therefore, intraarticular administration is unnecessary. The usual regimen has been 10 million units of penicillin G given intravenously, daily for 7 to 10 days. The need for such prolonged therapy has never been adequately documented. Certainly, many patients continue to have arthralgia, or even joint effusion, for 7 to 10 days or longer. An indication that less vigorous therapy might be adequate came from a study by Barr and Danielson [31], who treated 20 patients with disseminated gonorrhea, giving only 4.5 million units of penicillin parenterally, daily for 2 days, followed by 3 to 4 million units of penicillin V given by mouth daily for 10 days. Three patients received only 1 g of ampicillin orally, repeated 5 hours later. They saw no relapses. Blankenship and coworkers [53] treated 27 patients with gonococcal arthritis or tenosynovitis with 2.5 million units of aqueous crystalline penicillin G, given intravenously over 30-minute periods every 6 hours for 3 days. To two patients who were allergic to penicillin, they gave erythromycin glupeptate, 0.5 g intravenously every 6 hours for 3 days. Although seven patients had residual signs or symptoms, including joint effusions in four, all repeat cultures were negative. One patient had a recurrent effusion in his knee at the 2-week follow-up examination, but the joint fluid culture was sterile and 2 weeks later he was well. Thus, while the standard course of therapy is that outlined at the beginning of this section, the likelihood is that briefer treatment will prove adequate.

167. Dunn JP, Moses C: Correlation of serum lipids with uric acid and blood sugar in normal males. Metabolism 14:788–792, 1965

168. Duran-Reynals F: A necrotizing disease in rabbits affecting fatty and muscular tissues. Analogies with the Weber-Christian disease of humans. Yale J Biol Med 18:583–594, 1946

169. Dwyer JM, Bullock WE, Fields JP: Disturbance of the blood T:B lymphocyte ratio in lepromatous leprosy. Clinical and immunologic correlations. N Engl J Med 288:1036–1039, 1973

170. Dyer NH, Verbov JL, Dawson AM, Borrie PF, Stansfeld AG: Cutaneous polyarteritis nodosa associated with Crohn's disease. Lancet 1:648–650, 1970

171. Edeiken J, Hodes PJ: Roentgen Diagnosis of Diseases of Bone, Ed 2, Vol 2. Baltimore, The Williams and Wilkins Co., 1973, fig 1249, p 1142

172. Edozien JC, Udo UU, Young VR, Scrimshaw NS: Effects of high levels of yeast feeding on uric acid metabolism of young men. Nature (London) 228:180, 1970

173. Ehlers N, Kissmeyer-Nielsen F, Kjerbye KE, Lamm LU: HL-A27 in acute and chronic uveitis (letter to Editor). Lancet 1:99, 1974

174. Eisenberg H, Dubois EL, Sherwin RP, Balchum OJ: Diffuse interstitial lung disease in systemic lupus erythematosus. Ann Intern Med 79:37–45, 1973

175. Emmerson BT, Douglas W, Doherty RL, Feigl P: Serum urate concentrations in the Australian aboriginal. Ann Rheum Dis 28:150–156, 1969

176. Engel A, Burch TA: Chronic arthritis in the United States Health Examination Survey. Arthritis Rheum 10:61–62, 1967

177. Engel AG: Late-onset rod myopathy (a new syndrome?): light and electron microscopic observations in two cases. Mayo Clin Proc 41:713–741, 1966

178. Engel WK, Brooke MH, Nelson PG: Histochemical studies of denervated or tenotomized cat muscle: illustrating difficulties in relating experimental animal conditions to human neuromuscular diseases. Ann NY Acad Sci 138:160–185, 1966.

179. Epstein WV, Grausz H: Favorable outcome in diffuse proliferative glomerulonephritis of systemic lupus erythematosus. Arthritis Rheum 17:129–142, 1974

180. Erasmus LD: Scleroderma in gold-miners on the Witwatersrand with particular reference to pulmonary manifestations. S Afr J Lab Clin Med 3:209–231, 1957

181. Estes D, Christian CL: The natural history of systemic lupus erythematosus by prospective analysis. Medicine 50:85–95, 1971

182. Estes D, Larson DL: Systemic lupus erythematosus and pregnancy. Clin Obstet Gynecol 8:307–321, 1965

183. Evans JG, Prior IAM, Harvey HPB: Relation of serum uric acid to body bulk, haemoglobin, and alcohol intake in two South Pacific Polynesian populations. Ann Rheum Dis 27:319–325, 1968

184. Faes MH, Rosselle N: Radiation myopathy (letter to Editor). Lancet 1:1231, 1967

185. Falletta JM, Ramanujam N, Starling KA, Fernbach DJ: Ig-positive lymphocytes in Hodgkin's disease (letter to Editor). N Engl J Med 288:581–582, 1973

186. Fanelli GM Jr, Bohn D, Stafford S: Functional characteristics of renal urate transport in the *Cebus* monkey. Am J Physiol 218:627–636, 1970

187. Fanelli GM Jr, Bohn DL, Rcilly SS: Renal urate transport in the chimpanzee. Am J Physiol 220:613–620, 1971

188. Farmer RG, Gifford RW Jr, Hines EA Jr: Prognostic significance of Raynaud's phenomenon and other clinical characteristics of systemic scleroderma. A study of 271 cases. Circulation 21:1088–1095, 1960

189. Fauci AS, Wolff SM: Wegener's granulomatosis: studies in eighteen patients and a review of the literature. Medicine 52:535–561, 1973

190. Fauci AS, Wolff SM, Johnson JS: Effect of cyclophosphamide on the immune response in Wegener's granulomatosis. N Engl J Med 285:1493–1496, 1971

191. Feingold BF, with contributors: Introduction to Clinical Allergy. Springfield, Charles C Thomas, 1973

192. Feldman EB, Wallace SL: Serum lipids and lipoproteins in patients with gout without vascular disease (abstract). Arthritis Rheum 5:108, 1962

193. Feorino PM, Hierholzer JC, Norton WL: Viral isolation studies of inclusion positive biopsy from human connective tissue diseases. Arthritis Rheum 13:378–380, 1970

194. Ferris TF, Gorden P: Effect of angiotensin and norepinephrine upon urate clearance in man. Am J Med 44:359–365, 1968

195. Fessel WJ: The "antibrain" factors in psychiatric patients' sera. I. Further studies with a hemagglutination technique. Arch Gen Psychiatry 8:614–621, 1963

196. Fessel WJ: Dextran turbidity: acute distress-phase reaction. Nature (London) 205:771–773, 1965

197. Fessel WJ: Fat disorders and peripheral neuropathy. Brain 94:531–540, 1971

198. Fessel WJ: Interaction of multiple determinants of schizophrenia. A tentative synthesis and review. Arch Gen Psychiatry 11:1–18, 1964

199. Fessel WJ: Mental stress, blood proteins, and the hypothalamus. Experimental results showing effect of mental stress upon 4S and 19S proteins: speculation that the functional behavior disturbances may be expressions of a general metabolic disorder. Arch Gen Psychiatry 7:427–435, 1962

200. Fessel WJ: Myopathy of hypothyroidism. Ann Rheum Dis 27:590–596, 1968

201. Fessel WJ: Remote effects of benign neoplasms (letter to Editor). N Engl J Med 288:323, 1973

202. Fessel WJ, Pearson CM: Polymyalgia rheumatica and blindness. N Engl J Med 276:1403–1405, 1967

203. Fessel WJ, Raas MC: Autoimmunity in the pathogenesis of muscle disease. Neurology 18:1137–1139, 1968

204. Fessel WJ, Siegelaub AB, Johnson ES: Correlates and consequences of asymptomatic hyperuricemia. Arch Intern Med 132:44–54, 1973

205. Fessel WJ, Solomon GF: Psychosis and systemic lupus erythematosus. A review of the literature and case reports. Calif Med 92:266–270, 1960

206. Fessel WJ, Taylor JA, Johnson ES: Evaluating the complaint of muscle weakness. Simple quantitative clinical tests. In Canal N, Scarlato G, Eds: Muscle Diseases: Proceedings of an International Congress, Milan, May 1969. Excerpta Medica International Congress Series No. 199, pp 544–545

207. Finn R, Jones PO, Tweedie MCK, Hall SM, Dinsdale OF, Bourdillon RE: Frequency-distribution curve of uric acid in the general population. Lancet 2:185–187, 1966

208. Fishman RS, Sunderman FW: Band keratopathy in gout. Arch Ophthalmol 75:367–369, 1966

209. Flatz G: Genetic and constitutional influences on serum-uric-acid in a tropical rural population. Humangenetik 11:83–90, 1971

210. Foad BSI, Sheon RP, Kirsner AB: Systemic lupus erythematosus in the elderly. Arch Intern Med 130:743–746, 1972

211. Forbus WD: Granulomatous Inflammation; Its Nature, General Pathological Significance, and Clinical Character. Springfield, Charles C Thomas, 1949

212. Forrest JS, Brooks DL: Cyclic sciatica of endometriosis. JAMA 222: 1177–1178, 1972

213. Frame B, Heinze EG Jr, Block MA, Manson GA: Myopathy in primary hyperparathyroidism. Observations in three patients. Ann Intern Med 68:1022–1027, 1968

214. Frame B, Jackson CE, Reynolds WA, Umphrey JE: Hypercalcemia and skeletal effects in chronic hypervitaminosis A. Ann Intern Med 80:44–48, 1974

215. Franz DN, Iggo A: Dorsal root potentials and ventral root reflexes evoked by nonmyelinated fibers. Science 162:1140–1142, 1968

216. Fraser GM: The radiological manifestations of scleroderma (diffuse systemic sclerosis). Br J Dermatol 78:1–14, 1966

217. Fred HL, Eiband JM, Martincheck LA, Yow EM: More on gonococcal dermatitis. Arch Intern Med 115:191, 1965

218. Freedman DX, Fenichel G: Effect of midbrain lesion on experimental allergy. Arch Neurol Psychiatry 79:164–169, 1958

219. Freeman JM, Aron AM, Collard JE, MacKay MC: The emotional correlates of Sydenham's chorea. Pediatrics 35:42–49, 1965

220. Fresco R: Tubular (myxovirus-like) structures in glomerular deposits from case of lupus nephritis (abstract). Fed Proc 27:246, 1968

221. Fried FA, Vermeulen CW: Artificial uric acid concretions and observations on uric acid solubility and supersaturation. Invest Urol 2:131–144, 1964

222. Friedman GD, Siegelaub AB, Seltzer CC, Feldman R, Collen MF: Smoking habits and the leukocyte count. Arch Environ Health 26:137–143, 1973

223. Fries JF, Hoopes JE, Shulman LE: Reciprocal skin grafts in systemic sclerosis (scleroderma). Arthritis Rheum 14:571–578, 1971

224. Fries JF, Lindgren JA, Bull JM: Scleroderma-like lesions and the carcinoid syndrome. Arch Intern Med 131:550–553, 1973

225. Fries JF, Sharp GC, McDevitt HO, Holman HR: Cyclophosphamide therapy in systemic lupus erythematosus and polymyositis. Arthritis Rheum 16:154–162, 1973

226. Fries JF, Siegel RC: Testing the "preliminary criteria for classification of SLE". Ann Rheum Dis 32:171–177, 1973

227. Friis J, Svejgaard A: Salmonella arthritis and HL-A27 (letter to Editor). Lancet 1:1350, 1974

228. Frohnert PP, Sheps SG: Long-term follow-up study of periarteritis nodosa. Am J Med 43:8–14, 1967

229. Fudenberg HH: Immunologic deficiency, autoimmune disease, and lymphoma: observations, implications, and speculations. Arthritis Rheum 9:464–472, 1966

230. Fullmer HM, Siedler HD, Krooth RS, Kurland LT: A cutaneous disorder of connective tissue in amyotrophic lateral sclerosis. A histochemical study. Neurology 10:717–724, 1960

231. Gajdusek DC: Pneumocystis carinii—etiologic agent of interstitial plasma cell pneumonia of premature and young infants. Pediatrics 19:543–565, 1957

232. Gajl-Peczalska KJ, Lim SD, Jacobson RR, Good RA: B lymphocytes in lepromatous leprosy. N Engl J Med 288;1033–1035, 1973

233. Garcia W: Elevated creatine phosphokinase levels associated with large muscle mass. Another pitfall in evaluating the clinical significance of total serum CPK activity. JAMA 228:1395–1396, 1974

234. Garrod AB. Nature and Treatment of Gout and Rheumatic Gout. London, Walton & Maberly, 1859

235. Garsenstein M, Pollak VE, Kark RM: Systemic lupus erythematosus and pregnancy. N Engl J Med 267:165–169, 1962

236. Gelfand MC, Steinberg AD: Therapeutic studies in NZB/W mice. II. Relative efficacy of aza-thioprine, cyclophosphamide and methylprednisolone. Arthritis Rheum 15:247–252, 1972

237. Gelfand MC, Steinberg AD, Nagle R, Knepshield JH: Therapeutic studies in NZB/W mice. I. Synergy of azathioprine, cyclophosphamide and methylprednisolone in combination. Arthritis Rheum 15:239–246, 1972

238. Germuth FG Jr: A comparative histologic and immunologic study in rabbits of induced hypersensitivity of the serum sickness type. J Exp Med 97:257–282, 1953

239. Germuth FG Jr, Choi I-J, Taylor JJ, Rodriguez E: Antibasement membrane disease. I. The glomerular lesions of Goodpasture's disease and experimental disease in sheep. Johns Hopkins Med J 131:367–384, 1972

240. Gertler MM, Garn SM, Levine SA: Serum uric acid in relation to age and physique in health and in coronary heart disease. Ann Intern Med 34:1421–1431, 1951

241. Gertler MM, Oppenheimer BS: Serum uric acid levels in men and women past the age of 65 years. J Gerontol 8:465–471, 1953

242. Geschickter CF, Athanasiadou PA, O'Malley WE: The role of mucinolysis in collagen disease. Am J Clin Pathol 30:93–111, 1958

243. Gibson RW, Bross IDJ, Graham S, Lilienfeld AM, Schuman LM, Levin ML, Dowd JE: Leukemia in children exposed to multiple risk factors. N Engl J Med 279:906–909, 1968

244. Gifford RW Jr, Hines EA Jr, Craig W McK: Sympathectomy for Raynaud's phenomenon. Follow-up study of 70 women with Raynaud's disease and 54 women with secondary Raynaud's phenomenon. Circulation 17:5–13, 1958

245. Gilbert RK, Hazard JB: Regeneration in human skeletal muscle. J Pathol Bacteriol 89:503–512, 1965

246. Gillanders LA, Strachan RW, Blair DW: Temporal arteriography. A new technique for the investigation of giant cell arteritis and polymyalgia rheumatica. Ann Rheum Dis 28:267–269, 1969

247. Glueck CJ, Levy RI, Fredrickson DS: Acute tendinitis and arthritis, a presenting symptom of familial type II hyperlipoproteinemia. JAMA 206:2895–2897, 1968

248. Goldberg S, Glynn LE, Bywaters EGL: Anomaly of sedimentation rate in rheumatic diseases. Br Med J 1:202, 1952

249. Goldfine LJ, Stevens MB, Masi AT, Shulman LE: Clinical significance of the L. E.-cell phenomenon in rheumatoid arthritis. Ann Rheum Dis 24:153–160, 1965

250. Goldman JA, Glueck CJ, Abrams NR, Steiner P, Herman JH: Musculoskeletal disorders associated with type-IV hyperlipoproteinaemia. Lancet 2:449–452, 1972

251. Goldstein NP, Jones PH, Brown JR: Peripheral neuropathy after exposure to an ester of dichlorophenoxyacetic acid. JAMA 171:1306–1309, 1959

252. Gold therapy in rheumatoid arthritis: final report of a multicentre controlled trial arranged by the Research Sub-Committee of the Empire Rheumatism Council. Ann Rheum Dis 20:315–334, 1961

253. Gonick HC, Rubini ME, Gleason IO, Sommers SC: The renal lesion in gout. Ann Intern Med 62:667–674, 1965

254. Good AE: Acromegalic arthropathy. A case report. Arthritis Rheum 7:65–74, 1964

255. Good AE: Reiter's disease, ankylosing spondylitis and rheumatoid arthritis occurring within a single family. Arthritis Rheum 14:753–763, 1971

256. Goodman JR, Sylvester RA, Talal N, Tuffanelli DL: Virus-like structures in lymphocytes of patients with systemic and discoid lupus erythematosus. Ann Intern Med 79:396–402, 1973

257. Gorden P, Robertson GL, Seegmiller JE: Hyperuricemia, a concomitant of congenital vasopressin-resistant diabetes insipidus in the adult. N Engl J Med 284:1057–1060, 1971

258. Gordon AL, Yudell A: Cauda equina lesion associated with rheumatoid spondylitis. Ann Intern Med 78:555–557, 1973

259. Gordon DA, Stein JL, Broder I: The extra-articular features of rheumatoid arthritis. A systematic analysis of 127 cases. Am J Med 54:445–452, 1973

260. Gorham LW, Wright AW, Shultz HH, Maxon FC Jr: Disappearing bones: a rare form of massive osteolysis. Report of two cases, one with autopsy findings. Am J Med 17:674–682, 1954

261. Graham DT: Cutaneous vascular reactions in Raynaud's disease and in states of hostility, anxiety, and depression. Psychosom Med 17:200–207, 1955

262. Grahame R, Haslam RM, Scott JT: Sulphobromophthalein retention in gout and asymptomatic hyperuricemia. Ann Rheum Dis 27:19–26, 1968

263. Grainger RG: Discussion on the clinical and radiological aspects of sacro-iliac disease. Proc Roy Soc Med 50:854–858, 1957

264. Greenbaum D, Ross JH, Steinberg VL: Renal biopsy in gout. Br Med J 1:1502–1504, 1961

265. Greene ML, Glueck CJ, Fujimoto WY, Seegmiller JE: Benign symmetric lipomatosis (Launois-Bensaude adenolipomatosis) with gout and hyperlipoproteinemia. Am J Med 48:239–246, 1970

266. Greenfield JG, Shy GM, Alvord EC Jr, Berg L: An Atlas of Muscle Pathology in Neuromuscular Diseases. Edinburgh and London, E & S Livingstone, Ltd., 1957

267. Griggs RC, Leddy JP, Klemperer MR, Joynt RJ: Inflammatory myopathy and hereditary complement deficiency (abstract). Neurology 22:425, 1972

268. Groskloss HH: Fat embolism. Yale J Biol Med 8:59–91, 175–197, 1935; 8:297–315, 1936

269. Grumet FC, Coukell A, Bodmer JG, Bodmer WF, McDevitt HO: Histocompatibility (HL-A) antigens associated with systemic lupus erythematosus. A possible genetic predisposition to disease. N Engl J Med 285:193–196, 1971

270. Guckian JC, Perry JE: Granulomatous hepatitis of unknown etiology. An etiologic and functional evaluation. Am J Med 44:207–215, 1968

271. Guillain G: La myopathie consécutive à la fièvre typhoïde. Sem médicale 27:277–280, 1907

272. Gunn A, Keddie N: Some clinical observations on patients with gallstones. Lancet 2:239–241, 1972

273. Gutman AB, Yü TF: Renal function and gout. With a commentary on the renal regulation of urate excretion, and the role of the kidney in the pathogenesis of gout. Am J Med 23:600–622, 1957

274. Gutman AB, Yü TF, Berger L: Renal function in gout. III. Estimation of tubular secretion and reabsorption of uric acid by use of pyrazinamide (pyrazinoic acid). Am J Med 47:575–592, 1969

275. Györkey F, Min K-W, Sincovics JG, Györkey P: Systemic lupus erythematosus and myxovirus (letter to Editor). N Engl J Med 280:333, 1969

276. Haas DC: Treatment of polymyositis with immunosuppressive drugs. Neurology 23:55–62, 1973

277. Hadler NM, Franck WA, Bress NM, Robinson DR: Acute polyarticular gout. Am J Med 56:715–719, 1974

278. Hadler NM, Gerwin RD, Frank MM, Whitaker JN, Baker M, Decker JL: The fourth

component of complement in the cerebrospinal fluid in systemic lupus erythematosus. Arthritis Rheum 16:507–521, 1973

279. Hahn BH, Bagby MK, Hamilton TR, Osterland CK: Comparison of therapeutic and immunosuppressive effects of azathioprine, prednisolone and combined therapy in NZB/NZW mice. Arthritis Rheum 16:163–170, 1973

280. Hahn BH, Bagby MK, Osterland CK: Abnormalities of delayed hypersensitivity in systemic lupus erythematosus. Am J Med 55:25–31, 1973

281. Hall AP: Correlations among hyperuricemia, hypercholesterolemia, coronary disease and hypertension. Arthritis Rheum 8:846–852, 1965

282. Hall AP: Epidemiological consequences of hyperuricemia. In Kátona G, Gil JR, Eds: Panamerican Rheumatology. Proceedings of the Fourth Panamerican Congress of Rheumatology, Mexico D.F., October, 1967. Excerpta Medica International Congress Series 165:69–73, 1969

283. Hall AP, Barry PE, Dawber TR, McNamara PM: Epidemiology of gout and hyperuricemia. A long-term population study. Am J Med 42:27–37, 1967

284. Hamilton E, Williams R, Barlow KA, Smith PM: The arthropathy of idiopathic haemochromatosis. Q J Med 37:171–182, 1968

285. Hamrin B, Jonsson N, Landberg T: Arteritis in "polymyalgia rheumatica". Lancet 1:397–401, 1964

286. Hansen OE: Hyperuricemia in cerebral infarction. Acta Neurol Scand 41 (Suppl 13, Part I): 357–361, 1965

287. Harbeck RJ, Bardana EJ, Kohler PF, Carr RI: DNA:anti-DNA complexes: their detection in systemic lupus erythematosus sera. J Clin Invest 52:789–795, 1973

288. Hargraves MM: Discovery of the LE cell and its morphology. Mayo Clin Proc 44:579–599, 1969

289. Harris AW, Lynch GW, O'Hare JP: Periarteritis nodosa. Arch Intern Med 63;1163–1182, 1939

290. Harris DK, Adams WGF: Acro-osteolysis occurring in men engaged in the polymerization of vinyl chloride. Br Med J 3:712–714, 1967

291. Hartroft WS, Ridout JH: Pathogenesis of the cirrhosis produced by choline deficiency. Escape of lipid from fatty hepatic cysts into the biliary and vascular systems. Am J Pathol 27:951–968, 1951

292. Harvey AM: Auto-immune disease and the chronic biologic false-positive test for syphilis. JAMA 182:513–518, 1962

293. Haslock I: Arthritis and Crohn's disease. A family study. Ann Rheum Dis 32:479–486, 1973

294. Haslock I, Wright V: The musculo-skeletal complications of Crohn's disease. Medicine 52:217–225, 1973

295. Hasselbacher P, Le Roy EC: Serum DNA binding activity in healthy subjects and in rheumatic disease. Arthritis Rheum 17:63–71, 1974

296. Hauge M, Harvald B: Heredity in gout and hyperuricemia. Acta Med Scand 152:247–257, 1955

297. Hauser WA, Ferguson RH, Holley KE, Kurland LT: Epidemiological aspects of temporal arteritis in Rochester, Minn. (abstract). Neurology 19:291, 1969

298. Hay DR: Malignant carcinoid syndrome with scleroderma. NZ Med J 63:90–93, 1964

299. Hay ED: Skeletal-muscle regeneration. N Engl J Med 284;1033–1034, 1971

300. Haygood TA, Fessel WJ, Strange DA: Atheromatous microembolism simulating polymyositis. JAMA 203:423–425, 1968

301. Healey LA: Serum uric acid and achievement—an explanation (letter to Editor). JAMA 212:1960, 1970

302. Healey LA, Skeith MD, Decker JL, Bayani-Sioson PS: Hyperuricemia in Filipinos: interaction of heredity and environment. Am J Hum Genet 19:81–85, 1967

303. Healey LA, Wilske KR: Anemia as a presenting manifestation of giant cell arteritis. Arthritis Rheum 14:27–31, 1971

304. Hedberg H: Studies on synovial fluid in arthritis. I. The total complement activity. II. The occurrence of mononuclear cells with in vitro cytotoxic effect. Acta Med Scand (Suppl) 479:1–78, 1967

305. Heller H, Gafni J, Michaeli D, Shahin N, Sohar E, Ehrlich G, Karten I, Sokoloff L: The arthritis of familial Mediterranean fever (FMF). Arthritis Rheum 9:1–17, 1966

306. Henneman PH, Wallach S, Dempsey EF: The metabolic defect responsible for uric acid stone formation. J Clin Invest 41:537–542, 1962
307. Heptinstall RH: Pathology of the Kidney. Boston, Little, Brown and Co., 1966, pp 535–540
308. Herbst AL, Kurman RJ, Scully RE, Poskanzer DC: Clear-cell adenocarcinoma of the genital tract in young females. Registry report. N Engl J Med 287:1259–1264, 1972
309. Herman JB, Mount FW, Medalie JH, Groen JJ, Dublin TD, Neufeld NH, Riss E: Diabetes prevalence and serum uric acid. Observations among 10,000 men in a survey of ischemic heart disease in Israel. Diabetes 16:858–868, 1967
310. Herman JH, Hess EV: Immunopathologic studies in relapsing polychondritis (abstract). Arthritis Rheum 14:166, 1971
311. Hill DL, Barrows HS: Identical skeletal and cardiac muscle involvement in a case of fatal polymyositis. Arch Neurol 19:545–551, 1968
312. Hill RB Jr: Fatal fat embolism from steroid-induced fatty liver. N Engl J Med 265:318–320, 1961
313. Hollander JL, McCarty DJ Jr, Eds: Arthritis and Allied Conditions. A Textbook of Rheumatology. 8th ed., Philadelphia, Lea & Febiger, 1972
314. Hollenhorst RW, Brown JR, Wagener HP, Shick RM: Neurologic aspects of temporal arteritis. Neurology 10: 490–498, 1960
315. Hollinger FB, Sharp JT, Lidsky MD, Rawls WE: Antibodies to viral antigens in systemic lupus erythematosus. Arthritis Rheum 14:1–11, 1971
316. Holmes MC, Burnet FM: The natural history of autoimmune disease in NZB mice. A comparison with the pattern of human autoimmune manifestations. Ann Intern Med 59:265–276, 1963
317. Howe JR, Taren JA: Foramen magnum tumors. Pitfalls in diagnosis. JAMA 225:1061–1066, 1973
318. Hower J, Struck H, Tackmann W, Stolecke H: CPK activity in hypoparathyroidism (letter to Editor). N Engl J Med 287:1098, 1972
319. Huang C-T, Hennigar GR, Lyons HA: Pulmonary dysfunction in systemic lupus erythematosus. N Engl J Med 272:288–293, 1965
320. Hudgson P, Pearce GW, Walton JN: Pre-clinical muscular dystrophy: histopathological changes observed on muscle biopsy. Brain 90:565–576, 1967
321. Hughes JT, Esiri M, Oxbury JM, Whitty CWM: Chloroquine myopathy. Q J Med 40:85–93, 1971
322. Hughes RAC, Berry CL, Seifert M, Lessof MH: Relapsing polychondritis. Three cases with a clinico-pathological study and literature review. Q J Med 41:363–380, 1972
323. Hunder GG, Baker HL Jr, Rhoton AL Jr, Sheps SG, Ward LE: Superficial temporal arteriography in patients suspected of having temporal arteritis. Arthritis Rheum 15:561–570, 1972
324. Hunder GG, Disney TF, Ward LE: Polymyalgia rheumatica. Mayo Clin Proc 44:849–875, 1969
325. Hunder GG, Kelly PJ: Roentgenologic transient osteoporosis of the hip. A clinical syndrome? Ann Intern Med 68:539–552, 1968
326. Hunder GG, McDuffie FC: Hypocomplementemia in rheumatoid arthritis. Am J Med 54:461–472, 1973
327. Hunder GG, McDuffie FC, Hepper NGG: Pleural fluid complement in systemic lupus erythematosus and rheumatoid arthritis. Ann Intern Med 76:357–363, 1972
328. Hurd ER: Immunosuppressive and antiinflammatory properties of cyclophosphamide, azathioprine and methotrexate. Arthritis Rheum 16:84–88, 1973
329. Hurd ER, Dowdle W, Casey H, Ziff M: Virus antibody levels in systemic lupus erythematosus. Arthritis Rheum 15:267–274, 1972
330. Hurd ER, Eigenbrodt E, Worthen H, Strunk SS, Ziff M: Glomerular cytoplasmic tubular structures in renal biopsies of patients with systemic lupus erythematosus and other diseases. Arthritis Rheum 14:539–550, 1971
331. Hutchinson J: On the relation of certain diseases of the eye to gout. Trans Opthalmol Soc UK 5:1–30, 1884
332. Hutt MSR, Pinniger JL: Adrenal failure due to bilateral suprarenal infarction associated with systemic nodular panniculitis and endarteritis. J Clin Pathol 9:316–322, 1956
333. Isaacs H, Barlow MB: Malignant hyperpyrexia during anaesthesia: possible association with subclinical myopathy. Br Med J 1:275–277, 1970

334. Ishmael WK, Owens JN Jr, Payne RW, Honick MD: Diabetes mellitus in patients with gouty arthritis. JAMA 190:396–398, 1964

335. Isomäki HA, Takkunen H: Gout and hyperuricemia in a Finnish rural population. Acta Rheum Scand 15:112–120, 1969

336. Itabashi HH, Kökmen E: Chloroquine neuromyopathy. A reversible granulovacuolar myopathy. Arch Pathol 93:209–218, 1972

337. Jacoby RK, Jayson MIV, Cosh JA: Onset, early stages, and prognosis of rheumatoid arthritis: a clinical study of 100 patients with 11-year follow-up. Br Med J 2:96–100, 1973

338. James DG: Sarcoidosis—epitaph and prospect. In Levinský L, Macholda F, Eds: Fifth International Conference on Sarcoidosis. Praha, Universita Karlova, 1971, pp 647–650

339. Janković BD, Draškoci M, Paunović D, Popesković L: Suppression of experimental allergic encephalomyelitis in rats and chickens treated with reserpine. Nature (London) 204:1101–1102, 1964

340. Jardon OM, Burney DW, Fink RL: Hypophosphatasia in an adult. J Bone Joint Surg 52A:1477–1484, 1970

341. Jayson MIV, Salmon PR, Harrison WJ: Inflammatory bowel disease in ankylosing spondylitis. Gut 11:506–511, 1970

342. Jelliffe SE: Bodily organs and psychopathology. Am J Psychiatry 92:1051–1076, 1936

343. Jensen J, Blankenhorn DH, Chin HP, Sturgeon P, Ware AG: Serum lipids and serum uric acid in human twins. J Lipid Res 6:193–205, 1965

344. Jessar RA, Lamont-Havers RW, Ragan C: Natural history of lupus erythematosus disseminatus. Ann Intern Med 38:717–731, 1953

345. Jewesbury RC, Topley WWC: On certain changes occurring in the voluntary muscles in general diseases. J Pathol Bacteriol 17:432–453, 1912, 1913

346. JiJi RM, Firozvi T, Spurling CL: Chronic idiopathic thrombocytopenic purpura. Treatment with steroids and splenectomy. Arch Intern Med 132:380–383, 1973

347. Johnson RL, Fink CW, Ziff M: Lymphotoxin formation by lymphocytes and muscle in polymyositis. J Clin Invest 51:2435–2449, 1972

348. Johnson RT, Richardson EP: The neurological manifestations of systemic lupus erythematosus. A clinical-pathological study of 24 cases and review of the litlrature. Medicine 47:337–369, 1968

349. Johnsson T, Lavender JF, Hultin E, Rasmussen AF Jr: The influence of avoidance-learning stress on resistance to Coxsackie B virus in mice. J Immunol 91:569–575, 1963

350. Jones HB: A special consideration of the aging process, disease, and life expectancy. Adv Biol Med Phys 4:281–337, 1956

351. Jones JP Jr, Engleman EP, Najarian JS: Systemic fat embolism after renal homotransplantation and treatment with corticosteroids. N Engl J Med 273:1453–1458, 1965

352. Joslin EP, Root HF, White P, Marble A: The Treatment of Diabetes Mellitus, 9th ed. London, Lea, Kimpton, 1952

353. Kagen LJ: Immunofluorescent demonstration of myoglobin in the kidney. Case report and review of forty-three cases of myoglobinemia and myoglobinuria identified immunologically. Am J Med 48:649–653, 1970

354. Kagen LJ, Christian CL: Clinico-pathological studies of systemic lupus erythematosus (SLE) nephritis (abstract). Arthritis Rhcum 9:516, 1966

355. Kagen LJ, Kimball AC, Christian CL: Serologic evidence of toxoplasmosis among patients with polymyositis. Am J Med 56:186–191, 1974

356. Kakulas BA: In vitro destruction of skeletal muscle by sensitized cells. Nature (London) 210:1115–1118, 1966

357. Kakulas BA, Adams RD: Principles of myopathology as illustrated in the nutritional myopathy of the Rottnest Quokka (Setonix brachyurus). Ann NY Acad Sci 138:90–101, 1966

358. Kaley G, Weiner R: Prostaglandin E_1: A potential mediator of the inflammatory response. Ann NY Acad Sci 180:338–350, 1971

359. Kalliomäki JL, Laine VAI, Ruutsalo H-M: Effect of ergometric exercise on the activity in the serum of creatine phosphokinase, glutamate-oxaloacetate transaminase and aldolase in rheumatoid arthritis. Acta Rheum Scand 14:185–196, 1968

360. Kampmeier RH, Shapiro JL: Diffuse and sometimes recurrent course of diffuse arteritis. Observations and report of a patient observed for twenty-one years. Arch Intern Med 92:856–879, 1953

361. Kansu E, Özer FL, Akalin E, Güler Y, Zileli T, Tanman E, Kaplaman E, Müftüoğlu E: Behçet's syndrome with obstruction of the venae cavae. A report of seven cases. Q J Med 41:151–168, 1972

362. Kaplan SR, Hayslett JP, Calabresi P: Treatment of advanced Wegener's granulomatosis with azathioprine and duazomycin A. N Engl J Med 278:239–244, 1968

363. Kappas A, Jones HE, Roitt IM: Effects of steroid sex hormones on immunological phenomena. Nature (London) 198:902, 1963

364. Karat ABA, Karat S, Job CK, Furness MA: Acute exudative arthritis in leprosy—rheumatoid-arthritis-like syndrome in association with erythema nodosum leprosum. Br Med J 3:770–772, 1967

365. Kasdon EJ, Schlossman SF: An experimental model of pulmonary arterial granulomatous inflammation. Am J Pathol 71:365–374, 1973

366. Kasl S, Brooks GW, Rodgers WL: Serum uric acid and cholesterol in achievement behavior and motivation. II. The relationship to college attendance, extracurricular and social activities, and vocational aspirations. JAMA 213:1291–1299, 1970

367. Kasl SV, Brooks GW, Rodgers WL: Serum uric acid and cholesterol in achievement behavior and motivation. I. The relationship to ability, grades, test performance, and motivation. JAMA 213:1158–1164, 1970

368. Katsilambros N, Braaten J, Ferguson BD, Bradley RF: Muscular syndrome after clofibrate (letter to Editor). N Engl J Med 286:1110–1111, 1972

369. Kaufman JM, Greene ML, Seegmiller JE: Urine uric acid to creatinine ratio—a screening test for inherited disorders of purine metabolism. Phosphoribosyltransferase (PRT) deficiency in X-linked cerebral palsy and in a variant of gout. J Pediatr 73:583–592, 1968

370. Kavanaugh GJ, Svien HJ, Holman CB, Johnson RM: "Pseudoclaudication" syndrome produced by compression of the cauda equina. JAMA 206:2477–2481, 1968

371. Kawano K, Miller L, Kimmelstiel P: Virus-like structures in lupus erythematosus. N Engl J Med 281:1228–1229, 1969

372. Kellermeyer RW, Breckenridge RT: The inflammatory process in acute gouty arthritis. II. The presence of Hageman factor and plasma thromboplastin antecedent in synovial fluid. J Lab Clin Med 67:455–460, 1966

373. Kelley WN, Goldfinger SE, Hardy HL: Hyperuricemia in chronic beryllium disease. Ann Intern Med 70:977–983, 1969

374. Kelley WN, Greene ML, Rosenbloom FM, Henderson JF, Seegmiller JE: Hypoxanthine-guanine phosphoribosyltransferase deficiency in gout. Ann Intern Med 70:155–206, 1969

375. Kelley WN, Rosenbloom FM, Seegmiller JE, Howell RR: Excessive production of uric acid in type I glycogen storage disease. J Pediatr 72:488–496, 1968

376. Khachadurian AK: Migratory polyarthritis in familial hypercholesterolemia (type II hyperlipoproteinemia). Arthritis Rheum 11:385–393, 1968

377. Kibler RF, Nathan PW: Relief of pain and paresthesiae by nerve block distal to a lesion. J Neurol Neurosurg Psychiatry 23:91–98, 1960

378. Kimmelstiel P: Vascular occlusion and ischemic infarction in sickle cell disease. Am J Med Sci 216:11–19, 1948

379. Klein DC, Raisz LG: Prostaglandins: stimulation of bone resorption in tissue culture. Endocrinology 86:1436–1440, 1970

380. Klemperer P: The concept of collagen diseases. Am J Pathol 26:505–519, 1950

381. Klinkerfuss G, Bleisch V, Dioso NM, Perkoff GT: A spectrum of myopathy associated with alcoholism. II. Light and electron microscopic observations. Ann Intern Med 67:493–510, 1967

382. Knochel JP, Schlein EM: On the mechanism of rhabdomyolysis in potassium depletion. J Clin Invest 51: 1750–1758, 1972

383. Knowles HC Jr, Zeek PM, Blankenhorn MA: Studies on necrotizing angiitis. IV. Periarteritis nodosa and hypersensitivity angiitis. Arch Intern Med 92:789–805, 1953

384. Kocsis JJ, Hernandovich J, Silver MJ, Smith JB, Ingerman C: Duration of inhibition of platelet prostaglandin formation and aggregation by ingested aspirin or indomethacin. Prostaglandins 3:141–144, 1973

385. Koffler D, Sandson J, Carr R, Kunkel HG: Immunologic studies concerning the pulmonary lesions in Goodpasture's syndrome. Am J Pathol 54:293–305, 1969

386. Kolodny EH, Rebeiz JJ, Caviness VS Jr, Richardson EP Jr: Granulomatous angiitis of the central nervous system. Arch Neurol 19:510–524, 1968

387. Kontos HA: Myopathy associated with chronic colchicine toxicity. N Engl J Med 266:38–39, 1962

388. Korneva EA, Khai LM: [Effect of destruction of areas of the hypothalamic region on the process of immunogenesis.] Fiziol Zh SSSR 49:42–48, 1963

389. Koss MN, Chernack WJ, Griswold WR, McIntosh RM: The choroid plexus in acute serum sickness. Morphologic, ultrastructural, and immunohistologic studies. Arch Pathol 96:331–334, 1973

390. Kramer DW, Perilstein PK, deMedeiros A: Metabolic influences in vascular disorders with particular reference to cholesterol determinations in comparison with uric acid levels. Angiology 9:162–171, 1958

391. Křížek V: Serum uric acid in relation to body weight. Ann Rheum Dis 25:456–458, 1966

392. Kudrjashov BA, Kalishevska TM: Reflex nature of the physiological anticoagulating system. Nature (London) 196:647–649, 1962

393. Kugelberg E, Welander L: Heredofamilial juvenile muscular atrophy simulating muscular dystrophy. AMA Arch Neurol Psychiatry 75:500–509, 1956

394. Kurland LT, Hauser WA, Ferguson RH, Holley KE: Epidemiologic features of diffuse connective tissue disorders in Rochester, Minn., 1951 through 1967, with special reference to systemic lupus erythematosus. Mayo Clin Proc 44:649–663, 1969

395. Kurlander DJ, Kirsner JB: The association of chronic "nonspecific" inflammatory bowel disease with lupus erythematosus. Ann Intern Med 60:799–813, 1964

396. Laffin RJ, Bardawil WA, Pachas WN, McCarthy JS: Immunofluorescent studies on the occurrence of antinuclear factor in normal human serum. Am J Pathol 45:465–479, 1964

397. Lagercrantz R, Winberg J, Zetterström R: Extra-colonic manifestations in chronic ulcerative colitis. Acta Paediatr 47:675–687, 1958

398. Lajtha A: Amino acid and protein metabolism of the brain. V. Turnover of leucine in mouse tissues. J Neurochem 3:358–365, 1959

399. Lash JW, Holtzer H, Swift H: Regeneration of mature skeletal muscle. Anat Rec 128:679–697, 1957

400. Lawee D: Uric acid: the clinical application of 1000 unsolicited determinations. Can Med Assoc J 100:838–841, 1969

401. Lawrence JS: Geographical studies of rheumatoid arthritis. In Bennett PH, Wood PHN, Eds: Population Studies of the Rheumatic Diseases. Proceedings of the Third International Symposium, New York, June 5–10, 1966. International Congress Series No. 148. Amsterdam, Excerpta Medica Foundation, 1968, pp 45–54

402. Lawrence JS: Prevalence of rheumatoid arthritis. Ann Rheum Dis 20:11–17, 1961

403. Lawrence JS, Hewitt JV, Popert AJ: Gout and hyperuricaemia in the United Kingdom. In Kellgren JH, Jeffrey MR, Ball J, Eds: The Epidemiology of Chronic Rheumatism. Oxford, Blackwell, 1963, p 176

404. Lee SL, Blum L, Grishman E, Porush J: Guides to prognosis in systemic lupus erythematosus (SLE) (abstract). Arthritis Rheum 15:115–116, 1972

405. Lee SL, Rivero I, Siegel M: Activation of systemic lupus erythematosus by drugs. Arch Intern Med 117:620–626, 1966

406. Leeper RD, Benua RS, Brener JL, Rawson RW: Hyperuricemia in myxedema. J Clin Endocrinol Metab 20:1457–1466, 1960

407. Lehman EP, McNattin RF: Fat embolism. II. Incidence at postmortem. Arch Surg 17:179–189, 1928

408. Lehman EP, Moore RM: Fat embolism. Including experimental production without trauma. Arch Surg 14:621–662, 1927

409. Lellouch J, Schwartz D, Tran MH, Beaumont JL: The relationships between smoking and levels of serum urea and uric acid. Results of an epidemiological survey. J Chronic Dis 22:9–15, 1969

410. Lennane GAQ, Rose BS, Isdale IC: Gout in the Maori. Ann Rheum Dis 19:120–125, 1960

411. Lerner RA, Glassock RJ, Dixon FJ: The role of anti-glomerular basement membrane antibody in the pathogenesis of human glomerulonephritis. J Exp Med 126:989–1004, 1967

412. Lesch M, Nyhan WL: A familial disorder of uric acid metabolism and central nervous system function. Am J Med 36:561–570, 1964
413. Levin J, Conley CL: Thrombocytosis associated with malignant disease. Arch Intern Med 114:497–500, 1964
414. Levin MJ, Gardner P, Waldvogel FA: "Tropical" pyomyositis. An unusual infection due to *Staphylococcus aureus.* N Engl J Med 284:196–198, 1971
415. Levine S, Strebel R, Wenk EJ, Harman PJ: Suppression of experimental allergic encephalomyelitis by stress. Biol Med 109:294–298, 1962
416. Levy M: Aspirin use in patients with major upper gastrointestinal bleeding and peptic-ulcer disease. A report from the Boston Collaborative Drug Surveillance Program, Boston University Medical Center. N Engl J Med 290:1158–1162, 1974
417. Lewis BI, Sinton DW, Knott JR: Central nervous system involvement in disorders of collagen. Arch Intern Med 93:315–327, 1954
418. Lewis PD: Neuromuscular involvement in pituitary gigantism. Br Med J 2:499–500, 1972
419. Lewis T: Clinical observation and experiments relating to burning pain in the extremities, and to so-called "erythromelalgia" in particular. Clin Sci 1:175–211, 1933
420. Lewis T, Kellgren JH: Observations relating to referred pain, viscero-motor reflexes and other associated phenomena. Clin Sci 4:47–71, 1939
421. Lichtenstein LM, Gillespie E, Bourne HR, Henney CS: The effects of a series of prostaglandins on in vitro models of the allergic response and cellular immunity. Prostaglandins 2:519–528, 1972
422. Lidsky MD, Sharp JT, Billings S: Double-blind study of cyclophosphamide in rheumatoid arthritis. Arthritis Rheum 16:148–153, 1973
423. Lie TH, Rothfield NF: An evaluation of the preliminary criteria for the diagnosis of systemic lupus erythematosus. Arthritis Rheum 15:532–534, 1972
424. Lieber CS, Jones DP, Losowsky MS, Davidson CS: Interrelation of uric acid and ethanol metabolism in man. J Clin Invest 41:1863–1870, 1962
425. Lillington GA, Carr DT, Mayne JG: Rheumatoid pleurisy with effusion. Arch Intern Med 128:764–768, 1971
426. Lindström C, Wramsby H, Östberg G: Granulomatous arthritis in Crohn's disease. Gut 13:257–259, 1972
427. Locke S, Lawrence DG, Legg MA: Diabetic amyotrophy. Am J Med 34:775–785, 1963
428. Logan RG, Bandera JM, Mikkelsen WM, Duff IF: Polymyositis: a clinical study. Ann Intern Med 65:996–1007, 1966
429. Lotz M, Zisman E, Bartter FC: Evidence for a phosphorus-depletion syndrome in man. N Engl J Med 278:409–415, 1968
430. Lou HOC, Reske-Nielsen E: The central nervous system in Fabry's disease. A clinical, pathological, and biochemical investigation. Arch Neurol 25:351–359, 1971
431. Luk'yanenko VI: Mechanism of inhibition of anaphylactic reaction by narcosis. Biull Eks Biol Med 51:591–595, 1961 (English)
432. Lundin PM, Schelin U, Pellegrini G, Mellgren J: Plasma cell production in adaptation syndrome. Acta Pathol Microbiol Scand 35:339–356, 1954
433. Lynch MJG, Raphael SS, Dixon TP: Fat embolism in chronic alcoholism. Control study on incidence of fat embolism. AMA Arch Pathol 67:68–80, 1959
434. MacDonald RA, Robbins SL, Mallory GK: Dermal fibrosis following subcutaneous injections of serotonin creatine sulphate. Proc Soc Exp Biol Med 97:334–337, 1958
435. Mackay IR: Lupoid hepatitis and primary biliary cirrhosis: autoimmune diseases of the liver? Bull Rheum Dis 18:487–494, 1968
436. Mackay IR, Dwyer JM, Rowley MJ: Differing effects of azathioprine and cyclophosphamide on immune responses to flagellin in man. Arthritis Rheum 16:455–460, 1973
437. Maclachlan MJ, Rodnan GP, Cooper WM, Fennell RH Jr: Chronic active ("lupoid") hepatitis. A clinical, serological, and pathological study of 20 patients. Ann Intern Med 62:425–462, 1965
438. Maddock RK Jr, Stevens LE, Reemtsma K, Bloomer HA: Goodpasture's syndrome. Cessation of pulmonary hemorrhage after bilateral nephrectomy. Ann Intern Med 67:1258–1264, 1967
439. Mainland D, Sutcliffe MI: Hydroxychloroquine sulfate in rheumatoid arthritis, a six month, double-blind trial. Bull Rheum Dis 13:287–290, 1962

440. Mair WGP: Electron microscopic findings in biopsies from various myopathies. *In* Members of the Research Committee of the Muscular Dystrophy Group, Eds: Proceedings of the Third Symposium on Current Research in Muscular Dystrophy Held at the National Hospital, Queen Square, London WC1, 8th–9th January, 1965. London, Pitman Medical Publishing Co., Ltd., 1965, pp 164–180

441. Malaviya AN, Many A, Schwartz RS: Treatment of dermatomyositis with methotrexate. Lancet 2:485–488, 1968

442. Maldonado JE, Hanlon DG: Monocytosis: a current appraisal. Proc Mayo Clin 40:248–259, 1965

443. Mandel MJ, Carr RI, Weston WL, Sams WM Jr, Harbeck RJ, Krueger GG: Anti-native DNA antibodies in discoid lupus erythematosus. Arch Dermatol 106:668–670, 1972

444. Marinoff SC, Lempert P, Mandel EE: Association of hypercholesterolemia with hyperuricemia. A review of the literature. Chicago Med School Quarterly 22:135–142, 1962

445. Markowitz SS, McDonald CJ, Fethiere W, Kerzner MS: Occupational acroosteolysis. Arch Dermatol 106:219–223, 1972

446. Mason AA, Black S: Allergic skin responses abolished under treatment of asthma and hayfever by hypnosis. Lancet 1:877–880, 1958

447. Mastaglia FL, Currie S: Immunological and ultrastructural observations on the role of lymphoid cells in the pathogenesis of polymyositis. Acta Neuropathol 18:1–16, 1971

448. Mastaglia FL, Papadimitriou JM, Kakulas BA: Regeneration of muscle in Duchenne muscular dystrophy: an electron microscope study. J Neurol Sci 11:425–444, 1970

449. Mastaglia FL, Walton JN: Coxsackie virus-like particles in skeletal muscle from a case of polymyositis. J Neurol Sci 11:593–599, 1970

450. Mathews R, Williams H, Rickards W, Waterhouse I, Allan J: Sydenham's chorea: its relationship to rheumatic infection and psychological illness. Med J Aust 2:771–774, 1960

451. Matula G, Paterson PY: Spontaneous in vitro reduction of nitroblue tetrazolium by neutrophils of adult patients with bacterial infection. N Engl J Med 285:311–317, 1971

452. McArdle B: Myopathy due to a defect in muscle glycogen breakdown. Clin Sci 10:13–35, 1951

453. McCarty DJ Jr, Hogan JM, Gatter RA, Grossman M: Studies on pathological calcifications in human cartilage. I. Prevalence and types of crystal deposits in the menisci of two hundred fifteen cadavera. J Bone Joint Surg 48A:309–325, 1966

454. McClary AR, Meyer E, Weitzman EL: Observations on the role of the mechanism of depression in some patients with disseminated lupus erythematosus. Psychosom Med 17:311–321, 1955

455. McCombs RP: Systemic "allergic" vasculitis. Clinical and pathological relationships. JAMA 194:1059–1064, 1965

456. McCord CP: A new occupational disease is born. J Occup Med 12:234, 1970

457. McDevitt HO, Bodmer WF: HL-A, immune-response genes, and disease. Lancet 1:1269–1275, 1974

458. McFadyen IJ, Housley E, MacPherson AIS: Intraarterial reserpine administration in Raynaud syndrome. Arch Intern Med 132:526–528, 1973

459. McFarlin DE, Griggs RC: Treatment of inflammatory myopathies with azathioprine. Trans Am Neurol Assoc 93:244–246, 1968

460. McGregor HG: Psychological factor in rheumatic disease. Practitioner 143:627–636, 1939

461. McWilliams JR: Ocular findings in gout. Report of a case of conjunctival tophi. Am J Ophthalmol 35:1778–1783, 1952

462. Medical Research Council Report: Treatment of polyarteritis nodosa with cortisone: Results after three years. Br Med J 1:1399–1400, 1960

463. Medsger TA Jr, Masi AT, Rodnan GP, Benedek TG, Robinson H: Survival with systemic sclerosis (scleroderma). A life-table analysis of clinical and demographic factors in 309 patients. Ann Intern Med 75:369–376, 1971

464. Medsger TA Jr, Rodnan GP, Rabin B, Birnbaum N, Porter P: HL-A antigen 27 and psoriatic spondylitis (abstract). Arthritis Rheum 17:323, 1974

465. Melick RA, Henneman PH: Clinical and laboratory studies of 207 consecutive patients in a kidney-stone clinic. N Engl J Med 259:307–314, 1958

466. Mellors RC: Autoimmune disease in NZB/BL mice. II. Autoimmunity and malignant lymphoma. Blood 27:435–448, 1966

467. Mellors RC, Aoki T, Huebner RJ: Further implication of murine leukemia-like virus in the disorders of NZB mice. J Exp Med 129:1045–1062, 1968

468. Meltzer HY, Engel WK: Histochemical abnormalities of skeletal muscle in acutely psychotic patients. Part II. Arch Gen Psychiatry 23:492–502, 1970

469. Meltzer HY, Moline R: Muscle abnormalities in acute psychoses. Arch Gen Psychiatry 23:481–491, 1970

470, Meltzer HY, Moline R: Plasma enzymatic activity after exercise. Study of psychiatric patients and their relatives. Arch Gen Psychiatry 22:390–397, 1970

471. Melzack R, Wall PD: Pain mechanisms: a new theory. Science 150:971–979, 1965

472. Mesara BW, Brody GL, Oberman HA: "Pseudorheumatoid" subcutaneous nodules. Am J Clin Pathol 45:684–691, 1966

473. Meszaros WT: The regional manifestations of scleroderma. Radiology 70:313–325, 1958

474. Meyerowitz S, Jacox RF, Hess DW: Monozygotic twins discordant for rheumatoid arthritis: a genetic, clinical and psychological study of 8 sets. Arthritis Rheum 11:1–21, 1968

475. Meyerson LB, Meier GC: Cutaneous lesions in acroosteolysis. Arch Dermatol 106:224–227, 1972

476. Middleton PJ, Alexander RM, Szymanski MT: Severe myositis during recovery from influenza. Lancet 2:533–535, 1970

477. Mikkelsen WM: The possible association of hyperuricemia and/or gout with diabetes mellitus. Arthritis Rheum 8:853–864, 1965

478. Millet JAP: Psychoanalytic psychotherapy in Raynaud's disease. Psychosom Med 18:492–505, 1956

479. Milner RDG, Mitchinson MJ: Systemic Weber-Christian disease. J Clin Pathol 18:150–156, 1965

480. Mintz DH, Canary JJ, Carreon G, Kyle LH: Hyperuricemia in hyperparathyroidism. N Engl J Med 265:112–115, 1961

481. Mintz G, González-Angulo A, Fraga A: Ultrastructure of muscle in polymyositis. Am J Med 44:216–224, 1968

482. Mittelmann B, Wolff HG: Affective states and skin temperature: experimental study of subjects with "cold hands" and Raynaud's syndrome. Psychosom Med 1:271–292, 1939

483. Moll JMH, Wright V: Psoriatic arthritis. Semin Arthritis Rheum 3:55–78, 1973

484. Molnar Z, Stern WH, Stoltzner GH: Cytoplasmic tubular structures in pigmented villonodular synovitis. Arthritis Rheum 14:784–787, 1971

485. Monacelli M, Nazzaro P, Eds: International Symposium on Behçet's Disease, Rome, 1964. Basel, S. Karger, 1966, p 166

486. Mongan ES, Cass RM, Jacox RF, Vaughan JH: A study of the relation of seronegative and seropositive rheumatoid arthritis to each other and to necrotizing vasculitis. Am J Med 47:23–35, 1969

487. Moos RH: Personality factors associated with rheumatoid arthritis: a review. J Chronic Dis 17:41–55, 1964

488. Moos RH, Solomon GF: Personality correlates of the rapidity of progression of rheumatoid arthritis. Ann Rheum Dis 23:145–151, 1964

489. Moran CJ, Ryder G, Turk JL, Waters MFR: Evidence for circulating immune complexes in lepromatous leprosy. Lancet 2:572–573, 1972

490. Moran TJ: Cortisone-induced alterations in lipid metabolism. Morphologic and serologic observations in rabbits. Arch Pathol 73:300–312, 1962

491. Morris R, Metzger AL, Bluestone R, Terasaki PI: HL-A W27—a clue to the diagnosis and pathogenesis of Reiter's syndrome. N Engl J Med 290:554–556, 1974

492. Morris RI, Metzger AL, Bluestone R, Terasaki PI: HL-A W27—a useful discriminator in the arthropathies of inflammatory bowel disease. N Engl J Med 290:1117–1119, 1974

493. Moser C, Fessel WJ: Rheumatic manifestations of hypophosphatemia. Arch Intern Med 134:674–678, 1974

494. Moskowitz RW, Baggenstoss AH, Slocumb CH: Histopathologic classification of periarteritis nodosa: a study of 56 cases confirmed at necropsy. Proc Staff Meet Mayo Clin 38:345–357, 1963

495. Moskowitz RW, Katz D: Chondrocalcinosis and chondrocalsynovitis (pseudogout syndrome). Analysis of twenty-four cases. Am J Med 43:322–334, 1967

496. Mostofi FK, Engleman E: Fatal relapsing febrile nonsuppurative panniculitis. Arch Pathol 43:417–426, 1947

497. Mueller EF, Kasl SV, Brooks GW, Cobb S: Psychosocial correlates of serum urate levels. Psychol Bull 73:238–257, 1970

498. Muenter MD, Perry HO, Ludwig J: Chronic vitamin A intoxication in adults. Hepatic, neurologic and dermatologic complications. Am J Med 50:129–136, 1971

499. Mufson I: An etiology of scleroderma. Ann Intern Med 39:1219–1227, 1953

500. Mulder DW, Bastron JA, Lambert EH: Hyperinsulin neuronopathy. Neurology 6:627–635, 1956

501. Müller G: Quoted by Groskloss [268]

502. Müller R, Kugelberg E: Myopathy in Cushing's syndrome. J Neurol Neurosurg Psychiatry 22:314–319, 1959

503. Multicentre Trial Group: Controlled trial of D(-)penicillamine in severe rheumatoid arthritis. Lancet 1:275–280, 1973

504. Munsat TL, Baloh R, Pearson CM, Fowler W Jr: Serum enzyme alterations in neuromuscular disorders. JAMA 226:1536–1543, 1973

505. Munsat TL, Piper D, Cancilla P, Mednick J: Inflammatory myopathy with facioscapulohumeral distribution. Neurology 22:335–347, 1972

506. Mustard JF, Murphy EA, Ogryzlo MA, Smythe HA: Blood coagulation and platelet economy in subjects with primary gout. Can Med Assoc J 89:1207–1211, 1963

507. Myers AR, Epstein FH, Dodge HJ, Mikkelsen WM: The relationship of serum uric acid to risk factors in coronary heart disease. Am J Med 45:520–528, 1968

508. Nadler HL, Egan TJ: Deficiency of lysosomal acid phosphatase. A new familial metabolic disorder. N Engl J Med 282:302–307, 1970

509. Nakagawa S, Takayanagi N: Relapsing febrile nodular nonsuppurative panniculitis (Weber-Christian syndrome): report of a case with autopsy. Acta Pathol Jap 12:259–263, 1962

510. Namba T, Muguruma M: The role of skeletal muscle membrane in experimental myopathy. Neurology 22:611–618, 1972

511. Nanra RS, Kincaid-Smith P: Lupus nephritis: clinical course in relation to treatment. In Kincaid-Smith P, Mathew TH, Becker EL, Eds: Glomerulonephritis. Morphology, Natural History, and Treatment. New York, John Wiley and Sons, 1973, pp 1193–1210

512. Nelson JD: Antibiotic concentrations in septic joint effusions. N Engl J Med 284:349–353, 1971

513. Nesterov AI: The clinical course of Kashin-Beck disease. Arthritis Rheum 7:29–40, 1964

514. Newland H: Antagonism of the antithrombotic effect of warfarin by uric acid. Am J Med Sci 256:44–52, 1968

515. Nishikai M, Homma M: Anti-myoglobin antibody in polymyositis (letter to Editor). Lancet 2:1205–1206, 1972

516. Nobrega FT, Ferguson RH, Kurland LT, Hargraves MM: Lupus erythematosus in Rochester, Minnesota, 1950–1965: a preliminary study. In Bennett PH, Wood PHN, Eds: Population Studies of the Rheumatic Diseases. International Congress Series 148:259–266, 1968

517. Noonan CD, Taylor FB Jr, Engleman EP: Nodular rheumatoid disease of the lung with cavitation. Arthritis Rheum 6:232–240, 1963

518. Noordenbos W. Physiological correlates of clinical pain syndromes. In Soulairac A, Cahn J, Charpentier J, Eds: Pain: Proceedings of the International Symposium on Pain. London and New York, Academic Press, 1968, pp 465–475

519. Norris FH Jr, Dramov B, Calder CD, Johnson SG: Virus-like particles in myositis accompanying herpes zoster. Arch Neurol 21:25–31, 1969

520. Norton WL, Hurd ER, Lewis DC, Ziff M: Evidence of microvascular injury in scleroderma and systemic lupus erythematosus: Quantitative study of the microvascular bed. J Lab Clin Med 71:919–933, 1968

521. Nosanchuk JS, Naylor B: A unique cytologic picture in pleural fluid from patients with rheumatoid arthritis. Am J Clin Pathol 50:330–335, 1968

522. Novack SN, Pearson CM: Cyclophosphamide therapy in Wegener's granulomatosis. N Engl J Med 284:938–942, 1971

523. Nugent CA, Tyler FH: The renal excretion of uric acid in patients with gout and in nongouty subjects. J Clin Invest 38:1890–1898, 1959

524. Nuki G, Brooks R, Buchanan WW: The economics of arthritis. Bull Rheum Dis 23:726–733, 1972–1973

525. Nuzum JW Jr, Nuzum JW Sr: Polyarteritis nodosa. Statistical review of one hundred seventy-five cases from the literature and report of a "typical" case. Arch Intern Med 94:942–955, 1954

526. O'Brien WM, Burch TA, Bunim JJ: Genetics of hyperuricaemia in Blackfeet and Pima Indians. Ann Rheum Dis 25:117–119, 1966

527. O'Duffy JD, Carney JA, Deodhar S: Behçet's disease. Report of 10 cases, 3 with new manifestations. Ann Intern Med 75:561–570, 1971

528. Ogryzlo MA: Chronic inflammatory lesions of skeletal muscle in rheumatoid arthritis and in other diseases. Arch Pathol 46:301–312, 1948

529. Olefsky J, Kempson R, Jones H, Reaven G: "Tertiary" hyperparathyroidism and apparent "cure" of vitamin-D-resistant rickets after removal of an ossifying mesenchymal tumor of the pharynx. N Engl J Med 286:740–745, 1972

530. O'Sullivan JB: Gout in a New England town. A prevalence study in Sudbury, Massachusetts. Ann Rheum Dis 31:166–169, 1972

531. O'Sullivan JB, Cathcart ES: The prevalence of rheumatoid arthritis. Follow-up evaluation of the effect of criteria on rates in Sudbury, Massachusetts. Ann Intern Med 76:573–577, 1972

532. Otten HA, Boerma FW: Significance of the Waaler-Rose test, streptococcal agglutination, and antistreptolysin titre in the prognosis of rheumatoid arthritis. Ann Rheum Dis 18:24–28, 1959

533. Ouyang R, Mitchell DM, Rozdilsky B: Central nervous system involvement in rheumatoid disease. Report of a case. Neurology 17:1099–1105, 1967

534. Owens G, Sokal JE: Liver lipid as a source of embolic fat. J Appl Physiol 16:1100–1102, 1961

535. Pak Poy RK: Urinary pH in gout. Aust Ann Med 14:35–39, 1965

536. Panush RS, Alpert E, Schur PH: Absence of Australia antigen and antibody in patients with rheumatic diseases. Arthritis Rheum 14:782–783, 1971

537. Papamichail M, Holbrow EJ, Keith HI, Currey HLF: Subpopulations of human peripheral blood lymphocytes distinguished by combined rosette formation and membrane immuno-fluorescence. Lancet 2:64–66, 1972

538. Patterson CD, Harville WE, Pierce JA: Rheumatoid lung disease. Ann Intern Med 62:685–697, 1965

539. Patton JT: Skeletal changes in hypophosphataemic osteomalacia. In Jeliffe AM, Strickland B, Eds: European Association of Radiology, Symposium Ossium. Edinburgh and London, E & S Livingstone, 1970, pp 299–301

540. Pearce GW: Electron microscopy in the study of muscular dystrophy. Ann NY Acad Sci 138:138–150, 1966

541. Pearce GW, Pearce JMS, Walton JN: The Duchenne type muscular dystrophy: his-topathological studies of the carrier state. Brain 89:109–120, 1966

542. Pearce J, Aziz H: Uric acid and serum lipids in cerebrovascular disease. 2. Uric acid-plasma lipid correlations. J Neurol Neurosurg Psychiatry 33:88–91, 1970

543. Pearce JMS: Discussion of Prineas JW, Mason AS, Henson RA: Myopathy in metabolic bone disease. In Research Committee of Muscular Dystrophy Group, Eds: Third Symposium on Current Research in Muscular Dystrophy. London, Pitman Medical Publishing Co., Ltd., 1965, pp 55–56

544. Pearlstein RA, Kohn RR: Myosin and total protein turnover in denervated rat skeletal muscle. Am J Pathol 48:823–829, 1966

545. Pearson CM: Incidence and type of pathologic alterations observed in muscle in a routine autopsy survey. Neurology 9:757–766, 1959

546. Pearson CM: Polymyositis and dermatomyositis. Bull Rheum Dis 12:269–272, 1962

547. Penn AS, Rowland LP, Fraser DW: Drugs, coma, and myoglobinuria. Arch Neurol 26:336–343, 1972

548. Perkoff GT, Dioso MM, Bleisch V, Klinkerfuss G: A spectrum of myopathy associated with alcoholism. I. Clinical and laboratory features. Ann Intern Med 67:481–492, 1967

549. Perkoff GT, Hardy P, Velez-Garcia E: Reversible acute muscular syndrome in chronic alcoholism. N Engl J Med 274:1277–1285, 1966

550. Perkoff GT, Silber R, Tyler FH, Cartwright GE, Wintrobe MM: Studies in disorders of muscle. XII. Myopathy due to the administration of therapeutic amounts of 17-hydroxycorticosteroids. Am J Med 26:891–898, 1959

551. Perrotto JL, Warren KS: Inhibition of granuloma formation around *Schistosoma mansoni* eggs. IV. X-irradiation. Am J Pathol 56:279–291, 1969

552. Perry HO, Mayne JG: Psoriasis and Reiter's syndrome. Arch Dermatol 92:129–136, 1965

553. Person DA, Sharp JT, Rawls WE: A search for viruses and mycoplasmas in connective tissue diseases. Arthritis Rheum 16:677–687, 1973

554. Peters JP, Van Slyke DD: Quantitative Clinical Chemistry: Interpretations, Vol I, ed. 2. Baltimore, Williams and Wilkins, 1946, p 953

555. Petz LD, Sharp GC, Cooper NR, Irvin WS: Serum and cerebral spinal fluid complement and serum autoantibodies in systemic lupus erythematosus. Medicine 50:259–275, 1971

556. Phillips PE, Hirshaut Y: Epstein-Barr virus antibody levels in systemic lupus erythematosus. Arthritis Rheum 16:97–101, 1973

557. Pollack AD: Some observations on the pathology of systemic lupus erythematosus. *In* Baehr G, Klemperer P, Eds: A Mount Sinai Hospital Monograph on Systemic Lupus Erythematosus. New York, Grune & Stratton, 1959, pp 1–16

558. Popert AJ, Hewitt JV: Gout and hyperuricaemia in rural and urban populations. Ann Rheum Dis 21:154–163, 1962

559. Price HM, Pease DC, Pearson CM: Selective actin filament and Z-band degeneration induced by plasmocid. An electron microscopic study. Lab Invest 11:549–562, 1962

560. Prineas JW, Mason AS, Henson RA: Myopathy in metabolic bone disease. Br Med J 1:1034–1036, 1965

561. Prior IAM, Rose BS: Uric acid, gout and public health in the South Pacific. NZ Med J 65:295–300, 1966

562. Prior IAM, Rose BS, Harvey HPB, Davidson F: Hyperuricaemia, gout, and diabetic abnormality in Polynesian people. Lancet 1:333–338, 1966

563. Rachelefsky GS, Terasaki PI, Katz R, Stiehm ER: Increased prevalence of W27 in juvenile rheumatoid arthritis. N Engl J Med 290:892–893, 1974

564. Ragan C, Farrington E: The clinical features of rheumatoid arthritis. Prognostic indices. JAMA 181:663–667, 1962

565. Rahe RH, Arthur RJ: Stressful underwater demolition training. Serum urate and cholesterol variability. JAMA 202:1052–1054, 1967

566. Rahe RH, Rubin RT, Arthur RJ, Clark BR: Serum uric acid and cholesterol variability. A comprehensive view of underwater demolition team training. JAMA 206:2875–2880, 1968

567. Raitt JW: Wegener's granulomatosis: treatment with cytotoxic agents and adrenocorticoids. Ann Intern Med 74:344–356, 1971

568. Rakic MT, Valkenburg HA, Davidson RT, Engels JP, Mikkelsen WM, Neel JV, Duff IF: Observations on the natural history of hyperuricemia and gout. I. An eighteen year follow-up of nineteen gouty families. Am J Med 37:862–871, 1964

569. Ramsay ID: Muscle dysfunction in hyperthyroidism. Lancet 2:931–935, 1966

570. Rasmussen AF Jr, Spencer ES, Marsh JT: Decrease in susceptibility of mice to passive anaphylaxis following avoidance-learning stress. Proc Soc Exp Biol Med 100:878–879, 1959

571. Reingold IM, Escovitz WE: Metastatic cutaneous carcinoid. Report of a case of functioning malignant bronchial carcinoid. Arch Dermatol 82:971–975, 1960

572. Research Group on Neuromuscular Diseases, Subcommittee on Quantitation of Muscle Biopsy Findings: Quantitation of muscle biopsy findings. Appendix B to the minutes of the meeting in Montreal, Canada, Sept 21, 1967. J Neurol Sci 6:179–188, 1968

573. Research Sub-Committee of the Empire Rheumatism Council: Report. Relation of toxic reactions in gold therapy to improvement in rheumatoid arthritis. Ann Rheum Dis 20:335–340, 1961

574. Reynolds TB, Peters RL, Yamada S: Chronic active and lupoid hepatitis caused by a laxative, oxyphenisatin. N Engl J Med 285:813–820, 1971

575. Reznik M, Hansen JL: Mitochondria in degenerating and regenerating skeletal muscle. Arch Pathol 87:601–608, 1969

576. Richardson HB: Raynaud's phenomenon and scleroderma; a case report and psychodynamic formulation. Psychoanal Rev 42:24–38, 1955

577. Ridley DS, Jopling WH: Classification of leprosy according to immunity. A five-group system. Int J Lepr 34:255–273, 1966

578. Riedel: Quoted by Lehman and Moore [408]

579. Rieselbach RE, Sorensen LB, Shelp WD, Steele TH: Diminished renal urate secretion per nephron as a basis for primary gout. Ann Intern Med 73:359–366, 1970

580. Robins JM, Bookstein JJ: Regressing aneurysms in periarteritis nodosa. A report of 3 cases. Radiology 104:39–42, 1972

581. Robinson DR, Smith H, Levine L: Prostaglandin (PG) synthesis by human synovial cultures and its stimulation by colchicine (abstract). Arthritis Rheum 16:129, 1973

582. Rodarte JR, Garrison CO, Holley KE, Fontana RS: Whipple's disease simulating sarcoidosis: a case with unique clinical and histologic features. Arch Intern Med 129:479–482, 1972

583. Rodnan GP, Benedek TG, Medsger TA Jr, Cammarata RJ: The association of progressive systemic sclerosis (scleroderma) with coal miners' pneumoconiosis and other forms of silicosis. Ann Intern Med 66:323–334,1967

584. Romeo SG, Whalen RE, Tindall JP: Intra-arterial administration of reserpine. Its use in patients with Raynaud's disease or Raynaud's phenomenon. Arch Intern Med 125:825–829, 1970

585. Ropes MW, Bennett GA, Cobb S, Jacox R, Jessar RA: Proposed diagnostic criteria for rheumatoid arthritis. Bull Rheum Dis 7:121–124, 1956; Revision: Bull Rheum Dis 9:175–176, 1958

586. Rose AL, Walton JN: Polymyositis: a survey of 89 cases with particular reference to treatment and prognosis. Brain 89:747–768, 1966

587. Rose BS, Isdale IC: Gout and other arthritides in the Maori and European population in New Zealand. *In* Kellgren JH, Jeffrey MR, Ball J, Eds: The Epidemiology of Chronic Rheumatism. Oxford, Blackwell, 1963, p 156

588. Rose GA: The natural history of polyarteritis. Br Med J 2:1148–1152, 1957

589. Rose HM, Ragan C, Pearce E, Lipman MO: Differential agglutination of normal and sensitized sheep erythrocytes by sera of patients with rheumatoid arthritis. Proc Soc Exp Biol Med 68:1–6, 1948

590. Rosenberg AL, Bergstrom L, Troost T, Bartholomew BA: Hyperuricemia and neurologic deficits. A family study. N Engl J Med 282:992–997, 1970

591. Rosenthal SH, Lidsky MD, Sharp JT: Arthritis with nodules following ankylosing spondylitis. JAMA 206:2893–2894, 1968

592. Rowland LP, Greer M: Toxoplasmic polymyositis. Neurology 11:367–370, 1961

593. Rubin RT, Rahe RH, Clark BR, Arthur RJ: Serum uric acid, cholesterol, and cortisol levels. Interrelationships in normal men under stress. Arch Intern Med 125:815–819, 1970

594. Rudolph AH, Price EV: Penicillin reactions among patients in venereal disease clinics. A national survey. JAMA 223:499–501, 1973

595. Rumbaugh CL, Bergeron RT, Scanlan RL, Teal JS, Segall HD, Fang HCH, McCormick R: Cerebral vascular changes secondary to amphetamine abuse in the experimental animal. Radiology 101:345–351, 1971

596. Russell ML, Gordon DA, Ogryzlo MA, McPhedran RS: The cauda equina syndrome of ankylosing spondylitis. Ann Intern Med 78:551–554, 1973

597. Saha N, Banerjee B: Genetic influences on serum-uric-acid (letter to Editor). Lancet 2:911, 1969

598. Salisbury KW, Plotz PH, Holland PV, Steinberg AD, Peppercorn M: Serologic abnormalities in systemic lupus erythematosus associated with viral hepatitis and tuberculosis. Arthritis Rheum 16:406–410, 1973

599. Sambrook MA, Heron JR, Aber GM: Myopathy in association with primary hyperaldosteronism. J Neurol Neurosurg Psychiatry 35:202–207, 1972

600. Samter M, Beers RF: Concerning the nature of intolerance to aspirin. J Allergy 40:281–293, 1967

601. Santa T: Fine structure of the human skeletal muscle in myopathy. Arch Neurol 20:479–489, 1969

602. Saunders, Hamilton DJ: Lipaemia and fat embolism in the fatal dyspnoea and coma of diabetes. Edinburgh Med J 25:47–57, 1879

603. Schlosstein L, Terasaki PI, Bluestone R, Pearson CM: High association of an HL-A antigen, W27, with ankylosing spondylitis. N Engl J Med 288:704–706, 1973

604. Schneck SA, von Kaulla KN: Fibrinolysis and the nervous system. Neurology 11:959–969, 1961

605. Schoenfeld MR, Goldberger E: Serum cholesterol-uric acid correlations. Metabolism 12:714–717, 1963

606. Schraeder PL, Peters HA, Dahl DS: Polymyositis and penicillamine. Arch Neurol 27:456–457, 1972

607. Schumacher HR Jr: Hemochromatosis and arthritis. Arthritis Rheum 7:41–50, 1964

608. Sclater JG: An analysis of 388 cases of rheumatoid arthritis. Ann Rheum Dis 3:195–206, 1943

609. Scott ML: Studies on the interrelationship of selenium, vitamin E and sulfur amino acids in a nutritional myopathy of the chick. Ann NY Acad Sci 138:82–89, 1966

610. Scuderi CS: Fat embolism. Résumé of the literature plus some newer thoughts on diagnosis. Arch Surg 36:614–625, 1938

611. Seaman WE, Ishak KG, Plotz PH: Aspirin-induced hepatotoxicity in patients with systemic lupus erythematosus. Ann Intern Med 80:1–8, 1974

612. Selroos O: Thrombocytosis. Acta Med Scand 193:431–436, 1973

613. Selye H: Calciphylaxis. Chicago, University of Chicago Press, 1962

614. Selye H: The Pluricausal Cardiopathies. Springfield, Charles C Thomas, 1961

615. Shafiq SA, Gorycki MA, Milhorat AT: An electron microscopic study of regeneration and satellite cells in human muscle. Neurology 17:567–574, passim, 1967

616. Shafiq SA, Milhorat AT, Gorycki MA: Giant mitochondria in human muscle with inclusions. Arch Neurol 17:666–671, 1967

617. Shafiq SA, Sande MA, Carruthers RR, Killip T, Milhorat AT: Skeletal muscle in idiopathic cardiomyopathy. J Neurol Sci 15:303–320, 1972

618. Shafiroff BGP, Kau QY: Lipodystrophy of adipose areolar tissue in the retroperitoneal space. Surgery 59:696–702, 1966

619. Shagrin JW, Frame B, Duncan H: Polyarthritis in obese patients with intestinal bypass. Ann Intern Med 75:377–380, 1971

620. Shapiro JR, Klinenberg JR, Peck W, Goldfinger SE, Seegmiller JE: Hyperuricemia associated with obesity and intensified by caloric restriction (abstract). Arthritis Rheum 7-343, 1964

621. Sharon E, Kaplan D, Diamond HS: Exacerbation of systemic lupus erythematosus after withdrawal of azathioprine therapy. N Engl J Med 288:122–124,1973

622. Sharp GC, Irvin WS, Tan EM, Gould RG, Holman HR: Mixed connective tissue disease—an apparently distinct rheumatic disease syndrome associated with a specific antibody to an extractable nuclear antigen (ENA). Am J Med 52:148–159, 1972

623. Shearn MA: Sjögren's Syndrome. Chapter 7, Connective tissue, diseases associated with Sjögren's syndrome. Philadelphia, W. B. Saunders Co., 1971, pp 104–124

624. Shilkin KB, Chen BTM, Khoo OT: Rhabdomyolysis caused by hornet venom. Br Med J 1:156–157, 1972

625. Short CL, Bauer W: The course of rheumatoid arthritis in patients receiving simple medical and orthopedic measures. N Engl J Med 238:142–148, 1948

626. Shurtleff DB, Sparkes RS, Clawson DK, Guntheroth WG, Mottet NK: Hereditary osteolysis with hypertension and nephropathy. JAMA 188:363–368, 1964

627. Siegel M, Gwon N, Lee SL, Rivero I, Wong W: Survivorship in systemic lupus erythematosus: relationship to race and pregnancy. Arthritis Rheum 12:117–125, 1969

628. Siegel M, Holley HL, Lee SL: Epidemiologic studies on systemic lupus erythematosus. Comparative data for New York City and Jefferson County, Alabama, 1956–1965. Arthritis Rheum 13:802–811, 1970

629. Siegel M, Seelenfreund M: Racial and social factors in systemic lupus erythematosus. JAMA 191:77–80, 1965

630. Siegel RC, Fries JF: Double-blind, cross-over study of intraarterial reserpine and saline in scleroderma (abstract). Arthritis Rheum 15:454, 1972

631. Sigler JW, Bluhm GB, Duncan H, Sharp JT, Ensign DC, McCrum WR: Gold salts in the treatment of rheumatoid arthritis. A double-blind study. Ann Intern Med 80:21–26, 1974

632. Siltzbach LE, Duberstein JL: Arthritis in sarcoidosis. Clin Orthop 57:31–50, 1968

633. Simon EJ, Gross CS, Lessell IM: Turnover of muscle and liver proteins in mice with hereditary muscular dystrophy. Arch Biochem Biophys 96:41–46, 1962

634. Simon HB, Wolff SM: Granulomatous hepatitis and prolonged fever of unknown origin: a study of 13 patients. Medicine 52:1–21, 1973

635. Simon NM, Rovner RN, Berlin BS: Acute myoglobinuria associated with Type A2 (Hong Kong) influenza. JAMA 212:1704–1705, 1970.

636. Singer JM, Plotz CM: The latex fixation test. I. Application to the serologic diagnosis of rheumatoid arthritis. Am J Med 21:888–892, 1956

637. Skeith MD, Healey LA, Cutler RE: Urate excretion during mannitol and glucose diuresis. J Lab Clin Med 70:213–220, 1967

638. Smith JB, Willis AL: Aspirin selectively inhibits prostaglandin production in human platelets. Nature [New Biol] 231:235–237, 1971

639. Smith R, Stern G: Myopathy, osteomalacia and hyperparathyroidism. Brain 90:593–602, 1967

640. Smythe HA, Ogryzlo MA, McNeely DT, Murphy EA, Mustard JF: Platelet economy and blood coagulation in gout (abstract). Arthritis Rheum 5:322–323, 1962

641. Sobrevilla LA, Salazar F: High altitude hyperuricemia. Proc Soc Exp Biol Med 129:890–895, 1968

642. Sokoloff L, Bunim JJ: Vascular lesions in rheumatoid arthritis. J Chronic Dis 5:668–687, 1957

643. Sokoloff MC, Goldberg LS, Pearson CM: Treatment of corticosteroid-resistant polymyositis with methotrexate. Lancet 1:14–16, 1971

644. Solomon GF, Moos RH: Emotions, immunity, and disease. A speculative theoretical integration. Arch Gen Psychiatry 11:657–674, 1964

645. Somers JE, Winer N: Reversible myopathy and myotonia following administration of a hypocholesterolemia agent. Neurology 16:761–765, 1966

646. Somjen G: Sensory Coding in the Mammalian Nervous System. New York, Appleton-Century-Crofts, 1972, pp 259–260

647. Sondergaard J, Greaves MW: Prostaglandin E1: effect on human cutaneous vasculature and skin histamine. Br J Dermatol 84:424–428, 1971

648. Sones DA, McDuffie FC, Hunder GG: The clinical significance of the RA cell. Arthritis Rheum 11:400–406, 1968

649. Soren A: Joint affections in regional ileitis. Arch Intern Med 117:78–83, 1966

650. Sørensen LB: The elimination of uric acid in man studied by means of C¹⁴-labeled uric acid. Uricolysis. Scand J Clin Lab Invest 12 (Suppl 54):1–214, 1960

651. Sreter FA, Bauman ML, Gergely J, Luca N: Changes in muscle chemistry associated with stiffness and pain. Neurology 22:1172–1175, 1972

652. Stabile T: Cosmetics: Trick or Treat? New York, Hawthorn Books, 1966, p 127

653. Stavric B, Johnson WJ, Grice HC: Uric acid nephropathy: an experimental model. Proc Soc Exp Biol Med 130:512–516, 1969

654. Stecher PG, Ed: The Merck Index of Chemicals and Drugs. An Encyclopedia for Chemists, Pharmacists, Physicians, and Members of Allied Professions, 7th edition. Rahway, New Jersey, Merck & Co., Inc., 1960, p 834

655. Steele TH, Rieselbach RE: The renal mechanism for urate homeostasis in normal man. Am J Med 43:868–875, 1967

656. Steinberg AD, Kaltreider HB, Staples PJ, Goetzl EJ, Talal N, Decker JL: Cyclophosphamide in lupus nephritis: a controlled trial. Ann Intern Med 75:165–171, 1971

657. Steinberg AD, Plotz PH, Wolff SM, Wong VG, Agus SG, Decker JL: Cytotoxic drugs in treatment of nonmalignant diseases. Ann Intern Med 76:619–642, 1972

658. Steinberg B: Systemic nodular panniculitis. Am J Pathol 29:1059–1081, 1953

659. Stenger RJ, Spiro D, Scully RE, Shannon JM: Ultrastructural and physiologic alterations in ischemic skeletal muscle. Am J Pathol 40:1–20, 1962

660. Stevens MB, Hookman P, Siegel CI, Esterly JR, Shulman LE, Hendrix TR: Aperistalsis of the esophagus in patients with connective-tissue disorders and Raynaud's phenomenon. N Engl J Med 270:1218–1222, 1964

661. Stoeckle JD, Hardy HL, Weber AL: Chronic beryllium disease. Long-term follow-up of sixty cases and selective review of the literature. Am J Med 46:545–561, 1969

662. Straatsma BR: Ocular manifestations of Wegener's granulomatosis. Am J Ophthalmol 44:789–799, 1957

663. Striker GE, Kelly MR, Quadracci LJ, Scribner BH: The course of lupus nephritis. A clinical-pathological correlation of 50 patients. In Kincaid-Smith, Mathew, Becker, Eds [511], pp 1141–1166

664. Swineford O Jr, Bray WE Jr: Aspirin and the FDA. A critical review of the aspirin problem. Va Med Mon 98:128–132, 1971

665. Szenberg A, Warner NL: Immunological function of thymus and bursa of Fabricius. Dissociation of immunological responsiveness in fowls with a hormonally arrested developement of lymphoid tissues. Nature (London) 194:164–147, 1962

666. Szentiványi A, Filipp G: Anaphylaxis and the nervous system. II. Ann Allergy 16:143–151, 1958

667. Szentiványi A, Szekely J: Anaphylaxis and the nervous system. IV. Ann Allergy 16:389–392, 1958

668. Sztejnbok M, Stewart A, Diamond H, Kaplan D: Azathioprine in the treatment of systemic lupus erythematosus. Arthritis Rheum 14:639–645, 1971

669. Talal N: Immunologic and viral factors in the pathogenesis of systemic lupus erythematosus. Arthritis Rheum 13:887–894, 1970

670. Talbott JH, Lilienfeld A: Longevity in gout. Geriatrics 14:409–420, 1959

671. Talbott JH, Terplan KL: The kidney in gout. Medicine 39:405–467, 1960

672. Teilum G, Poulsen HE: Disseminated lupus erythematosus. Histopathology, morphogenesis, and relation to allergy. Arch Pathol 64:414–425, 1957

673. Telford ED, Simmons HT: Erythromelalgia. Br Med J 2:782–783, 1940

674. Thibierge M, Weissenbach MRJ: Une forme de concrétions calcaires sous-cutanées on relation avec la sclérodermie. Bull Soc Med Hop Paris 30:10–14, 1910

675. Thomas L: Reversible collapse of rabbit ears after intravenous papain, and prevention of recovery by cortisone. J Exp Med 104:245–252, 1956

676. Thomas L, Davidson M, McCluskey RT: Studies of PPLO infection. I. The production of cerebral polyarteritis by Mycoplasma gallisepticum in turkeys; the neurotoxic property of the Mycoplasma. J Exp Med 123:897–912, 1966

677. Thomas L, McCluskey RT, Potter JL, Weissmann G: Comparison of the effects of papain and vitamin A on cartilage. I. The effects in Rabbits. J Exp Med 111:705–718, 1960

678. Thompson M: Discussion on the clinical and radiological aspects of sacro-iliac disease. Proc Roy Soc Med 50:847–850, 1957

679. Thompson M, Bywaters EGL: Unilateral rheumatoid arthritis following hemiplegia. Ann Rheum Dis 21:370–377, 1962

680. Tomasi TB Jr, Fudenberg HH, Finby N: Possible relationship of rheumatoid factors and pulmonary disease. Am J Med 33:243–248, 1962

681. Tomlinson BE, Walton JN, Rebeiz JJ: The effects of ageing and of cachexia upon skeletal muscle. A histopathological study. J Neurol Sci 9:321–349, 1969

682. Torg JS, Steel HH: Essential osteolysis with nephropathy. A review of the literature and case report of an unusual syndrome. J Bone Joint Surg 50A:1629–1638, 1968

683. Townes AS, Sowa JM, Shulman LE: Controlled trial of cyclophosphamide in rheumatoid arthritis (RA): an 18-month double-blind crossover study (abstract). Arthritis Rheum 15:129–130, 1972

684. Traut EF, Knight AA, Szanto PB, Passerelli EW: Specific vascular changes in gout. JAMA 156:591–593, 1954

685. Trimble GX: Epidemic neuromyasthenia (letter to Editor). N Engl J Med 281:105–106, 1969

686. Trimble RB, Townes AS, Robinson H, Kaplan SB, Chandler RW, Hanissian AS, Masi AT: Preliminary criteria for the classification of systemic lupus erythematosus (SLE). Evaluation in early diagnosed SLE and rheumatoid arthritis. Arthritis Rheum 17:184–188, 1974

687. Tuffanelli DL, Winkelmann RK: Scleroderma and its relationship to the "collagenoses": dermatomyositis, lupus erythematosus, rheumatoid arthritis and Sjogren's syndrome. Am J Med Sci 243:133–146, 1962

688. Unanue ER, Benacerraf B: Immunologic events in experimental hypersensitivity granulomas. Am J Pathol 71:349–364, 1973

689. Urbánek K, Jansa P: Cellular inflammatory response. Findings in patients with neurological diseases. Arch Neurol 30:372–374, 1974

690. Urowitz MG, Gordon DA, Smythe HA, Pruzanski W, Ogryzlo MA: Azathioprine in rheumatoid arthritis. A double-blind, cross-over study. Arthritis Rheum 16:411–418, 1973

691. Van Wijngaarden GK, Bethlem J, Meijer AEFH, Hülsmann WCh, Feltkamp CA: Skeletal muscle disease with abnormal mitochondria. Brain 90:577–592, 1967

692. Varadi DP, Lawrence AM: Suppression of Raynaud's phenomenon by methyldopa. Arch Intern Med 124:13–18, 1969
693. Vaughan JH, Barnett EV, Sobel MV, Jacox RF: Intracytoplasmic inclusions of immunoglobulins in rheumatoid arthritis and other diseases. Arthritis Rheum 11:125–134, 1968
694. Velayos EE, Robinson H, Porciuncula FU, Masi AT: Clinical correlation analysis of 137 patients with Raynaud's phenomenon. Am J Med Sci 262:347–356, 1971.
695. Vessey SH: Effects of grouping on levels of circulating antibodies in mice. Proc Soc Exp Biol Med 115:252–255, 1964
696. Vicale CT: The diagnostic features of a muscular syndrome resulting from hyperparathyroidism, osteomalacia owing to renal tubular acidosis, and perhaps to related disorders of calcium metabolism. Trans Am Neurol Assoc 74:143–147, 1949
697. Vignos PH Jr, Bowling GF, Watkins MP: Polymyositis. Effect of corticosteroids on final result. Arch Intern Med 114:263–277, 1964
698. Vinyl chloride ban in pesticide sprays requested by EPA. Wall Street J 90:20, 1974 (Mar 29)
699. Viozzi FJ, Bluhm GB, Riddle JM, Barnhart MI: Coexistence of gout and arterial thrombosis (abstract). Arthritis Rheum 13:355–356, 1970
700. Waaler E: On the occurrence of a factor in human serum activating the specific agglutination of sheep blood corpuscles. Acta Pathol Microbiol Scand 17:172–188, 1940
701. Walker BE: A radioautographic study of muscle regeneration in dystrophic mice. Am J Pathol 41:41–53, 1962
702. Wall PD, Sweet WH: Temporary abolition of pain in man. Science 155:108–109, 1967
703. Wallace SL, Lattes R, Ragan C: Diagnostic significance of the muscle biopsy. Am J Med 25:600–610, 1958
704. Walton JN: Progressive muscular dystrophy: structural alterations in various stages and in carriers of Duchenne dystrophy. *In* Pearson CM, Mostofi FK, Eds: The Striated Muscle. Baltimore, Williams and Wilkins Co., 1973, pp 263–291
705. Walton JN, Adams JD: Polymyositis. Edinburgh and London, E & S Livingstone, Ltd., 1958
706. Walzer PD, Perl DP, Krogstad DJ, Rawson PG, Schultz MG: *Pneumocystis carinii* pneumonia in the United States. Epidemiologic, diagnostic, and clinical features. Ann Intern Med 80:83–93, 1974
707. Ward R, Stalker R: Sheep cell agglutination test in chronic interstitial pulmonary fibrosis. Ann Rheum Dis 24:246–256, 1965
708. Warren KS, Domingo EO, Cowan RBT: Granuloma formation around Schistosome eggs as a manifestation of delayed hypersensitivity. Am J Pathol 51:735–756, 1967
709. Wasserman F, Krosnick A, Tumen H: Necrotizing angiitis associated with chronic ulcerative colitis. Am J Med 17:736–743, 1954
710. Watts RWE, Scott JT, Chalmers RA, Bitensky L, Chayen J: Microscopic studies on skeletal muscle in gout patients treated with allopurinol. Q J Med 40:1–14, 1971
711. Wawrzynska-Pagowska J, Brzezinska B, Brzozowska M, Graff T, Juszczyk T, Michalski J, Pakula A, Piotrowska D, Wojcik-Seislowska M: Observations on the symptoms and signs of "early" rheumatoid arthritis in a prospective study. Acta Rheumatol Scand 16:99–105, 1970
712. Weinberger HW, Ropes MW, Kulka JP, Bauer W: Reiter's syndrome, clinical and pathologic observations. A long term study of 16 cases. Medicine 41:35–91, 1962
713. Weiss TE, Segaloff A, Moore C: Gout and diabetes. Metabolism 6:103–106, 1957
714. Welch KMA, Goldberg DM: Serum creatine phosphokinase in motor neuron disease. Neurology 22:697–701, 1972
715. Weve HTM: Over Keratitis Urica en Anderer Vormen van Tichtig Ooglijden. Rotterdam, W T Van Hengel, 1924
716. Whitaker JN, Engel WK: Vascular deposits of immunoglobulin and complement in idiopathic inflammatory myopathy. N Engl J Med 286:333–338, 1972
717. Whitcomb ME, Schwarz MI, Charles MA, Larson PH: Interstitial fibrosis after *Pneumocystis carinii* pneumonia. Ann Intern Med 73:761–765, 1970
718. Whitehouse FW, Cleary WJ Jr: Diabetes mellitus in patients with gout. JAMA 197:73–76, 1966
719. Wiedemann E, Rose HG, Schwartz E: Plasma lipoproteins, glucose tolerance and insulin response in primary gout. Am J Med 53:299–307, 1972
720. Wiernik PH: Amyloid joint disease. Medicine 51:465–497, 1972

721. Wigley RD, Coughman KG, Maule R; Polyarteritis nodosa: the natural history of a spontaneously occurring model in outbred mice. Aust Ann Med 19:319–327, 1970

722. Wilkinson M, Bywaters EGL: Clinical features and course of ankylosing spondylitis; as seen in a follow-up of 222 hospital referred cases. Ann Rheum Dis 17:209–228, 1958

723. Willerson JT, Thompson RH, Hookman P, Herdt J, Decker JL: Reserpine in Raynaud's disease and phenomenon. Short-term response to intra-arterial injection. Ann Intern Med 72:17–27, 1970

724. Willkens RF, Healey LA Jr: The nonspecificity of synovial leukocyte inclusions. J Lab Clin Med 68:628–635, 1966

725. Wilson CB, Smith RC: Goodpasture's syndrome associated with influenza A2 virus infection. Ann Intern Med 76:91–94, 1972

726. Wilson RH, McCormick WE, Tatum CF, Creech JL: Occupational acroosteolysis. Report of 31 cases. JAMA 201:577–581, 1967

727. Winkelmann RK, Mulder DW, Lambert EH, Howard FM Jr, Dressner GR: Course of dermatomyositis-polymyositis: comparison of untreated and cortisone-treated patients. Mayo Clin Proc 43:545–556, 1968

728. Wistar R Jr, Hildemann WH: Effect of stress on skin transplantation immunity in mice. Science 131:159–160, 1960

729. Wolf SM, Lusk W: Hypocalcemic myopathy. Bull Los Angeles Neurol Soc 37:167–177, 1972

730. Wolfe JD, Metzger AL, Goldstein RC: Aspirin hepatitis. Ann Intern Med 80:74–76, 1974

731. Wolfson WQ, Cohn C, Levine R, Hunt HD: Liver function and serum protein structure in gout. Ann Intern Med 30:598–614, 1949

732. Woodrow JC: HL-A 27 and Reiter's syndrome (letter to Editor). Lancet 2:671–672, 1973

733. Young DS, Thomas DW, Friedman RB, Pestaner LC: Effects of drugs on clinical laboratory tests. Clin Chem 18:1041–1303, 1972

734. Yourish N: Conjunctival tophi associated with gout. Arch Ophthalmol 50:370–371, 1953

735. Yu MK, Wright TL, Dettbarn W-D, Olson WH: Pargyline-induced myopathy with histochemical characteristics of Duchenne muscular dystrophy. Neurology 24:237–244, 1974

736. Yune HY, Vix VA, Klatte EC: Early fingertip changes in scleroderma. JAMA 215:1113–1116, 1971

737. Zakrividoroga ZS: [Data on the problem of nervous regulation of immunological reactions.] Zh Mikrobiol 32:14–17, 1961 (Rus)

738. Zarafonetis CJD, Lorber SH, Hanson SM: Association of functioning carcinoid syndrome and scleroderma. I. Case report. Am J Med Sci 236:1–14, 1958

739. Zeek PM: Periarteritis nodosa: a critical review. Am J Clin Pathol 22:777–790, 1952

740. Zeiders RS: T lymphocytes in rheumatic diseases (abstract). Arthritis Rheum 16:578, 1973

741. Zenker FA: Beiträge zur normalen und pathologischen Anatomie der Lunge. Dresden, J Brunsdorf, 1862

742. Zimmerman HJ: Aspirin-induced hepatic injury (Editorial). Ann Intern Med 80:103–105, 1974

743. Zurier RB, Ballas M: Prostaglandin E_1 (PGE_1) suppression of adjuvant arthritis histopathology. Arthritis Rheum 16:251–258, 1973

744. Zvaifler NJ: The immunopathology of joint inflammation in rheumatoid arthritis. Adv Immunol 16:265–336, 1973

745. Zvaifler NJ, Reefe WE, Black RL: Articular manifestations in primary hyperparathyroidism. Arthritis Rheum 5:237–249, 1962

746. Zweiman B, Kornblum J, Cornog J, Hildreth EA: The prognosis of lupus nephritis. Role of clinical-pathologic correlations. Ann Intern Med 69:441–462, 1968

Index